Individualized Care

Riitta Suhonen • Minna Stolt
Evridiki Papastavrou
Editors

Individualized Care

Theory, Measurement, Research
and Practice

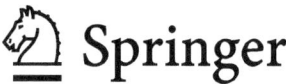 Springer

Editors
Riitta Suhonen
Department of Nursing Science
University of Turku
Turku
Finland

Minna Stolt
Department of Nursing Science
University of Turku
Turku
Finland

Evridiki Papastavrou
Department of Nursing
Cyprus University of Technology
Limassol
Cyprus

ISBN 978-3-030-07889-8   ISBN 978-3-319-89899-5   (eBook)
https://doi.org/10.1007/978-3-319-89899-5

Printed on acid-free paper

This Springer imprint is published by the registered company Springer International Publishing AG part of Springer Nature.
The registered company address is: Gewerbestrasse 11, 6330 Cham, Switzerland

Preface

The original idea of this book appeared in an international research meeting several years ago. Perhaps more than ever professional nurses, policymakers and educational experts and especially citizens speak about the need for individualised care and argue strongly for its presence in daily nursing care and healthcare services.

This contributed book is based on more than 20 years of research on patient individuality, care and services of the continuously changing healthcare system. It describes how research results can be used to respond to challenges on individuality in healthcare systems by providing a description of the concept, theory, measurement and research results about individualised nursing care from different perspectives. Especially service users', patients' or clients' points of view on care and health services are urgently needed in the process for restructuring care and services for individuals in addition to evidence-based practice.

This book describes the conceptualisation of the individualised nursing care phenomenon and the development process of the measuring instruments of that phenomenon in different contexts. It describes results about individualised nursing care from a variety of clinical contexts and explains factors associated with the perceptions and delivery of individualised nursing care from different points of view. This book may appeal to clinicians, nurses, practitioners and researchers from many fields.

This book provides an opportunity to collect different views on individualised nursing care and to examine its various dimensions: through a variety of approaches and contexts. This book is intended for researchers, theoreticians, students in different levels and professional nurses working bedside and leading nursing care and services.

This book is devoted to all nurses in different clinical contexts to remind us for the most cherished value in nursing care—the good for our patients.

Riitta Suhonen

Minna Stolt

Evridiki Papastavrou

Turku, Finland
Limassol, Cyprus

Acknowledgements

This book would not have been possible without a strong contribution of many people, especially all the authors who participated in writing the chapters of this book. In addition to writing, they have somehow participated in the creation of the conceptual, theoretical and empirical activities during the past 25 years, while knowledge about individualised nursing care; the instrumentation, namely the Individualised Care Scale; and its numerous translated and adapted versions have been created. In addition to the measurement, a large group of researchers have created important knowledge about the implementation of individualised nursing care for patients. The collaboration has given a possibility to share wider understanding about individualised care, nursing research and researcher networking.

We wish to express our sincere thanks to all the authors of this book but also to all those many nurse scientists, professional nurses and collaborators participating in the numerous international research studies during the years. We would like to thank all of you who during the last 25 years have changed your valuable thoughts, ideas and contributions for the benefit of individualised nursing care phenomenon.

Finally, we wish to thank our organisations for offering us a fruitful scene and possibilities for long-time commitment for research, international collaboration and scientific work. We wish to thank all universities that provided possibility for many researchers to join the network and invested in us with offering fruitful scientific environments. Special thanks to the University of Turku and the Cyprus University of Technology, which offered a special research environment for the editors.

We wish to thank several bodies that have funded the Individualised Care Project through the years. Especially we wish to thank the Finnish Cultural Federation, Kanta-Häme Hospital District (EVO budget), Health Care District of Forssa special grant-in-aid, Medical Research Fund, Tampere University Hospital, Hospital District of Southwest Finland/Turku University Hospital, Research Foundation for Nursing Education and Cyprus University of Technology.

Contents

Riitta Suhonen, RN, PhD is Professor in the University of Turku, Department of Nursing Science, Finland, and Director of Nursing (side position), Turku University Hospital, City of Turku, Welfare Division. She works as a professor and specialises in older people nursing science (gerontological nursing science) since 2011. Formerly, she has worked as a quality and development manager in a healthcare district and as a ward manager and registered nurse in surgical care unit. She is experienced in leading and participating in international cross-cultural studies and currently is a co-researcher in many projects. She has been a principal investigator and coordinator of the Individualised Care Project since 2002, which evaluates the realisation of individuality in patients' care from the point of view of patients and nurses in different clinical fields including national and international parts. Other research topics are nursing ethics, nursing education and nursing management. She teaches topics such as older people nursing care, research methodology, instrument development, academic writing, quantitative research methods in nursing science and research ethics. She has around 200 peer-reviewed scientific publications and is the board member of the European Academy of Nursing Science.

Minna Stolt is Docent and PhD (main subject nursing science) working currently as university teacher in the Department of Nursing Science in the University of Turku, Finland. Her professional background is in podiatry and research expertise in foot health. Moreover, she has research expertise in the evaluation of healthcare quality in the field of older people nursing research, ethics and competence of professionals. Her teaching profile includes instrument development, literature reviews and academic writing. She has published several scientific articles and presented her research in national and international conferences. In the field of societal interaction, she is an active advocate for foot health promotion in different age groups and has published plenty popular articles and two textbooks on this topic.

Evridiki Papastavrou holds a PhD and an MSc in Nursing, a BSc in Public Administration and is a Registered Nurse. She is an Associate Professor of Nursing at the School of Health Sciences, Cyprus University of Technology, and her research focuses on the concept of care and related concepts such as individualised care, the environment of care, rationing of care and the burden of care. She is the Chair of a COST Action Project and National Coordinator of 2 Erasmus Projects all funded by the European Union. She participates in other national and international research projects and is the author of several articles published in scientific journals.

About the Authors

Andreas Charalambous, RN, PhD (Oncology Nursing) has a clinical background in cancer care and has worked clinically and academically in Cyprus, the UK and Finland. He holds an Assistant Professor's position of Oncology and Palliative Care at the Cyprus University of Technology and a Docent's position at the University of Turku (Finland). He is an EONS Executive Board Member since 2013 and was elected as President-Elect in 2017. He is currently involved in the RECaN project of EONS and ECCO's Oncopolicy and Oncopolicy Executive Committees. He is involved in several national and international research programmes (i.e. EEPO, ICP, RANCARE) in various fields of care with specific interest in cancer and palliative care. He has published over 80 national and international publications in esteemed journals in the fields of cancer care, quality care, supportive care and integrative medicine. A major area of research interest includes the application of health technologies in specific cancer and dementia groups of patients.

Georgios Efstathiou holds a PhD in Nursing, an MSc in Health Studies and is a Registered Nurse. He is member of the Educational Sector of the Nursing Services of the Ministry of Health, Cyprus. His research and educational interests focus on infection control, the concept of care and the fundamentals of nursing. He has published in various national and international journals and given presentation in national and international conferences.

Marie Elf is an Associate Professor of healthcare architecture at the School of Education, Health and Social Studies at Dalarna University and Chalmers University of Technology, Sweden. Her research interests are design processes and the interaction between architecture and people with long-term disabilities.

Ann Gallagher, PhD, RN is Professor of Ethics and Care at the International Care Ethics Observatory, University of Surrey, UK. She is Editor of *Nursing Ethics* and a member of the Nuffield Council on Bioethics. At the time of writing, Ann was a Fulbright Scholar-in-Residence at the National Center for Bioethics in Research and Health Care at Tuskegee University, USA. Ann's research focuses on ethics as applied to health and social care. Her research areas include dignity in care, ethics education, slow ethics, professionalism and ethical aspects of professional regulation.

Michael Igoumenidis has studied Nursing (BSc) and Philosophy (BA) at the National and Kapodistrian University of Athens and holds a Master of Arts in Health Care Ethics and Law from the University of Manchester, School of Law, and a PhD from the same institution. He has published several articles related to health care, with an emphasis on ethical issues. He has participated in various health-related research projects, and he has presented much of his work in international conferences. He is currently an Assistant Professor at the Department of Nursing of the Technological Educational Institute of Western Greece.

Lena von Koch, PhD is professor in Karolinska Institutet, Sweden. She is a senior professor in health services research at Karolinska Institutet. Her overall research aim is to develop, evaluate and implement interventions to promote health for people living with long-term health conditions and their families.

Janika Koskenvuori, MSc (Biomedical Laboratory Scientist) is a doctoral candidate and a research assistant at the Department of Nursing Science at the University of Turku, Finland. Her research interests are in the field ethical health care and nursing.

Tella Jemina Lantta, PhD, RN works as a researcher at the University of Turku, Department of Nursing Science, Finland. Her clinical background is in adult psychiatric hospital care. Her research interests are especially in the area of violence prevention and management in mental health care.

Helena Leino-Kilpi is a professor and chair; Head of the Department, University of Turku, Faculty of Medicine, Department of Nursing Science; and Nurse director (part-time), Turku University Hospital. She is nationally and internationally well-known expert in the field of nursing and health sciences, a registered nurse with clinical expertise in surgical-intensive nursing care, MEd and PhD in nursing science. Her main teaching area is health care and nursing ethics. She has supervised more than 50 graduated PhDs in nursing science, has been chairing for years the Finnish National Doctoral Network in Nursing Science, taught research ethics in the European Academy of Nursing Science and is a member of the management board of the Baltic Sea Region Doctoral Network. Her research is in three main areas: health care and nursing ethics, clinical nursing and nursing education. Her research is strongly international, and she has published around 500 scientific, referee-based publications. She has expertise in international and national academic duties. She is Honorary Doctor in the University of Klaipeda (Lithuania), a Fellow of European Academy of Nursing Science and visiting professor in the University of Dublin Trinity College, Ireland.

Chryssoula Lemonidou, PhD has been qualified in Nursing at the National and Kapodistrian University of Athens (N.K.U.A) and the University of Pennsylvania, USA (Master of Science in Nursing). She holds a position as a Professor and Chair of the Department of Nursing at the N.K.U.A, Athens, Greece. She was representative of the Ministry of Health in the Advisory Committee on Training in Nursing of the European Commission and a member of the Committee on Nursing Education of the Central Council of Health in Greece. She also participates in various committees on legislation, development and evaluation of health programmes, etc. Her current research activities include collaboration with European and international institutions mainly in the area of ethics and patient care.

Susanna Nordin is a PhD and lecturer in nursing at the School of Education, Health and Social Studies at Dalarna University, Sweden. Her research focuses on the physical environment in residential care facilities for older people and how environmental aspects can affect persons living and working in these facilities.

Sunna Rannikko is a registered nurse and a public health nurse. She has clinical working experience as a nurse in a neurosurgical inpatient ward. She graduated as a Master of Nursing Science in 2016. From the year 2017, she has been a doctoral candidate at the Department of Nursing Science in the University of Turku, Finland. Her main research interests are nursing ethics, patients with neurological impairments and patients' lived experiences. In her doctoral thesis, she is constructing an ethical pathway of patients with stroke.

Beatriz Rodríguez-Martín is a PhD in Health and Social Research, an MSc in Health and Social Research, a BSc in Social Cultural Anthropology and a Registered Nurse. She is an Associate Professor of Gerontology and Research Methods at the University of Castilla-La Mancha (Faculty of Occupational Therapy, Speech Therapy and Nursing), Spain, and researcher at Health and Social Research Centre (CESS), University of Castilla-La Mancha. Her research work has focused on qualitative research in health, individualised care, patient health experience, health technology assessment, public health and social network. She participates in national and international research projects and has written several scientific articles.

Maritta Välimäki, PhD, Docent, RN is a professor at the Hong Kong Polytechnic University, School of Nursing (Hong Kong, China, SAR), and at the University of Turku, Department of Nursing Science, Finland. Välimäki is leading the Mental Health Care Research Team at the Hong Kong Polytechnic University. She is a Principal Investigator in a number of international and national research projects. Välimäki has authored more than 300 scholarly papers and a number of book chapters. Her research focuses on persons with serious mental illness, and she is interested in health technology and outcome research. She is an Editorial Board Member of the Schizophrenia group.

Stavros Vryonnides is a registered nurse holding a BSc degree in nursing, a diploma in nursing administration and a master's degree in business administration (MBA), and he is a doctoral student of the Cyprus University of Technology, Cyprus, Department of Nursing. His research focuses on how the ethical dimension of nursing and the ethical climate in nurses' workplace are related to missed nursing care, and he published some relevant articles in scientific journals. He currently works as an area nursing manager, responsible of all rural and urban healthcare centres of Limassol, and in addition, he is the Vice President of the managerial board of the Cyprus Nurses and Midwives Association (CYNMA).

Rueben C. Warren, DDS, MPH, Dr PH, MDiv is Professor of Bioethics and Director of the National Center Bioethics in Research and Health Care at Tuskegee University, USA. Adjunct appointments: Professor of Public Health, Medicine and Ethics, Interdenominational Theological Center; Clinical Professor, Department of Community Health/Preventive Medicine, Morehouse School of Medicine; Professor, Department of Behavioral Sciences and Health Education, Emory's Rollins School of Public Health; and Professor, Schools of Dentistry and Graduate Studies, Meharry Medical College. Dr. Warren is Dean Emeritus, School of Dentistry, Meharry Medical College.

Introduction

Riitta Suhonen, Minna Stolt, and Evridiki Papastavrou

This book is based on the long-lasting research efforts and international research collaboration (Individualised Care Project, ICProject) since the beginning of the 2000s. The ICProject commenced in 2000 as a doctoral study and later evolved to a research programme in the University of Turku, Department of Nursing Science, Turku, Finland. The aim of the ICProject was to identify and examine the nurse, patient and organisational factors associated with the provision of individualised care from both the patients' and nurses' perspectives in different care settings, to compare nurses' and patients' perceptions of individualised care and to examine the impact of individualised care on patient and nurse outcomes. The ICProject broadened in terms of the research contexts moving from an acute hospital context to older person long-term care, home care, sheltered housing and nursing homes and in primary healthcare centres. Individualised care is seen as an indicator of quality of nursing care and is associated with the organisational context, e.g. ethical climate, in which care is delivered. The research programme aims to produce and promote the use of research evidence about how the organisation and delivery of healthcare services contributes to improved health to ensure better strategic and patient outcomes and improved job satisfaction for nurses.

R. Suhonen (✉)
Department of Nursing Science, University of Turku, Turku University Hospital,
City of Turku, Welfare Division, Turku, Finland
e-mail: riisuh@utu.fi

M. Stolt
Department of Nursing Science, University of Turku, Turku, Finland
e-mail: minna.stolt@utu.fi

E. Papastavrou
School of Health Sciences, Department of Nursing, Cyprus University of Technology,
Limassol, Cyprus
e-mail: e.papastavrou@cut.ac.cy

© Springer International Publishing AG, part of Springer Nature 2019
R. Suhonen et al. (eds.), *Individualized Care*,
https://doi.org/10.1007/978-3-319-89899-5_1

The ICProject evolved into several studies, examining individualised care from the point of view of patients and professionals with two national studies, and two international studies including seven countries in acute care setting and one study in care settings for older people including several parts, such as the ICProject Elderly Study and the ICProject Organisational Study. These studies identified organisational factors, such as practice environment, job satisfaction and ethical climate, in relation to individualised patient care. Finally, many of these variables were joined and empirically tested in the sample of cancer patients in an international collaborative study.

This research programme includes the patients' and professionals' views on individualising care and identifies the environment provided by the organisation as a contributor to patient outcomes (Fig. 1.1). The interventions delivered by professionals are influenced by the patients, the professionals themselves and the environment in which care is delivered, which in turn affects the individualisation and quality of patient outcomes. Studies have now been conducted observing the process of individualised care delivery to determine which systems of care are the most influential for the improvement in patient care delivery and result in improved patient outcomes. The current research programme is called "Older Individuals' Health, Nursing and Services" and develops new knowledge and understanding of individual's health, nursing care and complex service systems for older individuals from the viewpoints of older individuals, professionals and organisations.

Several outcomes from the long-lasting research collaboration have been achieved. The theory of individualised care and factors related is generated based on the conceptual and theoretical examination of the phenomenon and empirically

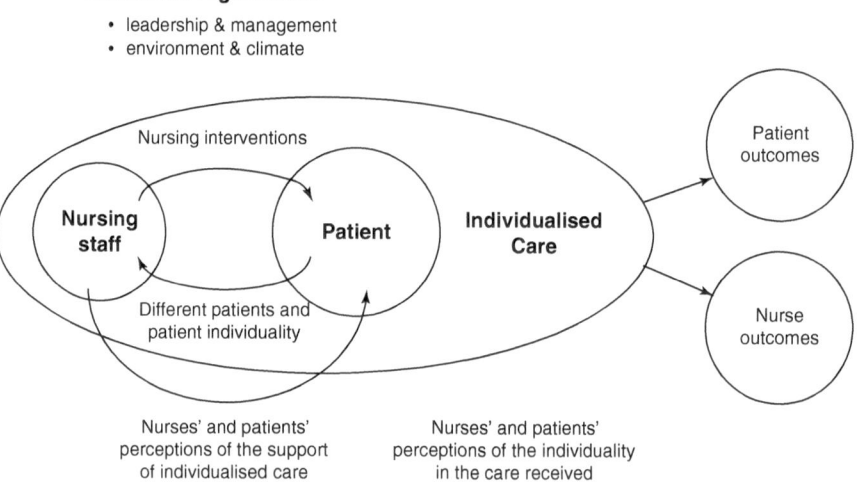

Fig. 1.1 Framework of the individualised care and factors associated

tested with the developed Individualised Care Scale, originated from the beginning of the 2000s. Both the patient and nurse versions were created and have been translated in several languages and cultures. Thus, the research interest in this topic has expanded rapidly, and the topic is timely and important at the moment.

This book includes four parts. The first part, the theoretical framework, describes the theoretical and philosophical framework of the individualised nursing care (Chap. 2), followed by the description of the content and the use and importance of the concept (Chap. 3), definitions of the concept of individualised nursing care through years (Chap. 4) and the ethical aspects of individualised care (Chap. 5). The second part, namely, the research framework, includes the aspects and the development of the instrument for the measurement of individualised care (Chap. 6), methods and processes for translation of the research instruments (Chap. 7), their validity and reliability (Chap. 8) as well as a description of the instruments developed for the measurement of individualised care and similar phenomenon (Chap. 9). The third part, research evidence on the delivery of individualised care, describes the results, the implementation and the maintenance of individualised care in different clinical contexts by giving examples of such care contexts. These include the maintenance of individualised care in operative surgical (Chap. 10), older people (Chap. 11), cancer (Chap. 12), mental and psychiatric (Chap. 13) and rehabilitation (Chap. 14) care settings. In addition, the third part includes a chapter about individual's foot health (Chap. 15) and factors associated with the maintenance of individualised care (Chap. 16). Finally, the fourth part, the organisational framework for the delivery of individualised care, includes the role of nursing interventions (Chap. 17) and nurse leadership (Chap. 18) in supporting individualised care delivery in clinical practice, highlighting also the importance of physical environment (Chap. 19) and ethical climate (Chap. 20). This book may appeal to clinicians, nurses, practitioners and researchers from many fields.

This book is focused on the concept of individualised care. No consensus exists about the use of the different terms, such as person-centred or tailored nursing care. This book continues to elaborate on the differences and similarities of the related concepts and sheds light on the use of these concepts in the theoretical and research literature as well as in clinical practice. However, the starting point here is the patients' point of view and their differences and individuality. Thus, the term individualised care is used here as patient's perception of being considered as an individual while being nursed and cared for in the healthcare system. All other viewpoints have been created around this cornerstone, patients' individuality and their individualised nursing care.

Part I

Theoretical Framework for Individualised Care

Theoretical and Philosophical Framework for Individualised Care

Michael Igoumenidis, Evridiki Papastavrou, and Chryssoula Lemonidou

Abstract

Individuality plays a central role in human existence. Its realisation varies greatly in different historical times and places. In modern societies it can often be under threat, under the influence of mass media and mass production, but its importance is recognised, and there have been constant efforts to enhance it. In health services, holistic care for individual patients has become a milestone goal. Individualised care can improve patient outcomes in an ethical and respectful way. Despite the difficulties posed by modern health-care delivery, an increasing number of studies ascertain the importance of individualised care. Based on the existing evidence, various health-care organisations recognise the need to enhance individualised care and implement various initiatives to do so. However, various economic constraints do not allow for wide implementation of individualised health interventions. Technological progress provides more opportunities than ever for individualised care, but limited health resources set a series of obstacles for its delivery. Further research in this field shall help towards embodying the best affordable individualised care in modern health delivery.

Keywords

Individualised care · Individuality concept · Humoral medicine · Personalised medicine · Patient advocacy

M. Igoumenidis (✉)
Department of Nursing, Technological Educational Institute of Western Greece, Patras, Greece
e-mail: migoumen@nurs.uoa.gr

E. Papastavrou
Department of Nursing, School of Health Sciences, Cyprus University of Technology, Limassol, Cyprus

C. Lemonidou
Department of Nursing, School of Health Sciences, National and Kapodistrian University of Athens, Athens, Greece

2.1   Introduction

Individualised care draws its importance from the concept of the individual, one of the most basic concepts in the history of humankind. To be sure, there are many ways to interpret such a concept. We are all individuals, in the arithmetic sense, insofar as each one of us possesses a distinct body. Also, we are all individuals in the biological sense; except for homozygote twins, who share the same genetic material, each one of us is the manifestation of a unique genetic plan, which entails different combinations of the thousands of genes that constitute the human genome. We are also individuals in a psychological sense: each one of us has a distinct personality, based on the multiple ways our brain can process sensory or rational information and adapt our behaviour accordingly. When our brain acquires self-conscience, we are also individuals in a deeper sense, because we understand our own individuality. However, this self-conscience, or knowledge of ourselves, functions in many ways within human society. The value of individuality and its place in our evolving societies have passed through many phases, and they have concerned some of the most important political and moral philosophers.

In what follows, we shall try to outline some basic points of the history of this concept, before concentrating on its modern significance and its relation to the importance of individualised care. We shall then describe an antithesis inherent to modern health-care delivery, that is, person-centred care versus managed care and health-care policies, based on economic criteria, and affecting groups of patients collectively rather than individual patients. Finally, we shall briefly discuss the ways in which individual health professionals become an integral part of individualised care.

2.2   Philosophical Approach of Individuality

Many insects, mammals, and birds tend to collaborate and form short-term or long-term groups, as group-living typically provides benefits to individual group members [1]. Sometimes these animal societies go to such extreme lengths that the concept of individuality loses any importance it may have. For instance, ant colonies and bee hives are strictly organised around their distinctive leaders, that is, the queen ant and the queen bee, respectively, and all the other ants and bees seem to function without any self-interest or self-awareness; the welfare of the group is paramount, leaving no room for individual variations and diversions. Human societies are more complex. Individuals collaborate for the greater good, but they also tend to differentiate themselves from others, shape distinct and evolving personalities, and often act on their own initiative. These expressions of individuality vary greatly in terms of intensity and diffusion in human societies, depending on cultural backgrounds, political regimes, and historical evolution. Throughout the ages, the concept of the individual has steadily been a subject of study and debate.

In ancient Greece, the Socratic tradition placed great emphasis on the worth of every individual. However, people at that time considered slavery to be natural and treated all women as naturally inferior to men. In *The Republic*, Plato goes one step further and holds the view that independence and individual freedom need to be constricted through state regulations to achieve a peaceful society [2]. On the other hand, Aristotle values each person's individuality by stating that good is an intermediate relative to us, which means that 'this is not one thing, nor is it the same for all' ([3], p. 1106a). Still, Aristotle had also developed a theory of natural slavery that was supposed to secure the morality of enslaving people [4]. It is obvious that today we cannot value individuality within the same context that great ancient thinkers did. The Christian tradition can also be considered as hostile to the concept of individual in many ways; a consistent analysis of this tradition and its relation to individuality is out of the scope of this chapter, but one can simply note that, even today, a Christian pastor's duty is to 'feed the flock' [5]. Individuality regained importance in the beginning of Renaissance, along with its emerging humanistic values, such as respect for human capabilities, and in parallel to the church's gradual loss of power and control over human lives.

Since the Renaissance, and especially during and after the age of Enlightenment, many philosophical approaches placed individuality at their core. Under the minimal state as put forward by John Locke and his followers, each individual has a right to decide what would become of himself and what he would do ([6], p. 171), while Thomas Hobbes rejects the notion of *summum bonum* (greatest good), arguing that 'good' is defined for each person individually, according to the person's desires ([7], p. 35). Purely egoistic approaches also emerged, such as Bernard Mandeville's idea that without private vices there exists no public benefit, as his *Fable of the Bees* implies [8]; a similar approach is adopted by Adam Smith in the *Wealth of Nations*, when he states that each person should act on their own motives, and society's *invisible hand* shall transfigure these individual selfish efforts to collective progress ([9], p. 456). Philosophical movements of the twentieth century such as existentialism (with its roots traced in nineteenth century's Kierkegaard and Nietzsche) focus on the person's responsibility, which entails individual rights as well as duties; as Sartre [10] has put it, man is condemned to be free.

This is a very important remark, considering the totalitarian regimes of the past century that influenced philosophical thought, some of which are still active worldwide. In totalitarian societies, people tend to shift their moral responsibility to higher authorities, like soldiers at war ([11], p. 47); by doing so, they lose their individual rights along with their duties, submitting to collective rights and duties for the greatest good. But even at peaceful times and in liberal societies, collective autonomy and individual autonomy may turn out to be inconsistent goals. In the nineteenth century, Max Weber had noted that the growing process of bureaucratisation put in jeopardy the individualistic life which he believed to be the core of the Western tradition ([12], p. 5). Indeed, the 'system' is another higher authority where individuals can shift their responsibilities. Both communism and capitalism, as the world's leading systems, are largely influenced by utilitarianism, the idea that right and good are to be defined by what produces greater benefits for the greater number of people; evidently, as Thomas Nagel notes, utilitarianism treats the desires and needs of distinct persons as if they were the desires and needs of a 'mass person' ([13], p. 134). Loss of individuality in bureaucratic societies is a recurring theme in many fictional works as well, mainly describing dystopias, such as Kafka's *The Trial*, Huxley's *Brave New World*, Orwell's *1984*, and Ayn Rand's *Anthem*, where people do not even have names and have forgotten words such as 'I' or 'ego'.

The struggle for individuality is real in modern societies, with mass media influencing most of human lives and bureaucratic mechanisms replacing human interactions. However, we also live in an era of self-realisation, and we place great value to individual autonomy. This may not be entirely evident under normal circumstances, because our busy way of living does not often leave much room for thought. But when we are reminded of our personal selves, our life goals, our beliefs, and our place within society, we consciously strive to be as autonomous, free, and unique as possible, and we expect from others to respect that. Discussing our health and facing health-related problems are great—albeit violent—opportunities for introspective reflection on our individual selves. Under this light, caring for each person as an individual acquires a very deep meaning.

2.3   The Importance of Seeing the Individuals

In the *Nicomachean Ethics*, Aristotle writes: 'Individual treatment is better than a common system, in education as in medicine. As a general rule rest and fasting are good for a fever, but they may not be best for a particular case… private attention gives more accurate results in particular cases, for the particular subject is more likely to get the treatment that suits him' ([3], p. 1180b). This view reflects the Hippocratic ideal, by and large focused on the holistic health-care model, applying standards that are still valid today [14]. In addition, the Hippocratic tradition influenced the practice of Western medicine until the second half of the nineteenth century, when biomedicine became accepted as orthodox by physicians, the public, and the state; until then, *humoral* medicine has held sway for many centuries ([15], p. 137). Humoral medicine is based on four 'humours' of the human body (blood, phlegm, yellow bile, and black bile) and the notion that, in each individual, every part of the body had a unique natural combination of these humours; when they were in balance, the body was healthy. Because this balance was different for each individual, the physician had to determine every patient's unique normal humoral condition [16]. Therefore, although humoral medicine was a mix of professional and lay theories that lacked a sound scientific basis, the emphasis was on the uniqueness of the sick individual ([15], p. 139).

Health care has made substantial progress since the era of Hippocrates, yet modern-day practitioners continue to be inspired by his commitment to the principle of beneficence—a duty to act in the individual patient's best interests [17]. Apart from physicians, the nursing profession has also evolved with the individual patient's interests as a compass to the right direction. For instance, the two first provisions of the American Nurses Association (ANA) Code of Ethics state that the nurse should practise with respect for the inherent dignity, worth, and unique attributes of every person and that the nurse's primary commitment is to the patient [18]; also, the two first provisions of the Nursing and Midwifery Council (NMC) Code for Nurses and Midwives demand to treat people as individuals and respond to their preferences [19]. These considerations are inherent to the nursing profession, in line with the holistic approach which entails care for the individual patient's personality traits beyond bodily functions, such as religious beliefs, cultural background, family status, or psychological reactions to disease and disability. But nurses go one step further, as they adopt patient advocacy duties, usually framed in individual patients [20].This means that, apart from caring for each patient as an individual, nurses also promote and protect each patient's individual rights. The significance of this duty is evident when one considers modern health-care delivery, highly specialised and fragmentary, driven by technological progress, increasingly bureaucratic and impersonal, and often hostile to individuality. We shall return to this issue in the next subchapter.

Despite the difficulties posed by modern health-care delivery, an increasing number of studies ascertain the importance of individualised care. Suhonen et al. [21] have developed a model which links individualised care to improved patient outcomes in terms of satisfaction, autonomy, and perceived health-related quality of life, noting that it can be used in further research related to individualised patient care advantages. Other researchers draw their attention to more specific patient outcomes. For instance, a recent study by Futier et al. [22] concludes that the risk of postoperative organ dysfunction for patients undergoing abdominal surgery was reduced with management strategies targeting an individualised systolic blood pressure, compared to standard management strategies. Other studies do not focus on indicating positive outcomes of individualised care, but rather on factors contributing to its effectiveness. In the field of nursing, Redfern [23] points out factors such as personal qualities of nurses, shared understanding of the goals of nursing care, levels of staffing, and effective leadership and management. As more reliable and widely used instruments to study individualised care are developed, it is expected that its evidence-based importance shall increase even further in the near future.

Based on the existing evidence, health-care organisations recognise the need to enhance individualised care and implement various initiatives to do so. For instance, UK's National Clinical Guideline Centre (NCGC) provides various recommendations to health-care professionals, such as to take into account domestic, social, and work situation of patients and avoid making assumptions based on their appearance or other personal characteristics ([24], p. 50). It is important to note that individualised care is also extended to individual patient education on how to manage their problems, since educational needs are different depending on patients' knowledge and attitude, as well as their specific diseases and health problems. Therefore, guidelines for patient education and empowerment also endorse the need for individualised counselling. For instance, the European League Against Rheumatism has issued recommendations for patient education for people with inflammatory arthritis, stating that it should be tailored to the individual patient's needs and citing many randomised controlled trials which indicate that individual counselling has beneficial health effects [25]. In sum, individualised care in its various aspects has become a universal trend in health-care delivery, with solid and augmenting evidence to back it up.

2.4   Individualised Care and Economic Constraints

It has thus been established that individualised care is important and that this is widely recognised. However, as noted above, this importance does not always take precedence over other considerations in modern health care. Resources are finite, while demand for health is infinite ([26], p. 19); therefore, there must be some kind of rationing. Policymakers try to allocate health resources in a just way, by considering the magnitude of the benefits that each health intervention produces, with respect to its cost. Expensive interventions that benefit small numbers of people tend to be low priorities compared to cheaper interventions that benefit great numbers of people. The doctrine of utilitarianism is manifest in the allocation of health-care resources. Policymakers decide about groups of patients than individual patients, with regulating bodies such as the UK's National Institute for Clinical Excellence (NICE) which sets the thresholds in terms of cost-effectiveness with regard to what health interventions can be reimbursed by the state [27]. The needs of individuals are important, but not as much as the greatest amount of good for the greatest number of people.

Apart from policymakers, who make decisions at a level of macro-allocation, there are also health-care professionals, who take decisions at a level of micro-allocation, but often bound by the policymakers' decisions and limitations. The traditional fundamental duty of health-care professionals to secure the individual patient's best interests and wishes must be balanced against the welfare of the health system in which they practise. Minogue [28] notes that physicians who view themselves as having ethical duties only to the individual patient are at odds with the new world of medicine; the physician, and every health-care professional for that matter, is both the agent of the patient and the agent of the health-care system. This means that no patient shall receive the best available care according to his individual needs if this is deemed unjust for society [29]. The state shall not reimburse the required interventions, so the only option for complete satisfaction of individual needs is an out-of-pocket payment or a private insurance contract, both at the expense of the patient. And, sometimes, even these options are not available for the individual. People with rare diseases may not get appropriate pharmacological treatment, because pharmaceutical companies do not invest in developing drugs for small target groups with little profit margin (orphan drugs). Therefore, even basic individual patient needs can be ignored by modern health-care systems.

On the other hand, one of the newest trends in health care is the field of *personalised medicine*, where decisions, interventions, and products are tailored to the individual patient's profile and needs, mainly based on his unique variation of the human genome. For instance, the FDA recently approved Kymriah©, a genetically engineered immunotherapy for leukaemia that alters a patient's own cells to fight cancer. This drug must be made individually for each patient, and it can cost as much as $475,000 [30]. Is it possible for any health-care system to afford costs of this size without reducing the budget for other interventions? If this new therapy is very effective and it cures leukaemia, then perhaps it makes sense, considering that all the other costs related to leukaemia's treatment shall be nullified. But this is not clear yet. The antithesis created by using cutting-edge technology in health care is evident in this case. Treatment can now be highly individualised; but this comes at a great financial cost, and it cannot be advanced in a just way—not yet at least—as it consumes health resources needed by other patients.

However, despite economic constraints and policymaking limitations, health-care professionals have many opportunities to practise individualised care, as the growing scientific evidence suggests. Inadequate staffing due to financial constraints may hinder these efforts, as well as the general structure of modern health-care facilities, with big hospitals that are economically viable replacing small regional units where health professionals and patients had more opportunities to better know each other. But other developments favour individualised care. Home-based nursing is such an example, with nurses and patients creating deeper professional relationships, thus facilitating individualised care interventions. And even within large hospitals, depending on the staff's commitment and willingness, there are many nursing actions that can be tailored to specific patients' needs. In general, small-scale individualised interventions which fall out of macro-allocation decisions need to be encouraged. To achieve this, it is not enough to refer to individual patients. Individualised care has two components: the individual patient on the one hand and the individual practitioner on the other.

2.5 Health Professionals' Individuality

Modern health professionals are expected to be competent in a wide variety of roles. These include those of manager, educator, computer specialist, bureaucrat, government (or medical insurance company) employee, technologist, writer, financial expert, businessman, judge, ethical expert, advocate for patients, family friend and confidant, as well as that of healer ([31], p. 68). Technological progress tends to remove modern health care from its anthropocentric mission, and many health professionals feel that their clinical autonomy is compromised as a result. Burnout symptoms, routinisation, and organisational cynicism increase among nurses and physicians who work in modern complex health-care settings [32], and empathy levels are in steady decline, even among nursing students who are exposed to patient encounters [33]. It would seem that health professionals' commitment and job satisfaction are in inverse proportion to their level of involvement in modern professional environments.

This finding represents a wider problem in today's health-care provision. Being recognised and treated as an individual is probably more important to a person when he becomes a patient, as he feels vulnerable and he tries to adapt to a new reality. Preserving the patient's autonomy has been set as a milestone goal for health-care systems worldwide. However, by focusing on patients' autonomy, health professionals often compromise their own. The patient's sense of individuality and the importance of his individualised care fail to be properly respected when health professionals ameliorate their own needs of professional individualism and self-realisation. To treat patients as individuals, practitioners must also be treated as individuals—before all else, they need to think of themselves as individuals and acknowledge that the care that each one of them is able to provide is unique. Patient empowerment cannot be achieved without health professional empowerment.

Conclusion

Each patient experiences health care in a unique and individual way, and so do health-care professionals. Proper individualised care needs to be based on both perspectives and at all periods of life. Ivan Illich, a pioneer critic of modern medicine, was especially concerned about massive health-care delivery in a homogenous way, even in patients' final hours: 'when hospitals draft all those who are in critical condition, they impose on society a new form of dying' ([34], p. 50). He recognised a continuous and universal demand for individuality, in health, illness, and death alike. Individualised care extends beyond mere differences in biological needs and symptoms, to different personalities and worldviews. However, the greatest good is often impossible without individual sacrifices. The quest to find a balance between social justice and individual needs in health care, or rather a *dynamic* balance, a mean that is relative to us in the words of Aristotle, must be continued. Modern medicine provides more opportunities than ever for individualised care, but it also sets a series of obstacles for its delivery. Health systems are still in transition; in due time, both patients and health professionals shall find the way to achieve this balance, in order for the best affordable individualised care to be provided.

References

1. Alexander R. The evolution of social behavior. Annu Rev Ecol Evol Syst. 1974;5:325–83.
2. Lear J. Inside and outside the Republic. Phronesis. 1992;37(2):184–215.
3. Aristotle. In: Rowe C, editor. Nicomachean ethics (trans.). New York: Oxford University Press; 2002.
4. Smith ND. Aristotle's theory of natural slavery. Phoenix. 1983;37(2):109–22.
5. Barrett M. The duty of a Pastor: John Owen on feeding the flock by diligent preaching of the word. Themelios. 2015;40(3):459–72.
6. Nozick R. Anarchy, state and utopia. New York: Basic Books; 1974.
7. Hampton J. Hobbes and the social contract tradition. Cambridge: Cambridge University Press; 1986.
8. Lamprecht SP. The fable of the bees. J Philos. 1926;23(21):561–79.
9. Smith A. An inquiry into the nature and causes of the wealth of nations. Oxford: Oxford University Press; 1976.
10. Sartre JP. Existentialism and humanism (trans. Mairet P). In: Priest S, editor. Jean-Paul Sartre: basic writings. London: Routledge; 2001.

11. Keijzer N. Military obedience. Alphen aan den Rijn: Sijthoff & Noordhoff; 1978.
12. Mommsen W. The age of bureaucracy: perspectives on the political sociology of Max Weber. Oxford: Basil Blackwell; 1974.
13. Nagel T. The possibility of altruism. Princeton: Princeton University Press; 2012.
14. Kleisiaris CF, Sfakianakis C, Papathanasiou IV. Health care practices in ancient Greece: the Hippocratic ideal. J Med Ethics Hist Med. 2014;7:6.
15. Greaves D. The healing tradition: reviving the soul of western medicine. Oxford: Radcliffe; 2004.
16. Jackson WA. A short guide to humoral medicine. Trends Pharmacol Sci. 2001;22(9):487–9.
17. Srinivasan M. From the editors' desk: Hippocrates and patient-centered medicine. J Gen Intern Med. 2012;27(2):135.
18. ANA. Code of ethics for nurses with interpretive statements. Silver Spring: American Nurses Association; 2015.
19. NMC. The code: professionals standards of practice and behaviour for nurses and midwives. London: Nursing and Midwifery Council; 2015.
20. Mahlin M. Individual patient advocacy, collective responsibility and activism within professional nursing associations. Nurs Ethics. 2010;17(2):247–54.
21. Suhonen R, Välimäki M, Katajisto J, Leino-Kilpi H. Provision of individualised care improves hospital patient outcomes: an explanatory model using LISREL. Int J Nurs Stud. 2007;44(2):197–207.
22. Futier E, Lefrant JY, Guinot PG, et al. Effect of individualized vs standard blood pressure management strategies on postoperative organ dysfunction among high-risk patients undergoing major surgery: a randomized clinical trial. JAMA. 2017;318(14):1346–57.
23. Redfern S. Individualised patient care: its meaning and practice in a general setting. NT Res. 1996;1(1):22–33.
24. NCGC. Patient experience in adult NHS services: improving the experience of care for people using adult NHS services. London: Royal College of Physicians; 2012.
25. Zangi HA, Ndosi M, Adams J, et al. EULAR recommendations for patient education for people with inflammatory arthritis. Ann Rheum Dis. 2015;74:954–62.
26. Daniels N. Just health care. Cambridge: Cambridge University Press; 1985.
27. McCabe C, Claxton K, Culyer AJ. The NICE cost-effectiveness threshold: what it is and what that means. PharmacoEconomics. 2008;26(9):733–44.
28. Minogue B. The two fundamental duties of the physician. Acad Med. 2000;75(5):431–42.
29. Waymack M. Health care as business: the ethic of Hippocrates versus the ethic of managed care. Bus Prof Ethics J. 1990;9:69–78.
30. Morrow T. Novartis's Kymriah: harnessing immune system comes with worry about reining in costs. Manag Care. 2017;26(10):28–30.
31. Helman CG. Culture, health and illness. 4th ed. Oxford: Reed Educational and Professional; 2000.
32. Volpe RL, Mohammed S, Hopkins M, et al. The negative impact of organizational cynicism on physicians and nurses. Health Care Manag. 2014;33(4):276–88.
33. Ward J, Cody J, Schaal M, Hojat M. The empathy enigma: an empirical study of decline in empathy among undergraduate nursing students. J Prof Nurs. 2012;28(1):34–40.
34. Illich I. Limits to medicine. Medical nemesis: the expropriation of health. Harmondsworth: Penguin Books; 1990.

Understanding the Basics and Importance of Individualised Nursing Care

Riitta Suhonen

Abstract

This chapter aims to describe the origin and history of the term individualised nursing care in general and as used in the nursing and nursing science literature. Furthermore, this chapter describes the research conducted on this topic over the past 60 years and how the concept itself has evolved during this time. The description is based on the development of professional nursing care and on the contexts, issues and ideologies to which the concept of individualised care has been linked. Finally, this chapter describes briefly why the topic is important in the healthcare context for individual clients or patients, professional nurses and organisations.

Keywords

Individualised care · Importance · Origin · History · Professional nursing
Nursing research · Development

3.1   The Origin of the Concept of Individualised Care

Individualised care has its origin in the word 'individual' as a noun or adjective. 'Individual' has been defined in terms of a single or particular person, distinguished from class or species, a human being as contrasted with social being, a particular person and being genetically individual [1]. These defining characteristics have a link to ontology, the origin and existence of an individual and the idea

R. Suhonen
Department of Nursing Science, University of Turku, Turku University Hospital and
City of Turku, Welfare Division, Turku, Finland
e-mail: riisuh@utu.fi

© Springer International Publishing AG, part of Springer Nature 2019   17
R. Suhonen et al. (eds.), *Individualized Care*,
https://doi.org/10.1007/978-3-319-89899-5_3

that each human being is different from others even after death. On the one hand, this definition links an individual strongly to the notion of human beings as species; on the other, it includes a link to the holistic constitution of the characteristics belonging to an individual. Later, the term 'individual' was defined in terms of a person who thinks or behaves in a different way from other people [2]. According to Kearns [3], 'person' is a moral and metaphysical category (p. 80) and 'can be applied to human beings and other entities that display certain characteristics' (p. 80). Kearns [3] also connects 'person' strongly with ethical consideration (see Chap. 5).

The origin of the word is in the medieval Latin word *individualis* and also in the Latin word *individuus*, meaning indivisible or inseparable [4]. The modern sense of individual was established from the seventeenth century onwards [5]. 'Extraordinary' became the modern meaning of individual [6], with the idea of freedom of thought and action for each individual person as the most important quality of society. However, the abstract notion of individualism needs to be distinguished from the idea of individuality, which refers to the development of different dispositions among individual humans as a result of interactions with their environment [6] containing both individual and social values.

Inspecting the word 'individuality' as a noun gives some more distinction to the concept of individualised care. Individuality has been defined, for example, in terms of 'different from other things, uniqueness' [7] or the qualities that distinguish one person or thing from all others and the condition of having separate existence [8]. These definitions suggest that individuality is the quality or characteristic that distinguishes one person from any other and the state of existing as an individual [9]. This term also connects the idea of individuality to the behavioural and cognitive development of individuals and their characteristics.

Adding an examination of the term 'individually' as an adverb makes the term more understandable from the point of view of interaction of at least two individuals and, in our context, takes it closer to clinical nursing practice. Individually means, for example, 'in an individual manner' [10], or 'one at a time or separately, personally and in an individual or personally unique manner' [11]. These definitions bring 'person' close to activities of individuals, particularly with reference to nursing care, and thus, the activity of a professional, when considering individualised nursing care. The care of an individual person needs to be individualised, having also an ethical or a moral ground, duty-based nursing care and consideration of an individual. Thus, the origin of the concept of individualised care, including aspects of the terms individual, individuality and individually, bounds nursing care on ethical grounds. This means nursing individuals and taking care of individuals. The ethical grounds are, for example, the domains of a person: dignity, privacy, autonomy and self-development.

Finally, there is a need for closer inspection of one more term, 'individualise' as a verb. The term to individualise means 'to treat or notice individually, particularise' [1] and 'an act of individualising' [12]. Collins COBUILD English language dictionary [7] defined individualisation as follows: 'If you individualise something, you make it different from other things and able to be recognised and identified'. In the 1990s, the dictionary definitions identified individual needs: to adapt to the needs of an individual [8]. Although the Oxford Dictionary of Nursing [13] defined the term to individualise as 'care that is planned to meet the particular needs of one patient, as opposed to a routine applied to all patients suffering from the same disease', the special meaning of the concept, based on Chinn and Kramer [14], has its roots in the 1970s: to treat or notice individually.

Based on the dictionaries, the noun 'individual' was not used synonymously with 'person', although it may be appropriate in situations where a single person is being considered in contrast to a group. However, the distinction between the different terms, namely, individual and person and individualised and personalised, has not been clear in the nursing literature.

3.2   Individualised Care in the Nursing Literature

The term 'individualised care' first appeared in the care literature in the early 1950s and has been used, for example, in the field of psychogeriatrics [15]. Clow [15] discussed ageing persons' needs to preserve their individual independence and personal identity. Furthermore, Clow [15] (p. 460) continued by writing that 'the greatest need of the ageing person is to feel that he is participating in the life rather than merely existing'. This was one of the first starting points recognising the need for individualised care of ageing people. It was also a starting point to suggest that there are many dimensions while analysing individuality in care and individualised care: whether it is an activity or a perception. For a while after that, it appeared rarely in the literature. In the 1960s, individualised care started to appear more often in the nursing literature, and the topic has been empirically studied since the 1970s in the discipline of nursing science.

Individual and individuality of a person have been regarded as one of the main concepts in many nursing theories. Nursing theorists linked individual, and thus individualised consideration of patients, in their theories (e.g. [16–19]). Although the theorists used the term 'patient-centred care' in their writings, they explained the content of the topic in a very similar way, meaning individual persons, their needs and nursing care activities performed in an individual manner. Myra Levine [18] wrote an epochal paper about what she believed about patient-centred care in which the individualisation of nursing care also gained a new basis and theoretical meaning in nursing science. Myra Levine [18] stated that patient-centred care lies on patient individuality and allowing that individuality to guide the care. She raised the importance of individualisation by stating 'that the entire structure of professional nursing rests on the ability of the practitioner to individualize care' (p. 54). However, she already knew at the time that the term itself had been substituted for the idea and was becoming a fantasy, not a reality. In more recent literature, Thompson et al. [20] also stated that especially health professionals may think of individualised care as an ideal as they consider the patient at the time instead of recognising and being able to analyse the reality. Thinking back to the 1960s, we may conclude individualisation of nursing care has a long tradition in nursing.

Today, based on empirical evidence, nursing scientists may ask the following question: Have we reached it? [21].

In the 1970s, nursing studies were focused on the nursing process, assessment techniques and the guidelines and principles of nursing activities, especially primary nursing [22–24] and care delivered by a named nurse [25]. At that time, primary nursing was frequently associated with individualised nursing care [22, 24–27]. This approach to care was already strongly linked with organisational merits, philosophies and achievements in the early 1970s [28, 29] although individualised approaches to care did not become a topical theme in discussions about healthcare systems in many Western countries until after the turn of the millennium (e.g. [30, 31]).

Concomitantly with the professionalisation of nursing, there was a strong focus on developing nursing care, activities, care processes and protocols to meet individual patients' needs and preferences, but for quite a while the development focused mostly on nursing from the nurses' point of view and on advancing professional nursing practice [28]. Van Servellen [26] suggested that individualised nursing care transforms standardised nursing procedures and activities into personally tailored care within the unique context of each patient's situation. Thus, one of the main strands of the research and literature in the area of individualised care was to try to understand the concept and professional nurses' experiences of the provision of such care [9, 32]. This intention coincides with the development of nursing education. In the early 1990s, there was a growing recognition of the importance of inclusion of individualised care planning in nursing education (e.g. [33]).

Individualised care may deal with the question on how care is organised, but the importance is based on patients' perspectives as informants. Although nurses reported adopting a patient-focused philosophy in their work, they also reported frustration and inability to notion was the missing imaginative element of communication between the professional and the patient. With lack of research and discussion of individualised nursing care from patients' or relatives' point of view, this element was largely neglected [34]. A new area in the research linked to the individualised care, knowing the patient [35, 36], can be considered a strong advancement for thinking about individuals.

A review by Suhonen et al. [32] pointed out the small amount of empirical research on the realisation, provision and maintenance of individualised care; in addition, only a minority of the studies were implement individualised care. Special methods and supervision to support the implementation of individualised care, especially care planning, emerged strongly in the first half of the 1990s. Papers focusing on patients' experiences of the care received (e.g. [37, 38]) made a contribution and fostered the development of a strong patient focus in empirical nursing research, followed by demands for the development of the quality of nursing practice. Thus, little knowledge from the patients' point of view was available until a marked increase in the volume of research and nursing literature on individualised care was seen in the latter half of the 1990s. A paper by Brown [39] contributed strongly to putting the patients' perspective in the front line of research. She wrote about tailoring nursing care to the individual client. A paper by Redfern [34] made a contribution by analysing nurses' perceptions of individualised care provision and the conditions under which it is successful. This paper was controversial in that it added circumstances as well as organisational and management variables to the examination of the topic. In the twentieth century, studies appeared focusing on the levels of nursing education and roles of nurses and also on their relation to management and organisational issues.

Several researchers in Europe (e.g. [34, 40, 41]) and in the United States (e.g. [42, 43]) have focused on researching individuality of care as perceived by the patient, followed by research on factors related to individualised nursing care [44]. Although the studies conducted in the late 1980s and the early 1990s were mostly qualitative in their nature, newly developed instruments and results derived with them were frequently reported. However, trying to understand patients' experiences and what they thought constituted good nursing care was important. Individualised care was frequently linked to good nursing care by patients. In their meta-synthesis of qualitative studies, Jakimowicz et al. [45] concluded that person-centred, individualised nursing care proved to consist of factors impacting patients' subjective experience.

A landmark of increasing interest in empirical research on the topic was the appearance of several instruments measuring individuality, recognition of individuality and perceptions of individuality in care (see Chap. 9). The number of studies on both patients' and nurses' perceptions of individuality in the care provided and received and on the support of individuality in care increased rapidly. Validated instruments made it possible to broaden the research on the factors associated and investigate the effects of individualised interventions [46–48]. Research on the factors associated with perceptions of individualised care from both the patients' and nurses' point of view increased in the twentieth century both nationally (e.g. [49, 50]) and internationally in multisite collaboration (e.g. [21, 51, 52]). A recent interesting addition to the research area is the investigation of the built environment in association with the provision of individualised nursing care [53].

3.3 The Importance of Individualised Care

The delivery of individualised nursing care is considered important for several reasons (Sect. 3.3). Individuality of care and services is essential for the realisation of healthcare quality [54], ethical obligations and the development of a deeper understanding of user perspectives necessary for healthcare, health policy development [54–56] and increasing patient choice [57, 58]. This topic is one of the most important priorities in research and healthcare [59] for several reasons: First, we have found over the years that individuality of care and services is considered important by patients and healthcare professionals (e.g. [60, 61]). Second, individually tailored interventions and care are effective in producing positive outcomes for both patients and professionals [46, 48, 61, 62] and are also cost-effective [63]. Third, individualised interventions are especially needed in the care of chronic conditions demanding long-term commitment or care (e.g. [64, 65]).

Individualised care has been considered as a form of person-centred care delivery and is accepted as best practice or golden standard. However, research evidence suggests that its implementation into actual care is far from complete. In addition, a considerable amount of evidence has been provided about the difficulties and shortcomings in the provision of individualised care, especially for older patients (Chap. 11) and in acute care settings (Chap. 10). On the one hand, nurses report not using individualised care in their day-to-day practice [66, 67], while on the other hand, they feel that they support patient individuality quite well [52]. However, patients have perceived that the care they have received has been individualised only to some extent [51]. Furthermore, patients' and professionals' perceptions of individualised nursing care have been found to differ [68].

As seen earlier in this chapter, individualised care has been linked to the development of professional nursing care practice and also to the development of the healthcare system. Individuality of care and services has been seen as the goal of care to reach positive outcomes. It has been the goal for the entire system, for example, in the restructuring of healthcare services [30, 69]. Despite widespread belief in the importance of individuality and individualised care and services, it has been found difficult to create a system in which all groups work together for the good of the patient [70].

Conclusion

This chapter sets out to begin the exploration of the conceptual base of individualised care and related terms. A key point developed in this chapter is the understanding of the variety in the use of the term as well as approaches to try to understand this phenomenon. The origin of the terms and special context in nursing and nursing science helps to shed light on the various developments in professional nursing over time. Individualised care has been an important topic in these developments. The examples given about the importance of such care show that this kind of care is beneficial not only for patients but also for professionals and healthcare organisations.

References

1. Wyld HC, editor. The universal dictionary of the English language. 2nd ed. London: Purnell & Sons; 1936.
2. Cambridge international dictionary of English. London: Cambridge University Press; 1995.
3. Kearns AJ. The concept of person. In: Scott PA, editor. Key concepts and issues in nursing ethics. Cham: Springer; 2017. p. 69–81.
4. Barnhard RK, editor. The Barnhart dictionary of etymology. London: H. W. Wilson; 1988.
5. Room A, editor. Adrian Room dictionary of changes in meaning. New York: Routledge and Kegan Paul; 1986.
6. Mascuch M. Origins of the individualist self. Cambridge/Bodmin: Polity/Hartnolls; 1997.
7. Collins COBUILD English language dictionary, 1st ed. Glasgow: W. Collins; 1987.
8. Webster's new encyclopedic dictionary, 3rd ed. Cologne: Könemann; 1994.
9. Suhonen R. Individualised care from the surgical patient's point of view. Developing and testing model. Annales Universitatis Turkuensis D 523, Painosalama, Turku. 2002.

10. Thatcher VS, McQueen A, editors. The new Webster dictionary of the English language. New York: Grolier; 1967.
11. The random house dictionary of the English language. New York: Random House; 1987.
12. Webster's third new international dictionary, 14th ed. Chicago: Donnelley & Sons, Lakeside Press; 1961.
13. McFerran TA, editor. Oxford dictionary of nursing. 3rd ed. Oxford: Oxford University Press; 1998.
14. Chinn PL, Kramer MK. Theory and nursing. A systematic approach. 4th ed. St. Louis: Mosby; 1995.
15. Clow HE. Individualising the care of the ageing. Am J Psychiatr. 1953;110:460–4.
16. Abdellah FG, Beland IL, Martin A, et al. Patient-centered approaches to nursing. New York: Macmillan; 1967.
17. Henderson V. The nature of nursing. New York: Macmillan; 1967.
18. Levine ME. This I believe about patient-centred care. Nurs Outlook. 1967;15(1):53–5.
19. Peplau HE. Interpersonal relationships in nursing. New York: G. P. Putnam; 1952.
20. Thompson IE, Melia KM, Boyd KM, et al. Nursing ethics. 5th ed. Edinburgh: Churchill Livingstone/Elsevier; 2006.
21. Charalambous A, Radwin L, Berg A, et al. Modelling trust in nurses, individualized care, nursing care quality and health-related quality of life: a path analysis. Int J Nurs Stud. 2016;61(1):176–86.
22. Evans L. Primary nursing—an alternative approach for midwives. Aust Coll Midwives Inc J. 1998;11(1):7–10.
23. Manthey M. The practice of primary nursing. Boston: Blackwell; 1980.
24. van Servellen G. The concept of individualized care in nursing practice. Nurs Health Care. 1982;3:482–5.
25. Turner H. Incorporating the named nurse concept into care. Prof Nurse. 1997;12(8):582–4.
26. van Servellen G. Nurses' perceptions of individualized care in nursing practise. West J Nurs Res. 1988;10(3):291–306.
27. van Servellen G. The individualised care index. In: Waltz C, Strickland O, editors. Measurement of nursing outcomes. Volume one, measuring client outcomes. New York: Springer; 1988. p. 499–522.
28. Clifford JC, Horvath KJ. Advancing professional nursing practice. Innovations at Boston's Beth Israel Hospital. New York: Springer; 1990.
29. Mackay C, Ault LD. A systematic approach to individualizing nursing care. J Nurs Adm. 1977;7(1):39–48.
30. DoH. Keeping it personal. In: Clinical case for change: repost by David Colin-Thomé. London: Department of Health; 2007.
31. OECD. Towards high-performing health systems. OECD health project. Paris: Organisation for Economic Co-operation and Development (OECD); 2004.
32. Suhonen R, Välimäki M, Leino-Kilpi H. "Individualised care" from patients', nurses' and relatives' perspective—a review of the literature. Int J Nurs Stud. 2002;39(6):645–54.
33. Thorell-Ekstrand I, Björvell H, Blanchard-Caesar L. Preceptorship in clinical nursing education in Sweden: aspects of quality assurance. Qual Assur Health Care. 1993;5(3):227–36.
34. Redfern S. Individualised patient care: its meaning and practice in a general setting. NT Res. 1996;1(1):22–33.
35. Jenny J, Logan J. Knowing the patient: one aspect of clinical knowledge. Image J Nurs Sch. 1992;24(4):254–8.
36. Tanner CA, Benner P, Chesla C, et al. The phenomenology of knowing the patient. Image J Nurs Sch. 1993;25(4):273–80.
37. Allyne J, Thomas VJ. The management of sickle cell crisis pain as experienced by patients and their carers. J Adv Nurs. 1994;19(4):725–32.
38. Oleson M, Heading C, McGlynn-Shadick K, et al. Quality of life in long stay institutions in England: nurse and resident perceptions. J Adv Nurs. 1994;20(1):23–32.

39. Brown S. Tailoring nursing care to the individual client. Empirical challenge of a theoretical concept. Res Nurs Health. 1992;15(1):39–46.
40. Suhonen R, Välimäki M, Katajisto J. Developing and testing an instrument for the measurement of individual care. J Adv Nurs. 2000;32(5):1253–63.
41. Suhonen R, Leino-Kilpi H, Välimäki M. Development and psychometric properties of the Individualised Care Scale. J Eval Clin Pract. 2005;11(1):7–20.
42. Radwin L, Alster K, Rubin KM. Development and testing of the oncology patients' perceptions of the quality of nursing care scale. Oncol Nurs Forum. 2003;30(2):283–90.
43. Schmidt LA. Patients' perceptions of nursing care in the hospital setting. J Adv Nurs. 2003;44(4):393–9.
44. Schmidt LA. Patients' perceptions of nurse staffing, nursing care, adverse events, and overall satisfaction with the hospital experience. Nurs Econ. 2004;22(6):295–306.
45. Jakimowicz S, Stirling C, Duddle M. An investigation of factors that impact patients' subjective experience of nurse-led clinics: a qualitative systematic review. J Clin Nurs. 2015;24(1):19–33.
46. Rebelo Botelho AM, Fonseca C, Suhonen R, et al. Intervenções de Enfermagem Individualizadas: Uma Revisão da Literatura. Individualised nursing interventions: a literature review (in English). Pensar Enfermagem. 2015;19(1):47–61.
47. Ryan P, Lauver R. The efficacy of tailored interventions. J Nurs Scholarsh. 2002;34(4):331–7.
48. Suhonen R, Välimäki M, Leino-Kilpi H. A review of outcomes of individualised nursing interventions on adult patients. J Clin Nurs. 2008;17(7):843–60.
49. Chappell NL, Reid RC, Gish JA. Staff-based measures of individualized care for persons with dementia in long-term care facilities. Dementia. 2007;6(4):527–47.
50. Suhonen R, Välimäki M, Katajisto J, et al. Provision of individualised care improves hospital patient outcomes: an explanatory model using LISREL. Int J Nurs Stud. 2007;44(2):197–207.
51. Suhonen R, Berg A, Idvall E, et al. Individualised care from the orthopaedic and trauma patients' perspective: an international comparative survey. Int J Nurs Stud. 2008;45(11):1586–97.
52. Suhonen R, Papastavrou E, Efstathiou G, et al. Nurses' perceptions of individualised care: an international comparison. J Adv Nurs. 2011;67(9):1895–907.
53. Sawamura K, Nakashima T, Nakanishi M. Provision of individualized care and built environment of nursing homes in Japan. Arch Gerontol Geriatr. 2013;56(3):416–24.
54. WHO. Towards people-centred health systems: an innovative approach for better health outcomes. WHO Regional office for Europe. Division of Health Systems and Public Health. 2013. http://www.euro.who.int/en/health-topics/Health-systems/public-health-services/publications/2013/towards-people-centred-health-systems-an-innovative-approach-for-better-health-outcomes. Accessed 11 Jan 2018.
55. OECD. Health at a Glance 2016: Europe. State of the Health in the EU Cycle. Paris: OECD; 2016. https://doi.org/10.1787/9789264265592-en.
56. WHO. Chronic diseases and health promotion. 2015. http://www.who.int/chp/about/strategy/chp_structure/en/. Accessed 11 Jan 2018.
57. European Commission. Impact of information on patients' choice within the context of the Directive 2011/24/EU of the European Parliament and of the Council on the application of patients' rights in cross-border healthcare. Final report. 2014. https://ec.europa.eu/.../cbhc_information_patientschoice_en.pdf. Accessed 11 Jan 2018.
58. The Health Care Act. 2010/1326. 2010. http://www.finlex.fi/fi/laki/kaannokset/2010/en20101326. Accessed 11 Jan 2018.
59. Nolte E, McKee M. Caring for people with chronic conditions. A health system perspective, European observatory on health systems and policies series. Glasgow: Bell and Bain; 2008.
60. Suhonen R, Välimäki M, Leino-Kilpi H. The driving and restraining forces that promote and impede the implementation of individualised nursing care: a literature review. Int J Nurs Stud. 2009;46(12):1637–49.
61. Suhonen R, Stolt M, Gustafsson M, et al. The associations between the ethical climate, the professional practice environment and individualised care in care settings for older people: a cross-sectional survey. J Adv Nurs. 2014;70(6):1356–68.

62. Schalk DMJ, Bijl LMP, Halfens RJG, et al. Interventions aimed at improving the nursing work environment: a systematic review. Implement Sci. 2010;5:34. https://doi.org/10.1186/1748-5908-5-34.
63. Olsson L-E, Hansson E, Ekman I, et al. A cost-effectiveness study of a patient-centered integrated care pathway. J Adv Nurs. 2009;65(8):1626–35.
64. Dorner B, Friedrich EK, Posthauer ME. Practice paper of the American Dietetic Association: individualized nutrition approaches for older adults in health care communities. J Am Diet Assoc. 2010;110(10):1554–63.
65. Spaling MA, Currie K, Strachan PH, et al. Improving support for heart failure patients: a systematic review to understand patients' perspectives on self-care. J Adv Nurs. 2015;71(11):2478–789.
66. Caspar S, O'Rourke N. The influence of care provider access to structural empowerment on individualized care in long-term-care facilities. J Gerontol B Psychol Sci Soc Sci. 2008;63B(4):S255–65.
67. Caspar S, O'Rourke N, Gutman GM. The differential influence of culture change models on long-term care staff empowerment and provision of individualized care. Can J Aging. 2009;28(2):165–75.
68. Suhonen R, Efstathiou G, Tsangari H, et al. Patients' and nurses' perceptions of individualised care: an international comparative study. J Clin Nurs. 2012;21(7-8):1155–67.
69. The Finnish SoHe reform. Regional government, health and social services reform. 2018. http://alueuudistus.fi/en/frontpage. Accessed 17 Jan 2018.
70. Kreindler S. The politics of patient-centred care. Health Expect. 2015;18(5):1139–50.

The Concept of Individualised Care

Riitta Suhonen and Andreas Charalambous

Abstract

The conceptual investigation of individualised care includes the meaning attributed to the term, the uses of the concept in nursing literature and the various proposed definitions of the concept found in the nursing literature. This chapter outlines the utilisation of the individualised care concept in nursing science literature but also in some other health disciplines. Furthermore, the development of the concept in regard to its different meanings and definitions used over time will be examined.

Keywords

Concept · Conceptualisation · Definition · Individualised care · Tailoring
Healthcare · Discipline

4.1   The Meaning of the Concept of Individualised Care

In the literature, the verbs individualising, personalising and tailoring have been used synonymously in the sense of acquiring and using a form of particularistic knowledge, or having knowledge about issues, circumstances or characteristics that

R. Suhonen (✉)
Department of Nursing Science, University of Turku, Turku University Hospital and
City of Turku, Welfare Division, Turku, Finland
e-mail: riisuh@utu.fi

A. Charalambous
Department of Nursing Science, Cyprus University of Technology, Limassol, Cyprus

University of Turku, Turku, Finland
e-mail: andreas.charalambous@cut.ac.cy

27
R. Suhonen et al. (eds.), *Individualized Care*,
https://doi.org/10.1007/978-3-319-89899-5_4

account for individual differences [1]. Although there is a difference, for example, between the two terms individualise and tailoring, authors have used them synonymously and interchangeably over the years in both clinical and theoretical nursing literature. Lauver et al. [2] state that "tailored interventions are based on assessment of multiple and individual characteristics (of a patient), each of which may have many values, interventions are matched and delivered from a predetermined specific protocol" (p. S31). The defined individualised interventions in terms of "highly customised, based on assessment of several characteristics of individuals… Guided by general guidelines, interventions evolve in interactions with participants in real time" (p. S31). Thus, Lauver et al. [2] conclude that the levels of specificity and complexity of individualised interventions (care) are much higher than are those for other kinds of patient-centred interventions" (p. S33).

In some work, tailoring has been seen as a sub-concept of individualised care, using tailoring as one conceptual specification for the individualisation of care [3]. For example, in terms of activities, nursing interventions, individualised and tailored interventions were considered as synonyms, but the level of depth in the definitions is different. Based on the definition by Cox [4, 5] in the Interaction Model of Client Health Behavior (IMCBH), tailoring was operationally defined in terms of attending to a client's singularity; discussing client singularity, clinical assessment and management content in association with the client; and carrying out interventions that are explicitly personalised to the individual. In some other work [6, 7], it was pointed out that the fundamental characteristics of patient-centred care were patient involvement in care and the individualisation of patient care, suggesting that individualisation may be a sub-concept of patient centeredness. This means that the concepts formulate a continuum where different characteristics vary.

"The third mode participial" of the term individualised care is also sometimes used synonymously with "tailored" and "client-centred" and also "personalised" and "person-centred" care [7–9]. All these terms convey the idea that the care provided takes into consideration individuals' needs, desires, experiences, preferences, behaviours, feelings, perceptions and understandings [7, 10–12]. Nevertheless, individualised care is typically used without a precise definition or consensus on a shared understanding [12]. In addition, there are differences in how the term is understood by patients [7, 11, 13] and by nurses [12, 14–16]; this is no doubt due to the only partially overlapping worlds of the two groups.

For example, the term patient-centred care has frequently been used in the context of organisation (healthcare services research [17–20]). This has usually referred to the client or patient contact inside the service system or organisation while aiming to view services from the patients' point of view. The term "tailored care" is especially used regarding the care of a group of patients (nursing [7, 21]), such as people in cardiac rehabilitation [21, 22] or people with type 2 diabetes [23], while more recently, the tailored model approach was introduced with elderly patients with depression in primary care [24].

When the terms tailoring or individualising have been used in the literature, they have usually referred to a professional nurse's activity or intervention (e.g. [8, 10]). Individualising or tailoring is a promising technique for encouraging greater performance of health-related behaviours ([25, 26], and is used a lot in health promotion literature. Tailored interventions are designated to be more individualised to personal characteristics, in contrast to standard or routine interventions where all patients receive the same type of care. A standardised, routine, "fit-for-all" view and depersonalised care are ideologically contrary terms for individualised care [1]. In such care, the person is seen in terms of the disease emitting signs and symptoms, on the basis of which a diagnosis can be made and appropriate treatment prescribed.

One question that seems to arise here is whether there is a common denominator underlying the concepts analysed above. To say the least, it seems that the concepts are informed or influenced (some to a greater and some to a lesser extent) by the theory of holism. A holistic nurse is a licensed nurse who takes a "mind-body-spirit-emotion-environment" approach to the practice of traditional nursing. By definition, nursing is informed by the holistic paradigm, as the nursing profession has traditionally viewed the person as a whole, concerned with the interrelationship of body, mind and spirit, promoting psychological and physiological well-being as well as fostering sociocultural relationships in an ever-changing economic environment of care ([27], p. 413). The close relationship between the nursing profession and the idea of "holism" is not new; it goes back to the 1970s with influences identified in the work of humanistic theorists such as Rogers [28] and Levine [29]. A central aspect to both of these theorists' work is viewing each patient as a unique human being with individual characteristics that need to be considered and addressed within the wholeness context.

4.2   The Use of the Concept of Individualised Care

The use of the term "individualised" care has different outputs in different fields of sciences close to nursing science. These may help to valorise the mixed use of the terms claimed to be views and definitions typical to a specific discipline but still having some similar elements. The context of each discipline in which the term has been used and defined offers a fruitful discussion for some shared understanding of the topic.

The term "individualised clinical assistance" has been used in the medical field, especially in the context of primary healthcare [30]. Weiner [30] argued that it is important to consider contextual factors that are unique to each patient and relevant to their care while making any decision. The paper by Weiner [30] highlighted the importance of the patient-physician encounter and focusing strongly on social systems together with clinical medical issues. In the medical field, with emphasis placed on the molecular and genetic level, personalised medicine appeared strongly in the literature in the twentieth century. Personalised medicine refers to the bio and genetic areas of medicine [31]. It is "a form of medicine that uses information about a person's genes, proteins, and environment to prevent, diagnose and treat disease" [32]. Personalised medicine has revolutionised cancer care in particular. Thus, personalised medicine focuses on improving the patient's situation by providing the right diagnosis leading to prevention or treatment at the right dose to the right patient at the right time. However, it should be acknowledged that the term "person-alised medicine" as it has been widely used focuses heavily on the physical dimen-sion of the person and does not embrace the person in its totality.

In social sciences, based on psychology, the term "personal psychosocial care" has been used (social gerontology [14]). Chappell et al. [14] criticised the use of the medical model especially in the care of older people as well as the strong focus on the therapeutic physical environments. Caspar and O'Rourke [33] argued that such specialised care is usually provider-driven instead of patient-driven. The psychoso-cial environment, which proved to be important in provision of individualised care, was largely neglected. However, when looking at empowerment, the formal care-giver's ability to provide individualised care becomes apparent [33].

Examination of the concept of person-centred care has been performed in the context of multi-disciplinary dementia care and in care facilities where the patients have been in danger of losing their identity due to the severe illness. Such contexts have highlighted the social dimension of care, the relationship between patient and professional [34]. This examination has helped scientists and their work and is strongly based on humanistic psychology [35]. Kitwood's idea on re-humanisation of dementia care strongly supports one research area in person-centred care [34]. In this area, person-centred care includes individuals' "experience" as perspective in addition to medical activity (referring to the medical model of disease, treatment and care), "subjectivity" (including experience of illness, daily activities, roles and social network) and "decision-making" about health, care and services (e.g. [18, 36]). A conceptual paper by Kitson et al. [37] synthesised literature from policy, medicine and nursing about patient-centred care, and they suggested three main themes: patient participation and involvement, the relationship between the patient and healthcare professional and the context where it is delivered. Adding to the paper of Kitson et al. [37], one would argue that an important aspect is missing from the three themes identified, namely, that of the process of tailoring the interventions to best meet the person's needs. It has been argued that care is often complex, mean-ing that many processes influence the outcomes in unpredictable ways. The Tailored Implementation for Chronic Diseases (TICD) collaborative research project imple-mented for patients with chronic diseases (mainly in primary care settings) comple-ments and highlights the knowledge on concepts and methods of tailoring interventions [38–40].

Finally, in nursing science, the term "individualised nursing care" has been con-sidered as a perception of the client (or healthcare consumer) or patient about the care provided [10, 41, 42], and it has received extensive attention in research by exploring different viewpoints and different contexts. This was deemed necessary in an effort to address the complexity of the concept but also to accommodate the vary-ing perceptions of those involved in delivering and receiving care (Chaps. 10, 11, 12, 13, 14 and 15).

A variety of uses and topics can be identified for the concept of individualised care in nursing science literature. The concept of individualised care has appeared as one of the principles of care of the nursing profession [43, 44]), especially in the nursing ethics literature (e.g. [45]). Furthermore, individualised care has been regarded as an approach or philosophy to nursing care [13, 46], goal of care [13, 47] and a golden standard of care. There is also a considerable amount of literature on individualised care as an element, indicator or component of nursing care quality [48–51]. In nursing practice, it has been defined in terms of a tool, method, intervention [52, 53], process or activities of nurses to obtain positive patient outcomes or a patient's perception of individuality in the received nursing care [49]. Individualised care has also been seen as an outcome of nursing care itself [54]. In the earliest framework, individualised care was defined in terms of organising or implementing care [15, 16].

4.3   Defining Individualised Care in Nursing Science

Several researchers have conceptualised, and later measured, the concept of individualised care. Some examples are given in Table 4.1. These definitions describe the time and view on how the concept itself has evolved over time (see Chap. 3). Some definitions describe the antecedents of the concept of individualised care while others provide exact attributes for the concept. The viewpoint to start the definition, whether for professional nurse, organisation or patient, provides a slightly different scope for the output.

4.3.1   Antecedents

In analysing the literature and defining the concept, *antecedents and consequences* for the concept may be found at the same analysis. There are three main antecedents that seem to be common over time to providing individualised nursing care in any case and irrespective of context. Firstly, there is a need for establishing a caring relationship in which the nurses assess and collect information about patients' preferences, needs and perceptions and one that entails respect to the person's unique identity (refer to Chap. 12). Secondly, there is a need for frequent contacts with the patient where the nurses fit (tailor or individualise) the information on nursing care interventions or rehabilitation activities in clinical settings, for example, to the patient's characteristics and situation, reactions to the patient's responses to a health concern and the physical and socio-environmental characteristics (e.g. [5]). Finally, the patients need to have possibilities to have decisional control, shared decision-making over their care intervention, referring to individuals' expectations of having the power to participate in making decisions to achieve informed preferences. Elwyn et al. [62] argue that shared decision-making is not simply information transfer to the patient; it extends towards honouring informed preferences, taking into consideration the principles of self-determination theory [63] and relational autonomy [64]. Within the nursing care context, shared decision-making becomes possible through patient-nurse interactions where nurses promote and commit to the patients, e.g. making space for patients to manifest their individuality.

Table 4.1 Examples of the definitions of individualised care in nursing literature

Definition	Context and viewpoint	Author
"Individualised nursing care, sometimes called patient-centred care, involves meeting the specific and comprehensive physical, psychological and social needs of each patient. A knowledge and understanding of the patient as an individual, as a member of a family and a resident of a community is a basis of this care"	Nursing care delivery, nursing process, organisational charting if care facilities and work are organised to support individualised care on a ward level	Mackay and Ault [55] (p. 39)
Tailoring of client-nurse interaction to the client's individuality represents a specification of the term individualisation of care [4] "Tailoring involves taking into account the client's individuality and allowing that individuality to determine interpersonal approaches and health-illness management actions" ([56], p. 43)	Cox's Interaction Model of Client Health Behavior Individualisation of care in an interaction	Cox [4] (p. 177) Brown [56] (p. 43)
An ideal aspect of nursing practice, patient right "… holds that all standardised procedures and care plans should be translated in terms of the unique peculiarity of each patient situation. Care is separate and distinct as it is applied to real, basic patient-family care; the right of the patient to protection of this uniqueness is ensured when a modality (of nursing care) stresses individuality of patients' responses to standardised treatment"	Meaning and essence of individualised care Specific nurse behaviours to promote individualised care Nursing activities	van Servellen [51] (p. 483) based on Marram (later van Servellen) et al. [57], van Servellen [15, 16]
"An interdisciplinary approach which acknowledge elders as unique persons and is practiced through consistent caring relationships"… includes four critical attributes: knowing the person, relationship (staff continuity and permanent assignment), choice (in decision-making and risk-taking) and resident participation and direction	Older ("frail elderly people") people care setting	Happ et al. [13] (p. 7)
A nursing practice based on the conception of the patient as a unique individual who deserves respect and who has a right to retain dignity… caring as an emotional response and caring as series of tending activities or tasks. Tending— attending to patients' nursing care needs, over and above practicing individualised patient care in the sense of concern for, and commitment to patients—is a process which unfolds from patients' admission	General nursing in hospital setting Principles and values, core practices and factors facilitating or limiting individualised patient care	Redfern [58] (p. 28–29)
"In ideology of the management of care of the patient on the basis of his unique needs, the objective being maximum independence from the necessity of such care"	Primary nurse care planning, organisational Hospital care	Waters and Easton [59] (p. 79–80) based on grant 1979

Table 4.1 (continued)

Definition	Context and viewpoint	Author
"Individualised care results when the nurse: Knows the patient as a unique individual, and Tailors nursing care to patient's experiences (including events associated with illness, home, work and leisure); behaviours (including physical indicators and preferred coping strategies); feelings; and perceptions (including meaning ascribed to experiences and interpretations of events)"	Framework for crafting and evaluating individualised care, whether nurses consider components of the definition as interventions are implemented Patient care, nurses' assessments	Radwin and Alster [7] (p. 62)
"Respecting individuality; Holistic care; Focusing on nursing needs; Promoting independence; Partnership and negotiation of care; and Equity and fairness"	Principles underpinning the philosophy of individualised care How nurses conceptualised and practiced individualised care	Gerrish [60] (p. 93)
The "Seeing the individual patient" category represents the individualised nature of nursing care experience"… "to be known as more than their diagnoses"… …"expected the nurses to treat them as a person". "patients' needs to be treated as unique individuals"	Hospitalised patients' perceptions of their nursing care Sub-concept for patients' perceptions of hospital care	Schmidt [61] (p. 395)

Likewise, Cox [4], Lauver et al. [8], Ryan and Lauver [65] and Lauver et al. [8] have noted that individualised care involves allowing the individuality of a patient to determine interpersonal approaches and nursing interventions. Because patients are different, a variety of interventions are required which define individualised care [66]. Therefore, the precise content of an individualised intervention is not determined prior to a nurse-patient interaction but develops during that interaction ([8], p. 251). In these circumstances nurses need to work from general guidelines rather than protocols so that the interventions evolve in interactions with patients in real time ([2], p. 31).

4.3.2 Defining Elements and Empirical Referents

In the Individualised Care Project (ICP), the term "individualised nursing care" was defined from the patients' point of view [10] as a perception of the patient or healthcare service user. Thus, the definition includes subject matters which patients can experience, see or recognise while being cared for (nursing activities performed at the bedside). Patients' perceptions and assessment of individuality on their care become possible when individualised care is set in the frame of patient-care provider interaction. Thus, the elements are set in the form that this interaction assumes. This meant the presence of nursing activities. Individualisation of care can be supported through specific nursing activities. While cared for with individualised activities, the patient can experience individuality in his/her care. Originally, individualised care was defined in terms of patients' views on how individuality was supported through specific nursing activities and how they experienced individuality in their own care [1, 42]. This definition was based on the deductive reasoning of the uses and definitions of the concept found in the literature (see Table 4.1) and also in qualitative research literature. As the literature at that time concentrated mainly on nurses' point of view or patients' perceptions of care in general, dictionary definitions were used to reveal the patient viewpoint. This definition includes two interpretations: the perception of how nurses support patient individuality by their activities and the perception (experience) of how their individuality is taken into account in care provision (maintenance of actual care). Both of these interpretations were included in the operationalisation of the concept for empirical research. The developed Individualised Care Scale comprised two parts:

> Individualised care is a type of nursing care delivery which takes into account patients' personal characteristics in their clinical situation (=condition), personal life situation and preferences and promoting patient participation and decision-making in his/her care (=decisional control) [1, 42].

Common themes in the individualised care literature have included the recognition of patients' individual clinical situation, personal life situation and decisional control over care (e.g. [5, 7, 13]). The criterion for identifying these themes (domains) was the frequency of the characteristics. Finally, the elements of the concept of individualised care were extracted through the selection of key statements by identifying and clustering similarities from mainly qualitative studies examining patients' perceptions (Table 4.2).

Table 4.2 Domains and elements of individualised nursing care

Patient's clinical situation	Patient's personal life situation	Patient's decisional control
Physical and psychological care needs, fears and anxieties	Life situation in general (employment, etc.)	Knowledge about illness and treatment/care
Abilities, capacities or resources	Cultural background, traditions	Making choices, having alternatives
Health condition	Daily activities, habits and preferences	Decision-making
Meaning of illness	Family involvement	Expressing own views, opinions, wishes and making proposals
Reactions or responses to illness	Earlier experiences of hospitalisation	
Feelings, affective states		

Conclusion

Over time, the concept of individualised care has triggered discussion and misunderstandings as to what it entails. Indeed, the context of healthcare, where the concept has mainly been championed, is a complex one that requires extensive study of the concept's antecedents, defining elements and empirical referents. However, one should acknowledge the limitations in any attempt to comprehensively attribute a conceptual definition to any given concept. Concepts are like ice cubes; just when you think you have grasped them, a lack of clarity results in their slipping beyond your grasp [27].

While the definitions of individualised care, tailored care and patient-centred care are not the same, they do share an important common attribute: their theoretical basis rests on the principles of holism which acknowledges that the human being, composed of a mind, body and soul integrated into an inseparable whole that is greater than the sum of the parts, is in constant interaction with the universe and all that it contains.

The complexity in seeking a comprehensive understanding of individualised care also lies on the varying viewpoints from where one can experience individuality. Primarily, there are two paramount viewpoints, that of the patient and the nurse. Bringing the concept of individualised nursing care from the patients' point of view was the main target of the initiatives taken by researchers in the Individualised Care Project and later continued by a wide network of nurse scientists throughout the world. However, individuality in patient care may also be assessed from other viewpoints, such as nurses' perceptions of the individuality of patient care. This enabled the development of the concept and especially the empirical research on the topic from different viewpoints.

Over the years, the model of care has moved to a more multidisciplinary and interdisciplinary approach, and future attempts to conceptualise and research the topic of individualised care need to accommodate this multi-professional landscape of care. Within this context the needs, preferences and expectations of the person need to be acknowledged by all the disciplines involved in the delivery of the care without the interventions of one's discipline neutralising those of another discipline. Tensions between the varying perspectives of individualised care can go beyond the conceptualisation of the concept to include differences in the realisation of the interventions that guide implementation practice. Primarily, the aim should be for these interventions to complement one another. Interventions need to be jointly developed to comprehensively capture the multidimensional aspects of the person and allowing the person to play an active role where decisions need to be made when aspiring to attain a shared-decision model.

References

1. Suhonen R. Individualised care from the surgical patient's point of view. Developing and testing model. Annales Universitatis Turkuensis D 523, Painosalama, Turku. 2002.
2. Lauver DR, Gross J, Ruff C, et al. Patient-centered interventions. Implications for incontinence. Nurs Res. 2004;53(6 Suppl):S30–5.

3. Brown S. Tailoring nursing care to the individual client. Empirical challenge of a theoretical concept. Res Nurs Health. 1992;15(1):39–46.
4. Cox CL. An interaction model of client health behavior: theoretical prescription for nursing. Adv Nurs Sci. 1982;5(1):41–56.
5. Cox CL, Roghmann KJ. Empirical test of the interaction model of client health behavior. Res Nurs Health. 1984;7(4):275–85.
6. Coulombe S, Radziszewski S, Meunier S, et al. Profiles of recovery from mood and anxiety disorders: a person-centered exploration of people's engagement in self-management. Front Psychol. 2016;7:584. https://doi.org/10.3389/fpsyg.2016.00584.
7. Radwin LE, Alster K. Individualised nursing care: an empirically generated definition. Int Nurs Rev. 2002;49(1):54–63.
8. Lauver DR, Ward SE, Heidrich SM, et al. Patient-centered interventions. Res Nurs Health. 2002;25(4):246–55.
9. O'Rourke N, Chappell NL, Caspar S. Measurement and analysis of individualized care inventory responses comparing long-term care nurses and care aides. Gerontologist. 2009;49(6):839–46.
10. Suhonen R, Välimäki M, Katajisto J. Developing and testing an instrument for the measurement of individual care. J Adv Nurs. 2000;32(5):1253–63.
11. Suhonen R, Schmidt LA, Radwin L. Measuring individualized nursing care: assessment of reliability and validity of three scales. J Adv Nurs. 2007;59(1):77–85.
12. Suhonen R, Gustafsson M-L, Katajisto J, et al. Individualised care scale–nurse version: a Finnish validation study. J Eval Clin Pract. 2010;16(1):145–54.
13. Happ MB, Williams CC, Strumpf NE, et al. Individualised care for frail elders: theory and practice. J Gerontol Nurs. 1996;22(3):6–14.
14. Chappell NL, Reid RC, Gish JA. Staff-based measures of individualized care for persons with dementia in long-term care facilities. Dementia. 2007;6(5):527–47.
15. van Servellen G. Nurses' perceptions of individualized care in nursing practise. West J Nurs Res. 1988;10(3):291–306.
16. van Servellen G. The individualised care index. In: Waltz C, Strickland O, editors. Measurement of nursing outcomes. Volume one, measuring client outcomes. New York: Springer; 1988. p. 499–522.
17. Jakimowicz S, Perry L. A concept analysis of patient-centred nursing in the intensive care unit. J Adv Nurs. 2015;71(7):1499–517.
18. McCormack B, McCance TV. Development of a framework for person-centred nursing. J Adv Nurs. 2006;56(5):472–9.
19. McCormack B, Karlsson B, Dewing J, et al. Exploring person-centredness: a qualitative meta-synthesis of four studies. Scand J Caring Sci. 2010;24(3):620–34.
20. Mead N, Bower P. Patient-centredness: a conceptual framework and review of the empirical literature. Soc Sci Med. 2000;51(7):1087–110.
21. Cossette S, Frasure-Smith N, Dupuis J, et al. Randomized controlled trial of tailored nursing interventions to improve cardiac rehabilitation enrolment. Nurs Res. 2012;61(2):111–20.
22. Johansson A, Adamson A, Ejdebäck J, et al. Evaluation of an individualised programme to promote self-care in sleep-activity in patients with coronary artery disease—a randomised intervention study. J Clin Nurs. 2014;23(19-20):2822–34.
23. Radhakrishnan K. The efficacy of tailored interventions for self-management outcomes of type 2 diabetes, hypertension or heart disease: a systematic review. J Adv Nurs. 2012;68(3):496–510.
24. Aakhus E, Granlund I, Odgaard-Jensen J, et al. A tailored intervention to implement guideline recommendations for elderly patients with depression in primary care: a pragmatic cluster randomised trial. Implement Sci. 2016;11:32. https://doi.org/10.1186/s13012-016-0397-3.
25. Rakowski W. The potential variances of tailoring in health behavior interventions. Ann Behav Med. 1999;21(4):284–9.
26. Suhonen R, Valimaki M, Leino-Kilpi H. A review of outcomes of individualised nursing interventions on adult patients. J Clin Nurs. 2008;17(7):843–60.
27. McEvoy L, Duffy A. Holistic practice—a concept analysis. Nurse Educ Pract. 2008;8(6):412–9.

28. Rogers ME. An introduction to the theoretical basis of nursing. Philadelphia: F. A. Davis; 1970.
29. Levine ME. Holistic nursing. Nurs Clin North Am. 1971;6:253–64.
30. Weiner SJ. Contextualizing medical decisions to individualize care. J Gen Intern Med. 2004;19(3):281–5.
31. European Commission. Towards personalised medicine. Research and innovation–health. 2012. https://ec.europa.eu/research/health/index.cfm?pg=policy&policyname=personalised. Accessed 17 Jan 2018.
32. NCI Dictionary of Cancer Terms. 2017. https://www.cancer.gov/publications/dictionaries/cancer-terms?cdrid=561717. Accessed 17 Jan 2018.
33. Caspar S, O'Rourke N. The influence of care provider access to structural empowerment on individualized care in long-term-care facilities. J Gerontol B Psychol Sci Soc Sci. 2008;63B(4):S255–65.
34. Kitwood T. Dementia reconsidered: the person comes first. Buckingham: Open University Press; 1997.
35. Rogers C. On becoming a person. New York: Houghton Mifflin; 1961.
36. Edvardsson D, Fetherstonhaugh D, Nay R, et al. Development and initial testing of the Person-centered Care Assessment Tool (P-CAT). Int Psychogeriatr. 2010;22(1):101–8.
37. Kitson A, Marshall A, Bassett K, et al. What are the core elements of patient-centered care? A narrative review and synthesis of the literature from health policy, medicine and nursing. J Adv Nurs. 2012;69(1):4–15.
38. Krause J, Van Lieshout J, Klomp R, et al. Identifying determinants of care for tailoring implementation in chronic diseases: an evaluation of different methods. Implement Sci. 2014;9:102. https://doi.org/10.1186/s13012-014-0102-3.
39. Wensing M, Huntink E, van Lieshout J, et al. Tailored implementation of evidence-based practice for patients with chronic diseases. PLoS One. 2014;9(7):e101981. https://doi.org/10.1371/journal.pone.0101981.
40. Wensing M. The Tailored Implementation in Chronic Diseases (TICD) project: introduction and main findings. Implement Sci. 2017;12(1):5. https://doi.org/10.1186/s13012-016-0536-x.
41. Charalambous A, Chappell NL, Katajisto J, et al. The conceptualization and measurement of individualized care. Geriatr Nurs. 2012;33(1):17–27.
42. Suhonen R, Leino-Kilpi H, Välimäki M. Development and psychometric properties of the Individualised Care Scale. J Eval Clin Pract. 2005;11(1):7–20.
43. Thompson IE, Melia KM, Boyd KM, et al. Nursing ethics. 5th ed. Edinburgh: Churchill Livingstone, Elsevier; 2006.
44. Levine ME. This I believe about patient-centered care. Nurs Outlook. 1967;15(1):53–5.
45. Davis AJ, Aroskar M. Ethical dilemmas and nursing practice. Norwalk: Appleton Century Crofts; 1983.
46. Wilson-Barnett J. Nursing values: exploring the clichés. J Adv Nurs. 1988;13(6):790–6.
47. Thomas LH. A comparison of the verbal interactions of qualified nurses and nursing auxiliaries in primary, team and functional nursing wards. Int J Nurs Stud. 1994;31(2):231–44.
48. Caspar S, Le A, McGilton KS. The responsive leadership intervention: improving leadership and individualized care in long-term care. Geriatr Nurs. 2017;38(6):559–66.
49. Radwin LE, Cabral HJ, Woodworth TS. Effects of race and language on patient-centered cancer nursing care and patient outcomes. J Health Care Poor Underserved. 2013;24(2):619–32.
50. Rose PM. Individualized care in the radiation oncology setting from the patients' and nurses' perspectives. Cancer Nurs. 2016;39(5):411–22.
51. van Servellen G. The concept of individualized care in nursing practice. Nurs Health Care. 1982;3:482–5.
52. Radwin LE, Cabral HJ, Wilkes G. Relationships between patient-centered cancer nursing interventions and desired health outcomes in the context of the health care system. Res Nurs Health. 2009;32(1):4–17.

53. Weldam SW, Lammers JJ, Zwakman M, et al. Nurses' perspectives of a new individualized nursing care intervention for COPD patients in primary care settings: a mixed method study. Appl Nurs Res. 2017;33:85–92. https://doi.org/10.1016/j.apnr.2016.
54. Annells M, Koch T. 'The real stuff': implications for nursing of assessing and measuring a terminally ill person's quality of life. J Clin Nurs. 2001;10(6):806–12.
55. Mackay C, Ault LD. A systematic approach to individualizing nursing care. J Nurs Adm. 1977;7(1):39–48.
56. Brown S. Communication strategies used by an expert nurse. Clin Nurs Res. 1994;3(1):43–56.
57. Marram G, Barrett M, Bevis E. Primary nursing—a model for individualised care. 2nd ed. St. Louis: C. V. Mosby; 1979.
58. Redfern S. Individualised patient care: its meaning and practice in a general setting. NT Res. 1996;1(1):22–33.
59. Waters KR, Easton N. Individualized care: is it possible to plan and carry out? J Adv Nurs. 1999;29(1):79–87.
60. Gerrish K. Individualized care: its conceptualization and practice within a multiethnic society. J Adv Nurs. 2000;32(1):91–9.
61. Schmidt LA. Patients' perceptions of nursing care in the hospital setting. J Adv Nurs. 2003;44(4):393–9.
62. Elwyn G, Frosch D, Thomson R, et al. Shared decision making: a model for clinical practice. J Gen Intern Med. 2012;27(10):1361–7.
63. Ryan RM, Deci EL. Self-determination theory and the facilitation of intrinsic motivation, social development, and well-being. Am Psychol. 2000;55(1):68–78.
64. Mackenzie C. Relational autonomy, normative authority and perfectionism. J Soc Philos. 2008;39(4):512–33.
65. Ryan P, Lauver DR. The efficacy of tailored interventions. J Nurs Scholarsh. 2002;34(3):331–7.
66. Radwin L. Oncology patients' perceptions of quality nursing care. Res Nurs Health. 2000;23(3):179–90.

Ann Gallagher and Rueben C. Warren

Abstract

The ethical underpinning of 'individualised care' seems obviously related to the value of autonomy. What is less clear is how individualised care compares with other models of care such as person-centred care and evidence-based care. Models of care with an ethical underpinning need also to integrate evidence to improve health-care outcomes. The facts must, therefore, inform the values and vice versa. What is too rarely considered is which values, in addition to autonomy, underpin individualised care so this is expanded to provide a sufficient model of care across contexts and cultures. Does individualised care, for example, have relevance to public health? Drawing on two practice scenarios relating to care in clinical and public health settings, we argue that individualised care is most helpfully contextualised within a model of 'integrative care' informed by an 'integrative ethics'. We develop a three-level model—individual, family and community—with scope to apply key ethical values. The approach we propose goes beyond a traditional autonomy-based model of individualised care towards an integrative bioethics with capacity to integrate the activities of advocacy, empowerment and activism.

Keywords

Individualised care · Person-centred care · Ethics · Public health · Integrative ethics

A. Gallagher (✉)
International Care Ethics Observatory, University of Surrey, Guildford, Surrey, UK
e-mail: a.gallagher@surrey.ac.uk

R. C. Warren
National Center for Bioethics in Research and Health Care,
Tuskegee University, Tuskegee, AL, USA

5.1   Introduction

The view that 'individualised care' is best suited to respond to the health needs of individual members of our communities is persuasive. How, for example, we respond to the total needs of an older person who chooses to refuse dialysis would seem to come under the umbrella of 'individualised care'. Similarly, how we engage with the health needs of a mother described as 'morbidly obese' who seeks medical help to have a second child would seem at first sight to be a good fit with this model of care. What is at stake, ethically, appears to be respect for autonomy and the individual's right to choose.

It is our view that 'individualised care' and related terms are not sufficient to respond to the holistic health needs of people across cultures and across care contexts. We argue for a three-level model of care underpinned by a pluralist and multidisciplinary approach to ethics. We are arguing, therefore, that 'individualised care' is but one component of what we should aspire to within an integrative model of care with a broader view of ethics across care contexts.

We build on previous work on 'integrative bioethics' [1] and draw on insights from ethics as applied to care and public health. We conclude by suggesting a tentative matrix with three levels of analysis—individual, family and community—and three ethical lenses which seem fit for purpose. To illuminate our discussion, we introduce two anonymized practice scenarios that highlight the limits of a sole focus on 'individualised care' and the value of an 'integrative model of care'. First, we engage with the meaning and ethical implications of individualised care and related models.

5.2   Individualised Care and Other Autonomy-Oriented Models of Care

A plethora of terms are used to refer to models of care that focus on responses to the needs of single care recipients, for example, personalised care [2], relationship-centred care [3], participant-centred care [4], consumer-directed care [5], person-centred care [6] and, the topic of this text, individualised care. Here we focus on two of the most common terms: person-centred care and individualised care. First, we engage with individualised care, the focus of this chapter and book.

It is not clear when the term 'individualised care' was first used, nor is it obvious how it can be distinguished from related models of care. It could be assumed that the shift in focus to individuals or persons was a reaction to care regimes which were institutionalised, routinised, depersonalised and oriented towards groups. It might be assumed also that the shift from depersonalised groups to focus on individuals was driven by attention to the many care scandals on both sides of the Atlantic. Reports of institutional neglect, abuse and exploitation can be traced back to previous decades in both the United Kingdom [7] and the United States, for example, the US Public Health Service Syphilis Study at Tuskegee [8]. It might also be suggested that legal and societal shifts to respect the moral status and rights of all people, regardless of their race/ethnicity, class, sex/gender, sexual orientation, disability or of...geographic location, served to challenge and change discriminatory and exploitative beliefs to some extent.

In nursing, the evolution of the 'nursing process' which dates back to the 1950s signalled a challenge to non-individualised medical care as it focused on holistic assessment, planning, implementation and evaluation. It also, crucially, draws on the nurse's reasoning and decision-making [9]. Alongside this is the rise of evidence-based practice in health care [10]. One of the editors of this volume co-wrote an article on the theme of individualised care and patient outcomes [11] and defined the phenomenon as 'a type of nursing care delivery which takes into account patients' personal characteristics and preferences promoting patient participation and decision-making in his or her care'. The authors go on to say that the 'patient's viewpoint' is operationalized in two ways: first, in the way the nursing intervention is 'tailored' to the patient's individual needs and, second, 'how well the patient's individuality is understood by the nursing staff'.

This is a good starting point for a discussion of individualised care in relation to nursing practice as it highlights a focus on the individual, the importance of getting to know the individual and of tailoring care interventions to his/her characteristics and preferences. The caveat of 'taking into account' suggests that there may be limits on individual choices, however, the overall ethical focus of this approach to care is on 'respect for autonomy'. We will discuss autonomy later. We next turn to some discussion of a well-known model of care that is similar to individualised care.

Whilst the origins of 'individualised care' are unclear, the history of person-centred care has been documented. American humanistic psychologist, Carl Rogers, is credited with the first use of 'person-centred' in relation to psychotherapy in the 1960s. He had previously used the term 'client-centred' therapy. American psychiatrist, George Engel, initiated a shift from a medical model to a biopsychosocial model which underpinned person-centred care. Health-care models in the United Kingdom and the United States embraced this development, and there are signs of the shift from the 1990s in policy and practice [12]. The role of person-centred dementia care is, however, credited to Thomas Kitwood at the University of Bradford in the United Kingdom in the late 1980s. Heerema [13] writes that a person-centred approach to people experiencing dementia involves a recognition that there is more to the individual than a diagnosis of dementia. She writes:

> A person-centred approach changes how we understand and respond to challenging behaviours in dementia. Person-centred care looks at behaviours as a way for the person with dementia to communicate his needs, and understands that figuring out what unmet need is causing the behaviours is key. Person-centred care also encourages and empowers the caregiver to understand the person with dementia as having personal beliefs, remaining abilities, life experiences and relationships that are important to them and contribute to who they are as a person. On a moment-by-moment basis, person-centred care strives to see the world through the eyes of the particular person with dementia.

In a report on the theme of 'person-centred care', the Health Foundation [12] opted to offer a four principles' framework rather than 'a concise but inevitably limited definition'. The foundation publication listed the following principles:

- Affording people's dignity, compassion and respect
- Offering coordinated care, support or treatment
- Offering personalised care, support or treatment
- Supporting people to recognise and develop their own strengths and abilities to enable them to live an independent and fulfilling life

Whilst these four principles are appealing from an ethical point of view, questions remain regarding definition so we can more clearly sketch the philosophical terrain within which to situate 'individualised care'. We might ask: What is meant by a person? What does person-centred really mean? and How might it be reconciled with 'family-centred care' or 'community-centred care'?

Readers may be aware that the term 'person' is contentious in philosophical terms. In short, on some views, not all humans are persons and some persons may be non-humans. The idea of 'personhood' has underpinned discussion of ethical issues at the beginning and end of life. Debates relating to abortion and embryo research and to withholding and withdrawing treatment and euthanasia, for example, have raised questions about the meaning and implications of personhood. Some philosophers argue that 'persons' are beings with intelligence, self-awareness and consciousness, and it is these qualities and the status of 'person' that bestow moral agency and rights (see, e.g. [14]).

A potential hazard of having strict criteria for 'personhood', as presented in some philosophical perspectives (e.g. intelligence, self-awareness, consciousness), is that some humans (neonates, those who are psychotic, have severe intellectual disabilities or are unconscious) will not count as 'persons'. The meaning of the term 'person' in 'person-centred care' needs then to be made clear and precision sought as to which perspectives on 'personhood' are ethically defensible and which are not. Kitwood's version of person-centred care [13], for example, does not adhere to traditional philosophical criteria for 'personhood' but rather focuses on the individual and who he/she is in the moment regardless of capacity.

Those perspectives on individual-focused care that are ethically defensible would include a holistic focus on the individual drawing on values that both individualised and person-centred care models could be said to have in common, namely, the value of autonomy and human dignity. So we have two individual-focused models of care which, whilst there are some different challenges with each, have a common orientation towards respecting choice and autonomy. But is respect for autonomy a sufficient basis in relation to these models?

5.3   From 'Traditional' to 'Relational' Autonomy

'Respect for autonomy' is one of the four principles of biomedical ethics [15] and, in its earliest iteration, was referred to as 'respect for persons'. In the Belmont report [16] 'respect for persons' was described as:

> Respect for persons incorporates at least two ethical convictions: first, that individuals should be treated as autonomous agents, and second, that persons with diminished autonomy are entitled to protection. The principle of respect for persons thus divides into two separate moral requirements: the requirement to acknowledge autonomy and the requirement to protect those with diminished autonomy.

Beauchamp and Childress [15] remind us of the Greek origins of autonomy as *autos* (self) and *nomos* (government or rule). The imperative to 'respect autonomy' involves rules relating to information-giving, consent and confidentiality. The constraints on autonomy are described as internal to the person (e.g. relating to limited mental capacity) and external (e.g. related to disempowering regimes or paternalism). Beauchamp and Childress [15] state that the two conditions necessary for autonomy are then 'liberty' (where the individual is free from 'controlling influences') and 'agency' (where the individual has capacity to make informed decisions). The paradigm of autonomy appears to be the rational freely choosing individual, and this is addressed directly by Beauchamp and Childress:

> […] in recent years, some feminists have sought both to affirm autonomy and revise individualistic or atomistic concepts of autonomy through ideas of "relational autonomy" that center on the conviction that "persons are socially embedded and that agents' identities are formed within the context of social relationships and shaped by a complex of intersecting social determinants, such as race, class, gender, and ethnicity". These accounts maintain that "oppressive socialization and oppressive social relationships" can impair autonomy. (p. 61, 2001 edition of Beauchamp and Childress)

As suggested here, feminist perspectives on autonomy enrich our ethical perspectives and contribute to a deepening of any analysis of individualised and related models of care. Mackenzie and Stoljar [17] discuss the importance of considering individuals as socially and historically embedded and of the need to think of autonomy as:

> A characteristic of agents who are emotional, embodied, desiring, creative, and feeling, as well as rational, creatures, and they highlight the ways in which agents are psychically internally differentiated and socially differentiated from others.

In discussing the role of self-trust and health care, McLeod and Sherwin (in [17], p. 259) point out that 'traditional autonomy theory' has focused on autonomy-inhibiting factors such as 'coercion, internal compulsion and ignorance'. They argue that another factor that compromises an individual's autonomy is by 'the forces of oppression'. They write (p. 259–260):

Oppression may itself involve dimensions of coercion, compulsion and ignorance, but it functions in complex and often largely invisible ways, affecting whole social groups rather than simply disrupting isolated individuals […] We understand relational autonomy to involve explicit recognition of the fact that autonomy is both defined and pursued in a social context significantly influences the opportunities an agent has to develop or express autonomy skills. In relational autonomy, it is necessary to explore an agent's social location if we hope to evaluate properly and respond appropriately to her ability to exercise autonomy.

The feminist critique of traditional forms of autonomy and the arguments for 'relational autonomy' suggest more meaningful approaches to models of individualised care that engage with less limiting and broader views of individuals. Individuals need to be considered within their social, political, historical and geographical context along with aspects of their individual identities (race, ethnicity, sex, gender, sexual orientation, class, age) and how these identities intersect need to be considered. So whereas the area of individual identity may well be captured by versions of 'individualised care', it is doubtful that the broader context of care will be addressed adequately.

We turn next to two anonymised practice scenarios which illustrate some of these conundrums. We will then consider some ways forward to respond combining relational autonomy and public health ethics perspectives into what we call an 'integrative care ethics' approach.

5.4   Two Care Scenarios: The Limitations of Autonomy-Focused 'Individualised Care'

5.4.1   Scenarios

1. Mrs. Gordon is 88 years old, a widow and a retired nurse. She has lived in a care home for 4 years and is in poor health. She has kidney failure and goes to a hospital for dialysis two times a week. Mrs. Gordon has a loving son (James) and a daughter-in-law (Lois) who visit her several times a week. The home caregivers are attentive and have come to know Mrs. Gordon very well. They have, they tell her son, come to think of her as 'family'. Mrs. Gordon tells James that she is now tired and plans to stop dialysis. Although sad to hear this news, James respects her choice. The home caregivers, on the other hand, do not understand her decision. They say 'but isn't she getting the best possible care here'? 'Stopping dialysis is suicide' and our job is to care.

2. Ms. Dixon is 30 years and has a BMI of 35. She talks with her physician about her plans to have a second child. Her physician reminds her that her first pregnancy was complicated by her weight and highlights the risks to mother and baby. Ms. Dixon points out that her son is just fine and a 'chunky' 5 year old. Ms. Dixon's partner, Johua Grant, is also overweight, has high blood pressure and is not motivated to change his lifestyle. The family is on a low income and live in a rural area, and the nearest hospital is 30 miles away. They have limited access

to fresh fruit and vegetables and opt for cheaper, less healthy food options for themselves and their 5-year-old son. Mr. Grant is a painter and decorator and is regularly exposed to toxins in the materials he uses, and this could also have an impact on his fertility.

5.5 Towards an Integrative Model of Care

The ethical issues in both scenarios are not straightforward. The first observation is that both involve individuals in relationships with others—in families and in local and global communities. Mrs. Gordon has been a nurse and has, it seems, very good relationships with her family and the care home staff. It seems likely that her decision to discontinue dialysis was well considered, and there was no evidence of coercion, compulsion or ignorance. Her decision can, then, be considered autonomous in the traditional sense. However, there are other considerations. The quality of these relationships is important, and, in addition to autonomy, an underpinning value must be 'care'.

Tronto's [18] four phases of care are helpful in considering the aspects and attitudes involved in the care of Mrs. Gordon. First, 'caring about'—this involves the attitudes of 'attentiveness' and recognising the care needs of others. Minimally, there is a triadic relationship here amongst Mrs. Gordon, her family and the home caregivers. Minimally, there needs to be consideration of their care needs. The second phase is 'taking care of', and this relates primarily to the family of Mrs. Gordon who, we assume, take 'responsibility' and have made arrangements in collaboration with her, to have care provided both in the care home and in the hospital, where she receives her dialysis. The third phase of 'caregiving' directly involves Mrs. Gordon's formal caregivers. They demonstrate 'competence' in care. The fourth phase of care is care receiving and relates to the 'responsiveness' of the care recipient in relation to care provided. It involves being recognised and appreciated for care delivered (see Gallagher in Scott [19]).

The scenario suggests that the care received by Mrs. Gordon was attentive and competent and responsibility was taken by the family, the caregivers and also by Mrs. Gordon herself. She has made a decision that she no longer wishes to have dialysis, and this decision will lead to her death. It is understandable that the caregivers may feel that the care given has not been fully appreciated as Mrs. Gordon no longer wishes to live. Mrs. Gordon's decision is upsetting to the care home staff and perhaps may even be viewed as an affront to their caregiving mission. What needs to be made clear to them is that her decision does not come from any dissatisfaction with her care—in fact, she too has viewed the care home staff as 'family'—but rather that she is tired of living and suffering and views her dialysis as burdensome. Both Mrs. Gordon and her family need to make it clear that the care received has been greatly appreciated and that Mrs. Gordon's decision is unrelated to this. Nevertheless, it needs to be remembered that in this triadic care relationship structure, all are in need of care and no one should feel abandoned [20].

The situation of Ms. Dixon and her family introduces a range of additional ethical issues. This is not just a scenario relating to one person's decision to try for another baby but rather an issue with significant public health dimensions. The issue of obesity is a significant public health challenge and has been described as 'a risk factor for several health conditions, including diabetes, stroke, some cancers and lung and liver problems' [21]. At the time of writing, figures from the World Obesity Foundation (WOF) reported that there will be 2.7 billion people who are overweight and obese and many of these will need medical care. The WOF estimate is that 34% of people in the United States are obese with this set to rise to 41% by 2025. In the United Kingdom, 27% of people are estimated to be obese with this rising to 34% by 2025 [22]. A headline from the Boseley article is that:

> Without action the annual worldwide obesity bill will reach $1.2tn in 2025 with 46% of the cost falling on the US.

The general adult obesity rate varies by race, and ethnicity with the highest age-adjusted rate of obesity is 48.1% in the Black population [23].

It is pointed out that the causes of obesity are 'complex and there are no simple solutions'. The role of 'obesogenic' environments presents obstacles in promoting healthy lifestyles and can be said to 'cause obesity'. Responsibility for the rise of obesity is attributed to a number of stakeholders, for example, the corporate social responsibility of the food and drinks industries, the role of government and public services and the role of 'civic society and individuals' [21]. The Nuffield Council on Bioethics proposes an ethical framework for public health with elements that befit both of our scenarios, most importantly, the role of autonomy, health as a value, equality of health outcomes, equality 'of opportunity and access' (to health services and health-conducive environments) and the 'value of community'. By the latter is meant:

> [...] the value of belonging to a society in which each person's welfare, that of the whole community, matters to everyone. This value is central in the justification of both the goal of reducing health inequalities and the limitation on individual consent when it obstructs important health benefits. Public health often depends on universal programmes which need to be endorsed collectively if they are to be successfully implemented. ([21], p. 33)

Public health ethics, then, necessarily involves engagement with respect for individual autonomy and also with the collective. This is framed as a libertarian versus a collectivist position [21].

The idea of personal responsibility for health is controversial. Wikler [24] puts it this way:

> These claims of personal responsibility for health are sometimes answered jointly and peremptorily with one or both of a pair of rebuttals. One rebuttal is that such claims involve nothing more than "blaming the victim". The other rebuttal is that the policy consequences of recognition of personal responsibility for health would violate individual privacy.

It seems we have then a quandary as to how to think about and respond to the predicament of Ms. Dixon and her family. On the one hand, taking into account her social and political disadvantage initiatives that promote personal responsibility could be viewed as "victim blaming" or, on the other hand, as intrusive and violating the privacy of the family. Assuming a punitive approach to health promotion in relation to obesity is unlikely to reap positive benefits and could and should be reconsidered. A solidarity-based approach offers an alternative:

> [...] it would be preferable to call for active and healthy lifestyles in a positive way, as joyful ways of living. And many people respond positively to the argument that more active lifestyles are one factor that helps support the shared commitment of helping each other via a public health care system [25].

Returning to the discussion of relational autonomy, it becomes clear that a focus solely on Ms. Dixon as an individual is inadequate. There needs also to be consideration of her 'social location'. If, for example, she is African-American and living in a deprived part of the United States, she is likely to have experienced oppression [17] and disadvantage from her race, class, gender and history. Patricia Hill Collins [26] writes of how African-American women have to fight against prejudicial discourses of themselves as 'mammies, matriarchs, and welfare mothers' ([27], p. 38).

So whilst the physician who is having a conversation with Ms. Dixon may be listening and giving advice on an individual basis, she needs to go beyond 'individualised care' to consider Ms. Dixon in relation to her intersecting identities and in relation to all of the complexity which comes from her 'social location'. An 'integrated model of care' enables caregivers and policymakers to engage with the individual features of the person and also with the wide range of factors that contribute to health status that is necessary. This is a perspective on ethics that is helpful for both caregiving *and* public health activities.

5.6   Towards an Integrative Care Ethics: Sketching the Terrain

The two scenarios suggest that focusing on individuals, with too little regard for their family and community situation, is limiting. Whilst a holistic focus on the needs of care recipients—their biopsychosocial functioning—is important, there needs also to be a wider and deeper engagement with their 'social location'. The perspective of 'integrative bioethics' is particularly illuminating here. Sodeke [1] writes:

> Integrative bioethics is the science of life struggles, survival, and flourishing, particularly the environment of the United States where the seeds of race, ethnicity, gender, class, culture and spirituality have flourished (for good or ill). Essential to the public's realization of a humanly lived life is good health and health behaviours [...] We surmised that an integrative bioethical blending of historical, practical, and ethical considerations of issues, behaviours and actions is necessary to ensure defensible and appropriate responses, social policy and law.

Table 5.1 An integrative ethics of care

Levels	Individual	Family	Community
Values	Relational autonomy Care Empathy	Utility Equity Non-abandonment	Social justice Sustainability Solidarity
Focus of activity	Advocacy	Empowerment	Activism

The content of this is open for discussion; however, our engagement with the scenarios of Mrs. Gordon and Ms. Dixon and with literature relating to integrative ethics suggest a tentative matrix along the following lines (Table 5.1):

Three A's of bioethics have been suggested as academia, advocacy and activism [28]. There is much in bioethics 'academia' that can throw light on the two scenarios, most particularly insights from the four principles of biomedical ethics [15], from virtue ethics [29] and from care ethics (e.g. [18]) in particular.

We have illustrated how the traditional view of the principle of respect for autonomy is limited and how a *relational autonomy* perspective provides a broader view. The three other principles, from Beauchamp and Childress [15], have potential to expand our analysis, particularly as we consider ethical issues that relate to the family in caregiving and public health. Those principles are beneficence (do good) and non-maleficence (do no harm) which come together as the principle of *utility*. Here we need to weigh the benefits and harms of actions and omissions for all concerned—family and caregivers alike. The principle of justice is the fourth principle and reminds us of issues of fairness and equality in the distribution of resources. We have labelled this as '*social justice*' as this has wider implications and a more adequate response to oppression and historical and social injustice.

It can be argued that 'care' is relevant to all three levels in the matrix and, indeed, Joan Tronto considers care as essentially social and political. She writes:

> To recognize the value of care calls into question the structure of values in our society. Care is not a parochial concern of women, a type of secondary moral question, or the work of the least well off in society. Care is a central concern of human life. It is time that we began to change our political and social institutions to reflect this truth ([18], p. 180).

The care we have in mind in relation to the two scenarios involves attentiveness which underpins the virtue of empathy and requires listening and moral imagination to truly engage with the predicament of care recipients. The philosopher Iris Murdoch [30] writes of looking with a 'just and loving eye', and this, we think, captures the essence of empathy. This involves a commitment to understand the perspectives of care recipients, family members and communities and the motivation to never abandon. It is our view that the value of *non-abandonment* [20] needs to be highlighted when there is too little appreciation of the lived experience of care recipients and, perhaps, when there is fear either of death (as in the scenario of Mrs. Gordon) or of medical failure (as in the scenario of the Dixon/Grant family).

The values of *sustainability* and *solidarity* are included on the matrix to emphasise the importance of taking a longer view of caregiving and public health activities. Sustainability relates primarily to *community* at a local and global level. The United Nations' Sustainable Development Goals [31] has 17 critical aspirations. Three that are most relevant to the scenario of Ms. Dixon are good health and well-being ('promote health lives and promote well-being for all at all ages), gender equality ('achieve gender equality and empower all women and girls') and reduced inequalities ('within and among countries'). There is much to be gained from cross-cultural engagement, particularly in the areas of end-of-life care and in responding to challenges that impact on health and well-being such as obesity.

Regarding the value of *solidarity*, this has a long history and dates back to the nineteenth-century France. Auguste Comte argued that solidarity was the antidote to increasing atomisation and individualisation of society and this needed to have less priority than collective well-being and social concerns [25]. The Nuffield Council report on the value of solidarity suggests that much discussion of *solidarity* in bioethics focuses on one of two meanings: as a descriptive term referring to the perceived reality of social cohesion in a particular context or group, for example, in terms of shared goals and bonds, and as a prescriptive terms which call for more social cohesion and support whereby solidarity takes on a political role. An understanding of solidarity suggested in the Nuffield Council support is as follows:

> [...] solidarity signifies shared practices reflecting a collective commitment to carry 'costs' (financial, social, emotional or otherwise) to assist others [...] a practice and not merely as an inner sentiment or an abstract value. As such it requires actions. Motivations, feelings such as empathy etc. are not sufficient to satisfy this understanding of solidarity, unless they manifest themselves in acts.

This resonates with the three A's of bioethics referred to above and suggests both the impetus to support political activism to remedy injustice, to promote the empowerment of the family by providing information and enabling to them to avail of community resources and also to engage in an informed advocacy. Advocacy, in this context, is using scientific evidence to guide individualised care. When the science is incomplete, caution should be exercised. Activism emphasises vigorous action and is consistent with the overall value of *utility* bringing together principles of beneficence and non-maleficence which underpin direct caregiving and public health activities.

Conclusion

The social-cultural context in which individualised care is provided must be explored if positive and sustained health outcomes at the levels of the individual, family or community are expected. Health can be described as a relationship, a dynamic interplay, between the physical, social, psychological and spiritual elements that create the well-being of the individual and/or group in their physical and social environment [32]. It is a dynamic interface between one's self and one's 'social location'.

Individualised care, whilst focusing on individuals, is unlikely to be effective if the individual is isolated from the group, be it from a family or a community. Hence our argument is for an integrative model of care. The group has an underestimated influence on the health of the individual. People seldom are healthy or ill in isolation [33]. With the advent of the Genome Project, personalised medicine can now target care based on the specific genomic mapping of individuals. Epidemiology provides the scientific foundation from which evidence-based care is delivered and from which individualised care must also rely.

There are many ethical lenses through which to view individualised care and the two scenarios. We have tentatively sketched the terrain for an integrative model of care underpinned by an integrative ethics. We derived insights from the four principles of biomedical ethics, from care and feminist ethics and from the public health ethics literature. We also suggested the relevance of virtue ethics in relation to the ethical qualities of the caregiver [29]. The study of public health ethics requires the practitioner to effectively conceptualise and operate with an appreciation of the tension of individual rights and collective interest [34].

We cannot claim to have developed a complete account of ethics in relation to an integrative model of care. We do, however, hope that we have raised some questions and stimulated reflection about the adequacy of individualised care as ordinarily understood.

References

1. Sodeke SO. Tuskegee University experience challenges conventional wisdom: is integrative bioethics practice the new ethics for the public's health? J Health Care Poor Underserved. 2012;23(4 Suppl):15–33.
2. Department of Health. Personalised care planning: information sheet 1. 2011. https://www.gov.uk/government/uploads/system/uploads/attachment_data/file/215946/dh_124048.pdf. Accessed 25 Feb 2018.
3. My Home Life. Relationship-centred care. 2017. http://myhomelife.org.uk/good-practice/relationship-centred-care/. Accessed 28 Mar 2018.
4. Oregan Health Authority (undated) Patient Centered Services (PCS). See https://www.oregan.gov/OHA/PH/HEALTHYPEOPLEFAMILIES/WIC/Pages/orwl/aspx.
5. Australian Government. What is consumer directed care? Information for home care package providers. Department of Social Services. https://www.myagedcare.gov.au/. Accessed 28 Mar 2018.
6. Royal College of Nursing. What person-centred care means: first steps for health care assistants. http://rcnhca.org.uk/sample-page/what-person-centred-care-means/. Accessed 28 Mar 2018.
7. Hutchison JS. Scandals in health-care: their impact on health policy and nursing. Nurs Inq. 2015;23(1):32–41.
8. Katz RV, Warren RC. The search for the legacy of the USPHS syphilis study at Tuskegee. Lanham: Lexington; 2011.
9. Frauman AC, Skelly AH. Evolution of the nursing process. Clin Excell Nurse Pract. 1999;3(4):238–44.
10. Greenhalgh T. How to implement evidence-based healthcare. Wiley. 2017. http://www.wiley.com/WileyCDA/WileyTitle/productCd-1119238528.html. Accessed 28 Mar 2018.
11. Suhonen R, Valimaki M, Katajisto J, et al. Provision of individualized care improves hospital patient outcomes: an explanatory model using LISREL. Int J Nurs Stud. 2007;44(2):197–207.
12. Health Foundation. Person-centred care made simple. 2014. http://www.health.org.uk/sites/health/files/PersonCentredCareMadeSimple.pdf. Accessed 28 Mar 2018.
13. Heerema E. Thomas Kitwood's person-centred care for dementia. 2017. https://www.verywell.com/what-is-person-centered-care-in-dementia-97737. Accessed 28 Mar 2018.

14. Anderson D. What is a person? Consortium on Cognitive Science Instruction. 2000. http://www.mind.ilstu.edu/curriculum/what_is_a_person/what_is_a_person.php. Accessed 25 Feb 2018.
15. Beauchamp TL, Childress JF. Principles of biomedical ethics. 7th ed. New York: Oxford University Press; 2013.
16. The Belmont report. The National Commission for the Protection of Human Subjects of Biomedical and Behavioural Research. 1979. https://videocast.nih.gov/pdf/ohrp_appendix_belmont_report_vol_2.pdf. Accessed 28 Mar 2018.
17. Mackenzie C, Stoljar N. Relational autonomy: feminist perspectives on autonomy, agency and the social self. New York: Oxford University Press; 2000. p. 35–51.
18. Tronto JC. Moral boundaries: a political argument for an ethic of care. New York: Routledge; 1993.
19. Gallagher A. Care ethics and nursing practice. In: Scott A, editor. Key concepts and issues in nursing ethics. Cham: Springer; 2017. p. 55–68.
20. Martinsen EH. Caring in medicine: from a gentleman's care to 'a more sophisticated sense of human independence'. In: Olthuis G, Kohlen H, Keier J, editors. Moral boundaries redrawn: the significance of Joan Tronto's argument for political theory, professional ethics and care as practice. Leuven: Peeters; 2014. p. 113–32.
21. Nuffield Council on Bioethics. Public health: ethical issues. 2007. http://nuffieldbioethics.org/project/public-health. Accessed 28 Mar 2018.
22. Boseley S. Global cost of obesity-related illness to hit $1.2tn a year from 2015. The Guardian newspaper. 2017. https://www.theguardian.com/society/2017/oct/10/treating-obesity-related-illness-will-cost-12tn-a-year-from-2025-experts-warn. Accessed 28 Mar 2018.
23. Centers for Disease Control and Prevention Adult Obesity Facts, 2017. See https://www.cdc.gov/obesity/data/adult.html.
24. Wikler D. Who should be blamed for being sick? In: Bayer R, Gostin LO, Jennings B, et al., editors. Public health ethics: theory, policy and practice. New York: Oxford University Press; 2007.
25. Nuffield Council on Bioethics. Solidarity: reflections on an emerging concept in bioethics. 2007. http://nuffieldbioethics.org/project/solidarity. Accessed 28 Mar 2018.
26. Collins PH. Black feminist thought: knowledge, consciousness and the politics of empowerment. New York: Routledge; 1991.
27. Friedman M. Autonomy, social disruption and women. In: Mackenzie C, Stoljar N, editors. Relational autonomy: feminist perspectives on autonomy, agency and the social self. New York: Oxford University Press; 2000. p. 35–51.
28. Arbeit M. What are we ready to risk? Academia, advocacy, and activism. 2015. http://sexedtransforms.blogspot.com/2015/05/what-are-we-ready-to-risk-academia.html. Accessed 25 Feb 2018.
29. Banks SJ, Gallagher A. Ethics in professional life: virtues for health and social care. Basingstoke: Palgrave; 2009.
30. Murdoch I. The sovereignty of good. Abingdon: Routledge; 1971.
31. United Nations. Sustainable development goals. 2016. https://sustainabledevelopment.un.org/sdgs. Accessed 28 Mar 2018.
32. Warren RC. Towards new models. Section introduction. In: De La Cancela V, Lau Chin J, Jenkins YM, editors. Community health psychology, empowerment for diverse communities. New York: Routledge; 1998. p. 219.
33. Warren RC. The social context of faith and health. In: Warren RC, HCJ L, Zulfiqar AA, editors. The health behavioural change imperative: theoretical, educational and practice dimensions. New York: Kluwer Academic/Plenum; 2002.
34. Bayer R, Beauchamp DE. Public health ethics: new ethics for the public's health. Oxford: Oxford University Press; 2007.

Part II

Research Framework: Measuring Individualised Care

Measuring Individualised Care

Riitta Suhonen and Chryssoula Lemonidou

Abstract

Scale construction is a complex procedure. There must be firm evidence of the need for developing an instrument to measure a particular phenomenon important to nursing practice. This chapter outlines the development of the Individualised Care Scales (ICS), both the patient and nurse versions. A detailed explanation of the process for developing the ICS-Patient version will be given using the existing literature. Methodological references have been updated for researcher purposes. Furthermore, this chapter gives an overview of the use of the instrument in several international collaborative studies as well as in national studies. A variety of researchers have used the ICS and produced different translations and adaptations of the scales. This chapter may help those who may use the instrument in the future to understand the development process.

Keywords

Measurement · Instrument · Instrumentation · Individualised Care Scale Scale

R. Suhonen (✉)
Department of Nursing Science, Turku University Hospital and City of Turku, Welfare Division, University of Turku, Turku, Finland
e-mail: riisuh@utu.fi

C. Lemonidou
Faculty of Nursing, University of Athens, Athens, Greece
e-mail: clemonid@nurs.uoa.gr

6.1   The Individualised Care Scale: Self-Assessment Instrument for Hospitalised Patients

Developing an instrument for research purposes is a long process and should follow systematic theoretical and methodological steps ensuring the validity and reliability of future measurements. Measuring individualised care, an abstract concept, requires suitable instruments, measures or scales. Scales are a more precise means of measuring phenomena than are questionnaires with open-ended questions. Instruments or measures include a set of questions or items and scales for selecting an appropriate option for the respondent. Scaling is based on mathematical logic and a theory-based process, such as the classic test theory [1]. Measuring individualised care from the patients' point of views originated in the middle of the 1990s in Finland, where the starting point of the Individualised Care Scale [2, 3] can be located. The ICS-Patient was originally developed in the Finnish language [2–4]. As suitable measures for the purpose were not found in the scientific databases, there was a need to develop one. Developing a valid and reliable instrument, which is also practical and acceptable by research informants, needs to follow specific protocols [5, 6] and forms a process including series of methods for the step-by-step development of the measure.

In addition to being valid and reliable, an instrument needs to have some other qualities as well. In order to be useful, the ICS instrument also had to meet the following criteria: (a) as a form of self-assessment, the scale had to be brief in order to minimise response burden; (b) as it was intended for use by hospital patients, they should be able to complete it reliably after a brief period of care; (c) it should reflect the degree to which patients felt their individuality was met; and (d) it was to be influenced as little as possible by sociodemographic and respondent characteristics and be as sensitive as possible to the phenomenon measured, (e) be culturally sensitive and (f) be at the educational level of the potential subjects.

The original Individualised Care Scale (ICS) is a bipartite, self-report measure for patients. It is composed of two dimensions: (1) patients' views (perceptions) on how individuality was supported through specific nursing interventions (17 items in the last version) and (2) how they perceived individuality in their own care (17 items in the last version). Both parts consist of three subscales eliciting information on (1) individual patient characteristics in the clinical situation caused by the hospitalisation (clinical situation; 7 items), (2) the patient's personal life situation (personal life situation; 4 items) and (3) decisional control over care (decisional control; 6 items). Each item is rated on a scale reflecting the patient's level of agreement or disagreement with the statement.

Scoring on the ICS is based straightforwardly on the assigned points on the scale. The response format uses a five-point Likert scale (1 = fully disagree, 2 = disagree, 3 = neither disagree nor agree, 4 = agree, 5 = fully agree). As the items of the ICS are on an ordinal level of measurement, descriptive statistics includes the frequencies and percentages of each option category. However, based on the theoretical definition, the ICS includes three subscales, and the corresponding sum-variables, namely, clinical situation, personal life situation and decisional control, can be formed based on the definition and its operationalisation. Scale item construction results in a summative score that is averaged to obtain an overall score. The higher the score, the more support is provided through nursing interventions to individualised care and the higher the degree of individuality in care perceived by the patients.

6.2   Development of the ICS

The current, widely known version of the ICS is its third shortened modification. The items were constructed in accordance with the guidelines set out in the methodological literature at the time of the development (e.g. [5, 7]). The *first* step in the instrument development is to create the operational definition (derived from the conceptual work done) for the concept items to measure the concept under consideration, focusing on the concept and its possible parts (see Chap. 4). Based on a detailed review of the literature, we identified the essential content to be covered by the scales, and a pool of 115 items was developed. The *second* step is to validate the developed items based on expert review panels ensuring the relevance and clarity of the items. Such procedures support content validity [8]. The items intended for the ICS were first reduced to 93 and then to 43 items based on two nursing experts' reviews and preliminary piloting [2], keeping in mind the defined domains of individualised care. These expert reviews considered the clarity, accuracy, appropriateness and relevance [9] of the items on a dichotomous and a four-point scale, in addition to technical flaws in item construction, wording and redundancy, grammar or appearance of bias. In deleting the items, the main focus was on the shift from theoretical to operational definition [10]. After the items had been developed, we carefully planned how they would be ordered. In addition, instructions to the subject on how to respond to the statements were included at the beginning of the scale.

The *third* step included the use of the newly developed scale. The first version of the ICS instrument was ready for the first pilot and data collection in a sample of 203 general hospital patients [3]. This data were used for evaluating the construct validity of the ICS. A more precise concept analysis was also performed to validate the content of the concept of individualised care [4]. These research activities concluded to examine patients' views of the support of individuality through nursing activities (part A) and then the perceptions about individuality in the care provided (part B). Thus, the second version of the ICS comprised 40 items (ICS-A 20 items and ICS-B 20 items) and was developed on the basis of the results of statistical analyses in a sample of 203 hospital patients [2, 3]. Each item was rated on a scale reflecting the patient's level of agreement or disagreement with the statement (from 1 = never to 5 = always). After the second phase, the scaling was returned to be the rating of agreement on a five-point Likert-type scale.

The ICS was pretested twice [3, 4] in conditions similar to those anticipated in subsequent studies before using the instrument in collecting the research data (see [5, 7, 11]). In addition, three of the empirical data sets collected (see below) were used to examine the content and construct validity of the ICS in two surgical patient samples ($n = 279$, $n = 450$) [12, 13]. Based on the statistical procedures (principal component analysis and item analysis), the number and content of the items were deleted and trimmed so that each item loaded on theoretically and empirically identifiable factors (see [14, 15]). Hypothesis testing was conducted in analysing the parts, the subscales in association with each other and in relation to the whole ICS. Finally, the construct validity of the ICS-Patient was confirmed using LISREL procedures [12]. Confirmatory factor analysis procedures can be used to test whether a set of factors are correlated, supporting construct validity of the scale.

The *fourth* step was to use the scale in new samples in addition to surgical patients in operative units. The Individualised Care Scale was used nationally to continue the validation and also the investigation of the factors related [16–19]. In a sample of hospitalised patients ($n = 861$), factors related to patients [16], nurses, care environment and organisation variables were determined [18]. In addition, criterion-related validity of the ICS was assessed using Schmidt's Perceptions of Nursing Care Scale (SPNCS) subscale "Seeing the Individual Patient" [19, 20] and the Oncology Patient's Perceptions of the Quality of Nursing Care Scale (OPPQNCS) "Individualisation" subscales together with the ICS [19, 21].

The *fifth* and final step, to produce the current ICS 34-item version (part A ICS-A 17 items; part B ICS-B 17 items), was taken in preparing the international collaborative study in four European countries in addition to the United States. Some semantic difficulties were faced while preparing the ICS items for use in the Greek, English and Swedish languages [22–25]. Thus, two items were merged in two subscales: patients' views of the support of individuality through nursing activities (part A) and then the perceptions about individuality in the care provided (part B), to clearly differentiate the items [26–28]. A series of statistical procedures was used to assess the construct and content validity of the translated versions as well as examination of the internal consistency [28]. The use of the scales in different countries and languages has provided valuable information about the topic, methodology and provision of individualised care in clinical practice (e.g. [29–31]). Rasch analysis, an alternative approach for classical theory testing representing the use of the item response theory, provided strong evidence about the ability of the different language versions to detect patients' perceptions of individualised care quite similarly [32].

Starting from 2005, the ICS-Nurse was also developed on the basis of the ICS-Patient aiming to analyse individualised nursing care from professional nurses' point of view [27]. The Nurse version is based on similar questions as the patient version, but the questions have been set from the nurses' point of view: The extent to which they have supported patient's individuality (ICS-Nurse part A) and their perceptions of how the care they provided in their last work shift was individualised or took patients' individuality into account (ICS-Nurse part B). When assessing individualised care, nurses are to assess the care they provided in terms of to what extent they supported patient individuality and how they actually managed to provide individualised care for the patients during their latest work shift. The Individualised Care Scale-Nurse version was developed in a sample of 544 nurses in the Finnish health-care system including somatic and psychiatric hospital settings and primary health-care settings [27]. The ICS-Nurse has followed a similar process for validation and was firstly used in national contexts, followed by a seven-country comparative cross-sectional survey (*n* = 1163) study in Cyprus, Greece, Finland, Portugal, Sweden, Turkey and the United States [33]. The data were collected from 34 acute hospitals and 91 orthopaedic surgical units. Since that study, the ICS-Nurse has been used in older people care settings [34–36].

6.3   The Available Validated Versions of the ICS

Based on the published articles and the work done by the international researcher groups, the ICS has become a frequently used and well-known instrument for measuring individualised nursing care in different health-care contexts and organisations. The use of the scales has provided important information about the topic throughout the world as well as on patients' and nurses' perceptions on the care experience. In addition, the empirical research done in different countries have produced a wide understanding about patient-, nurse- and organisation-related factors and their associations with the perceptions. A list of different versions was constructed based on the references found in the electronic databases or work or citations sent by the authors (Table 6.1).

In addition to the versions listed in Table 6.1, research projects are under way in many countries including Malaysia, Singapore, Switzerland, Oman, Japan, Saudi-Arabia, Slovakia and France.

6.4   Permissions to Use the ICS

Permission to use the Individualised Care Scale (ICS) (Nurse and Patient version) for non-commercial, research purposes is granted by the copyright holder. The instructions for the instrument may be edited as appropriate for the sample(s) that will be used. It is possible to use any demographic information the user wishes. However, the wording of the items and the scaling options may not be changed without permission by the copyright holder. Semantic and language validation is naturally forwarded. Any edited versions of the instrument will remain the copyright holder's property, and a copy of the edited version should be provided for the records.

The instrument itself may not be duplicated or reproduced in any publications because of owned right for publication of the journal and university series. A copy of or information about any published manuscripts or abstracts of presentations that reference the ICS are appreciated for the archives. For the time being, all published work must contain the following credit:

ICS-Patient: Suhonen R, Leino-Kilpi H and Välimäki M. 2005. Development and psychometric properties of the Individualised Care Scale. Journal of Evaluation in Clinical Practice 11(1), 7–20 [13].

Table 6.1 Available versions of the Individualised Care Scale

Country, language	Version	Context	Reference	Researcher
Australia (English)	ICS-patient	Radiation oncology	[37]	Rose, Pauline
	ICS-nurse	Radiation oncology	[37]	Rose, Pauline
Belgium (Flemish)	ICS-patient	Hospital	[38]	IBenC project
Belgium (Flanders)	ICS-nurse		[38, 39]	IBenC project
Canada (English)	ICS-patient	Orthopaedic	[40]	Petroz, Ursula
China (Chinese)	ICS-patient	Hospital	[41]	Yi, Kai-gui
Cyprus (Greek)	ICS-patient	Surgical, acute care Cancer units	[35, 42–45]	Papastavrou, Evridiki
	ICS-nurse	Orthopaedic Surgical units	[33, 43, 46, 47],	Papastavrou, Evridiki
Czech Republic (Czech language)	ICS-patient	Surgical units	[43, 44, 47]	Jarosova, Darja
	ICS-nurse	Surgical units	[43, 47]	Jarosova, Darja
Finland (Finnish)	ICS-patient	Surgical units Hospital units Cancer units	[13, 17–19, 45]	Suhonen, Riitta
	ICS-nurse	Surgical Hospital Older people care settings	[27, 28, 34]	Suhonen, Riitta
Germany (German)	ICS-patient	Hospital	[48, 49]	Pöhler, A 2010 Köberich, Stefan
Greece (Greek)	ICS-patient	Orthopaedic units Cancer units	[26, 28, 32, 35, 45]	Lemonidou, Chryssoula, Kalafati Maria
	ICS-nurse	Orthopaedic units	[33]	Lemonidou, Chryssoula
Hungary (Hungarian)	ICS-patient	Surgical units	[43, 44, 47]	Balogh, Zoltan
	ICS-nurse	Surgical units	[43, 47]	Balogh, Zoltan
Iran (Persian)	ICS-patient	Internal medicine and surgical units	[50]	Rasooli, Aleha Sayyed; Shahbazpoor, Mahnaz
Italy (Italian)	ICS-patient	Hospital patients	[51]	Rovetta, Fabrizio
Portugal (Portuguese)	ICS-patient	Internal medicine and surgical units	[52, 53]	Amaral, AF
	ICS-nurse	Orthopaedic	[33, 47]	Da Luz, Deolinda
South Korea (Korean)	ICS-patient	Internal medical units	[54]	Yang, In-Suk
Spain (Spanish)	ICS-patient	Public hospital	[55]	Rodriques-Martin, Beatriz
	ICS-nurse		Unpubl. manuscript	Rodriques-Martin, Beatriz

Table 6.1 (continued)

Country, language	Version	Context	Reference	Researcher
Sweden (Swedish)	ICS-patient	Orthopaedic Cancer units	[26, 28, 29, 45]	Berg, Agneta; Idvall, Ewa
	ICS-nurse	Orthopaedic	[33, 56]	Berg, Agneta; Idvall, Ewa
Turkey (Turkish)	ICS-patient	Neurosurgical and orthopaedic Orthopaedic and traumatology Internal medicine and surgical Orthopaedic surgery	[57–61]	Acaroglu, Rengin
	ICS-nurse	Orthopaedic Intensive, internal medicine and surgical units	[33, 57, 62]	Acaroglu, Rengin
The Netherlands (Dutch)	ICS-patient	Hospital		Heinen, Maud
	ICS-nurse	Home care settings for elderly		Van Eenoo, Lisa IBenC project
UK (British English)	ICS-patient	Orthopaedic	[26, 28, 31]	Land, Lucy
	ICS-nurse		[33]	Land, Lucy
USA (American English)	ICS-patient	Orthopaedic Out-patient physical therapy	[28]	Schmidt, Lee
	ICS-nurse	Orthopaedic	[33]	Sousa, Valmi D

ICS-Nurse: Suhonen R, Gustafsson M-L, Katajisto J, Välimäki M and Leino-Kilpi H. 2010. Individualised Care Scale-Nurse version: A Finnish validation study. Journal of Evaluation in Clinical Practice 16(1), 145–154 [27].

Researchers interested in using the Individualised Care Scales may register their studies and ask permission for the ICS on the website of the University of Turku, Department of Nursing Science: http://www.utu.fi/en/units/med/units/hoitotiede/research/projects/older-individuals/ICS/Pages/permission.aspx.

Conclusion

This chapter has outlined the process of developing the Individualised Care Scales. This information about the process and many procedures and methods used in the development of instruments may help early career researchers to develop instruments for nursing research for investigation of abstract concepts. The information derived through scales and questionnaires is similar to that obtained by interview, but scales are a more precise means of measuring phenomena than questionnaires. Although scales tend to have less depth compared to an interview, questions are presented in a consistent manner, and there is less opportunity for bias in measurement. Results derived from surveys using questionnaires are generalisable and useful for the development of care and services, hereF the individuality of nursing care.

The Individualised Care Scales were designed to determine patients' facts, from the viewpoint of patients and nurses, about individuality of care, and these scales have been distributed in national and international patient populations and nurses. Although the questions on the scales appear easy to design, they required considerable theoretical effort and statistical procedures. In determining the concept under investigation, the researcher shapes the view in which the topic will appear. It is good to remember that what you measure is what you get. Therefore, it is of utmost importance that the measurement tool is precise and accurate, capturing the content of the phenomenon and nothing else. In addition, reliability, i.e. consistent results over and over again, is an important quality of the measurement tool.

At the moment, the ICS has been translated into several languages and has been used in many countries. The topic is receiving increasing attention both in clinical practice and research. Both of the versions, the ICS-Patient and the ICS-Nurse, have proven validity and reliability, showing good psychometric properties in particular.

References

1. Nunnally JC, Bernstein IH. Psychometric theory. 3rd ed. New York: McGraw-Hill; 1994.
2. Suhonen ., valimäki M, Katajisto J. Individualized care in a Finnish healthcare organization. J Clin Nurs. 2000;9(2):218–27.
3. Suhonen R, Välimäki M, Katajisto J. Developing and testing an instrument for the measurement of individual care. J Adv Nurs. 2000;32(5):1253–63.
4. Suhonen R. Individualised care from the surgical patient's point of view. Developing and testing model. Turku: Annales Universitatis Turkuensis; 2002.
5. DeVellis R. Scale development: theory and applications. 3rd ed. Newbury Park: NT Sage; 2012.
6. Rattray J, Jones MC. Essential elements of questionnaire design and development. J Clin Nurs. 2007;16(2):234–43.
7. Priest J, McColl E, Thomas L, et al. Developing and refining a new measurement tool. Nurse Res. 1995;2(1):69–81.
8. DeVon HA, Block ME, Moyle-Wright P, et al. A psychometric toolbox for testing validity and reliability. J Nurs Scholarsh. 2007;39(2):155–64.
9. Lynn MR. Determination and quantification of content validity. Nurs Res. 1986;35(6):382–5.
10. Strickland OL. Deleting items during instrument development - some caveats. J Nurs Meas. 2000;8(1):103–4.
11. Jacobson SF. Evaluating instruments for use in clinical nursing research. In: Frank-Stromborg M, Olsen SJ, editors. Instruments for clinical health-care research. 2nd ed. Boston: Jones & Bartlett Publishers; 1997. p. 3–19.
12. Suhonen R, Välimäki M, Leino-Kilpi H, et al. Testing the individualised care model. Scand J Caring Sci. 2004;18(1):27–36.
13. Suhonen R, Leino-Kilpi H, Valimaki M. Development and psychometric properties of the individualized care scale. J Eval Clin Pract. 2005;11(1):7–20.
14. Ferketich S. Internal consistency estimates of reliability. Res Nurs Health. 1990;13(6):437–40.

15. Ferketich S. Focus on psychometrics. Aspects of item analysis. Res Nurs Health. 1991;14(2):165–8.
16. Suhonen R, Välimäki M, Katajisto J, et al. Patient characteristics in relation to perceptions of how individualised care is delivered - research into the sensitivity of the individualised care scale (ICS). J Prof Nurs. 2006;22(4):253–61.
17. Suhonen R, Välimäki M, Katajisto J, et al. Provision of individualised care improves hospital patient outcomes: an explanatory model using LISREL. Int J Nurs Stud. 2007;44(2):197–207.
18. Suhonen R, Välimäki M, Katajisto J, et al. Hospitals' organizational factors and patients' perceptions of individualized nursing care. J Nurs Manag. 2007;15(2):197–206.
19. Suhonen R, Schmidt LA, Radwin L. Measuring individualized nursing care: assessment of reliability and validity of three scales. J Adv Nurs. 2007;59(1):77–85.
20. Schmidt LA. The development and testing of a measure of patient satisfaction with nursing care. Diss Abstr Int. 2001;63(03):1325B. (UMI No. AAT3008198).
21. Radwin L, Alster K, Rubin KM. Developments and testing of the oncology patients' perceptions of the quality of nursing care scale. Oncol Nurs Forum. 2003;30(2):283–90.
22. Beck CT, Bernal H, Froman R. Methods to document semantic equivalence of a translated scale. Res Nurs Health. 2003;26(1):64–73.
23. Hilton A, Skrutkowski M. Translating instruments into other languages: development and testing process. Cancer Nurs. 2002;25(1):1–7.
24. Maneesriwongul W, Dixon JK. Instrument translation process: a methods review. J Adv Nurs. 2004;48(2):175–86.
25. Sousa VD, Rojjanasrirat W. Translation, adaptation and validation of instruments or scales for use in cross-cultural health care research: a clear and user-friendly guideline. J Eval Clin Pract. 2011;17(2):268–74.
26. Suhonen R, Berg A, Idvall E, et al. Individualised care from the orthopaedic and trauma patients' perspective: an international comparative survey. Int J Nurs Stud. 2008;45(11):1586–97.
27. Suhonen R, Gustafsson ML, Katajisto J, et al. Individualized care scale - nurse version: a Finnish validation study. J Eval Clin Pract. 2010;16(1):145–54.
28. Suhonen R, Berg A, Idvall E, et al. Adapting the individualized care scale for cross-cultural comparison. Scand J Caring Sci. 2010;24(2):392–403.
29. Berg A, Suhonen R, Idvall E. A survey of orthopaedic patients' assessment of care using the individualised care scale. J Orthop Nurs. 2007;11(3–4):185–93.
30. Kalafati M, Lemonidou C, Dedousis P, et al. Hospitalized orthopedic patients' view on individualized nursing care. Nurs Care Res. 2007;18(1):15–25.
31. Land L, Suhonen R. Orthopaedic and trauma patients' perceptions of individualized care. Int Nurs Rev. 2009;56(1):131–7.
32. Suhonen R, Schmidt LA, Katajisto J, et al. Cross-cultural validity of the individualised care scale - a Rasch model analysis. J Clin Nurs. 2013;22(5–6):648–60.
33. Suhonen R, Papastavrou E, Efstathiou G, et al. Nurses' perceptions of individualized care: an international comparison. J Adv Nurs. 2011;67(9):1895–907.
34. Charalambous A, Chappell NL, Katajisto J, et al. The conceptualization and measurement of individualized care. Geriatr Nurs. 2012;33(1):17–27.
35. Suhonen R, Stolt M, Puro M, et al. Individuality in older people's care – challenges for the development of nursing and nursing management. J Nurs Manag. 2011;19(7):883–96.
36. Suhonen R, Alikleemola P, Katajisto J, et al. Nurses' perceptions of individualised care in long-term care institutions. J Clin Nurs. 2012;21(7–8):1178–88.
37. Rose PM. Individualized care in the radiation oncology setting from the patients' and nurses' perspectives. Cancer Nurs. 2016;39(5):411–22.
38. Malfait S, Eeckloo K, Lust E, et al. Feasibility, appropriateness, meaningfulness and effectiveness of patient participation at bedside shift reporting: mixed-method research protocol. J Adv Nurs. 2017;73(2):482–94.
39. Van Eenoo L, van der Roest H, van Hout H, et al. Quality of care and job satisfaction in the European home care setting: research protocol. Int J Integr Care. 2016;16(3):14. https://doi.org/10.5334/ijic.2519.

40. Petroz U, Kennedy D, Webster F, et al. Patients' perceptions of individualized care: evaluating psychometric properties and results of the individualized care scale. Can J Nurs Res. 2011;43(2):80–100.
41. Yi K-G, Ding S-Q, Zhong Z-Q, et al. Translation, revision and assessment of reliability and validity of the individualized care scale–patient version. Chin J Nurs. 2017;52:373–6.
42. Charalambous A, Radwin L, Berg A, et al. An international study of hospitalized cancer patients' health status, nursing care quality, perceived individuality in care and trust in nurses: a path analysis. Int J Nurs Stud. 2016;61(1):176–86.
43. Papastavrou E, Efstathiou G, Tsangari H, et al. Patients' decisional control over care: a cross-national comparison from both the patients' and nurses' points of view. Scand J Caring Sci. 2016;30(1):26–36.
44. Suhonen R, Papastavrou E, Efstathiou G, et al. Patient satisfaction as an outcome of individualised nursing care. Scand J Caring Sci. 2012;26(2):372–80.
45. Suhonen R, Charalambous A, Berg A, et al. Hospitalised cancer patients' perceptions of individualised nursing care in four European countries. Eur J Cancer Care (Engl). 2018;27(1):112. https://doi.org/10.1111/ecc.12525.
46. Idvall E, Berg A, Katajisto J, et al. Nurses' sociodemographic background and assessments of individualized care. J Nurs Scholarsh. 2012;44(3):284–93.
47. Suhonen R, Efstathiou G, Tsangari H, et al. Patients' and nurses' perceptions of individualised care: an international comparative study. J Clin Nurs. 2011;21(7–8):1155–67.
48. Köberich S, Feuchtinger J, Farin E. Factors influencing hospitalized patients perception of individualized nursing care - a cross-sectional study. BMC Nurs. 2016;15:14. https://doi.org/10.1186/s12912-016-0137-7.
49. Köberich S, Suhonen R, Feuchtinger J. The German version of the individualized care scale - assessing validity and reliability. Patient Prefer Adherence. 2015;9:483–94.
50. Rasooli A, Zamanzadeh V, Rahmani A, et al. Patients' point of view about nurses' support of individualized nursing care in training hospitals affiliated with tabriz university of medical sciences. J Caring Sci. 2013;2(3):203–9.
51. Rovetta F, Giordano A, Manara DF. The measurement of individualized care: translation and validation semantics of individualized care scale. Prof Inferm. 2012;65(1):39–45.
52. Amaral A, Ferreira P, Suhonen R. Translation and validation of the individualized care scale. Int J Caring Sci. 2014;7(1):90–101.
53. Amaral A, Fereira P, Cardoso M. Implementation of the nursing role effectiveness model. Int J Caring Sci. 2014;7:757–70.
54. Yang IS. Individualized care, satisfaction with nursing care and health-related quality of life-focusing on heart disease. Korean J Women Health. 2008;9(1):37–56.
55. Rodriques-Martin B, Martin-Martin R, Suhonen R. Individualized care scale-patient: a Spanish validation study. Nurs Ethics. 2018 Jan 1:969733018769351. https://doi.org/10.1177/0969733018769351.
56. Berg A, Idvall E, Katajisto J, et al. A comparison between orthopaedic nurses' and patients' perception of individualised care. Int J Orthop Trauma Nurs. 2012;16(3):136–46.
57. Acaroglu R, Sendir M. Bireyselleştirilmiş Bakımı Değerlendirme Skalaları (The scales for assessment of individualized care). İ.Ü.F.N. Hem Derg. 2012;1:10–6.
58. Acaroglu R, Suhonen R, Sendir M, et al. Reliability and validity of Turkish version of the individualised care scale. J Clin Nurs. 2011;20(1–2):136–45.
59. Ceylan B, Eser I. Assessment of individualized nursing care in hospitalized patients in a university hospital in Turkey. J Nurs Manag. 2016;24(7):954–61.
60. Gurdogan E, Findik U, Arslan B. Patients' perception of individualized care and satisfaction with nursing care levels in Turkey. Int J Caring Sci. 2015;8(2):369–75.
61. Tekin F, Findik UY. Level of perception of individualized care and satisfaction with nursing in orthopaedic surgery patients. Orthop Nurs. 2015;34(6):371–4.
62. Can S, Acaroglou R. Hemşirelerin Mesleki Değerlerinin Bireyselleştirilmiş (Relation of professional values of the nurses with their individualized care perceptions). İ.Ü.F.N. Hem Derg. 2015;1:32–40.

Translation, Adaptation and Validation Process of Research Instruments

7

Georgios Efstathiou

Abstract

The process of translating, adapting and validating research instruments or scales is crucial for international research projects, as it will facilitate safe comparisons. Versions of research instruments or scales in different languages need to be reliable and valid but also have semantic equivalence between them. This is very important since diversity among people worldwide exists. It is particularly important for nursing research due to the different definitions widely given for the same concept. This chapter focusses on the most common methodological approaches that can be used by researchers who want to translate, adapt and validate a research instrument or scale into a different language.

Keywords
Adaptation · Instrument · Scale · Translation · Validation

7.1 Introduction

Nursing care's complex and diverse content and meaning have received a lot of attention in recent years. Global economic crisis, understaffing and lack of resources created a need for the development of an international understanding of the different aspects of nursing care in order to allow a common meaning of nursing and facilitate the exchange of knowledge from one culture to another. This has led to the need of measuring and investigating nursing and its dimensions. Various concepts of nursing care (e.g. individualised care) have been studied nationally and

G. Efstathiou
Nursing Services, Ministry Of Health, Nicosia, Cyprus
e-mail: george.efstathiou@cytanet.com.cy

© Springer International Publishing AG, part of Springer Nature 2019
R. Suhonen et al. (eds.), *Individualized Care*,
https://doi.org/10.1007/978-3-319-89899-5_7

internationally, aiming to create a theoretical framework that will assist nurses to improve their practice and enhance patient satisfaction [1–3]. To achieve this, nursing researchers worldwide collaborate in a number of international projects, producing a huge number of data for analysis. The need for collaboration, comparison and transferability of findings from one culture to another has increased the necessity of using common, reliable and valid research instruments or scales [4]. Therefore, there is a need for understanding the process for achieving conceptual equivalence among translated research instruments or scales [5].

7.2   Translation of Research Instruments or Scales

Cross-cultural equivalence of translated versions of a research instrument or scale with the original one is important to achieve, since the findings from settings in different countries need to be compared and discussed. The translated research instrument or scale needs to measure the same theoretical concept with the original one in order to conclude to equivalence of the same instrument or scale in different cultural settings. In this way, similarity on how the theoretical construct of the instrument or scale is understood and interpreted is achieved.

The translation process aims to achieve equivalence between the original version and the translated version of a research instrument or scale [6]. This process follows certain steps, ensuring that comparisons among different cultural setting are safe [5, 7, 8].

7.2.1   Forward Translation

The original research instrument or scale (the instrument or scale in the original language—OL) needs to be translated into the target language (TL). Translation begins with a *forward translation* of the instrument or scale from the OL to the TL. The forward translation should be done by independent translators (at least two) who should be fluent in both languages (bilingual) and ideally having knowledge and experience of the culture of both languages [9]. Background on nursing would also be preferable by one of the translators since this will allow the capture of the nursing concept and terminology included in the research instrument or scale. Non-clinical aspects (e.g. when a research instrument or scale will be used among patients) will be better captured by a second translator whose background is not nursing/clinical. The translators produce two independent translations that allow comparisons on how word and phrases have been translated.

7.2.2   Synthesis of Translated Versions (TL)

Both translations are examined by a third translator who compares the original research instrument or scale (in the OL) with both translated versions in the TL. After discussing with the first two translators and resolving any discrepancies, the third translator synthesises the two translated versions into one. The participation of the research team/principal investigator is vital in this stage, to resolve any issues arising during both phases of translation.

7.2.3 Backward Translation (Blind)

The synthesised new version of the translated instrument/scale (in the TL) is translated back to the OL by two independent translators, with similar characteristics as those described above. Both translators (TL and OL) are unaware (blind) of the original version of the research instrument or scale in the OL. Two backward translations are produced in this stage [5, 9].

7.2.4 Synthesis of Translated Versions (OL)

An expert review committee, consisted of members of the research team/principal investigator, nurses familiar with research methodology and the topic under study, all translators and if possible the developer of the original version of the research instrument or scale (in the OL), discuss the two backward translated versions. The committee's aim is to resolve any ambiguities between the two backward translated versions, compare them with the original version (OL) and then synthesise a pre-final backward version. The pre-final version should have conceptual, semantic and content equivalence with the original version of the research instrument or scale. Any disagreements or discrepancies (in terms of wording, structure and understanding) should be resolved at this stage and achieve a consensus regarding the pre-final version.

Consensus is necessary to be achieved during the process of synthesising the new versions (in TL and OL). If consensus cannot be achieved, then the stages of translating should be repeated as many times as needed to achieve agreement regarding the pre-final version [5].

7.2.5 Pretest of Synthesised Translated Version: Cognitive Debriefing and Cultural Equivalence

The pre-final version of the translated instrument or scale needs to be further examined among people whose TL is their mother language (tongue). This cognitive debriefing allows researchers to evaluate the clarity of instructions and content and ideally is done among individuals in which the translated instrument/scale is meant to be used. At a first stage, a sample between 10 and 40 persons is asked to read the research instrument or scale as well as any instructions. Each participant is asked to express its opinion regarding the clarity (understanding) of the instrument or scale and of the instructions (clear or unclear) and to provide further suggestions, if needed. Items within the instrument or scale, which are indicated by more of the 20% of the above sample as unclear, need to be further examined. Changes are made prior to proceeding to further assessment of the translated version [5].

At a later stage, a purposive sample of experts on the subject under study (e.g. on concept and construct of the measured field and target population) is recruited. The experts (ideally 8–10 persons whose mother language is the same with the TL of the translated instrument or scale) form an evaluation committee, and each member, separately, repeats the above process (evaluation of instructions and clarity of items). In this way, the experts' committee evaluates the *conceptual equivalence* of the research instrument or scale. Once again, items within the instrument or scale, which are indicated by more of the 20% of the above committee as unclear, need to be further examined [10], based on suggestions that the committee may provide. Conceptual equivalence is achieved when the expert's committee is confident that the translated version's construct is equivalent with the original one.

The panel of experts proceeds with calculation of a content validity index (CVI), both at item level (I-CVI) and instrument or scale level (S-CVI)—*content equivalence*. The members of the panel rate each item, for example, as (1) *not relevant*, (2) *somewhat relevant*, (3) *quite relevant* and (4) *highly relevant*. Items rated as not relevant or somewhat relevant need further consideration and evaluation. In general, values of equal or above 0.8 for CVI, I-CVI and S-CVI are considered as acceptable [5, 11]. Experts should continue examining the CVI—making alterations to items that were rated as not relevant or somewhat relevant—until acceptable level of CVI value is achieved [5].

In order to examine the equivalence of different translated versions, international researchers may have group discussions to resolve any discrepancies. These group meetings may give the chance for changes and also content and meaning improvement, in order to produce *semantic equivalence* and maximise safe comparisons.

7.3 Psychometric Testing

In order to produce the final version of a translated instrument or scale, researchers may run some psychometric tests. These tests can be used to measure the equivalence between the translated and the original versions, by testing how well the translated version corresponds the properties of the original one. This process requires the distribution of the translated version to a sample of the target population (based on the research aims). Depending on the psychometric approaches and tests that are planned, sample may vary from 5–10 subjects per item of the research instrument or scale, for internal consistency tests and exploratory factor analysis, to over 300 subjects—for confirmatory factor analysis [12]. Power analysis can also be used to estimate the appropriate sample.

The most frequent psychometric approaches are:

1. *Internal consistency reliability* measures the extent to which the items included in a research instrument or scale correlate. Cronbach's alpha is frequently used to estimate a scale's reliability, with the lowest acceptable level for scale reli-

ability being alpha of 0.7 [13, 14]. Further analysis of data may also include item-to-item and item-to-total correlations. Low levels of internal consistency reliability of the translated version, compared to higher levels of the original version, may indicate the need for re-examining the translation process or testing the appropriateness of item inclusion.

2. *Stability over time (test-retest reliability)* tests the stability of an instrument over a period of a time. It requires the administration of an instrument or scale twice among the same subjects under study, with an interval of at least 2 weeks. Pearson's correlation is frequently used to compare the responses of both administrations; high level of significant correlation indicates stability of the instrument or scale over time [11, 13].

3. *Validity*

   (a) *Construct validity* tests the extent to which an instrument or scale actually measures what is supposed to measure. It is performed by comparing the instrument or the scale with other tests that (1) measure the same thing (concept) (therefore their outcomes when compared should correlate (convergent validity)) or (2) measure different things (concepts) (therefore their outcomes when compared should not be related (discriminant or divergent validity)) [15].

   (b) *Criterion validity* tests the extent to which the outcomes of the instrument or scale correlate with other measure, which is considered as valid. This other measure is often referred as a gold standard; however it may not always exist. Criterion validity is divided into (1) predictive validity, in which the instrument or scale is tested if it can predict future outcomes (changes), and (2) concurrent validity, in which the outcomes of the instrument or scale correspond to those of another valid one (measuring the same concept) [15].

   (c) *Factor structure (exploratory factor analysis)*, in which a number of dimensions of the concept under study are extracted and the items of the instrument or scale are grouped in factors. Each factor represents a dimension of the concept that the instrument or scale measures and includes items that are consistent with each other. A factor is considered strong if it incorporates at least three items; items not included in a strong factor can be discarded or semantically included in another factor. Factorial equivalence between the translated and the original version indicates that both measure the same dimensions/concept.

4. *Model fit (confirmatory factor analysis)*, a test where the factor structure of a research instrument or scale is verified. In this case, the factor structure produced from an exploratory factor analysis is confirmed or rejected, and an attempt to describe how well a proposed model is made. This can be used to test if the factor structure of the translated version fits to the theoretical model of the original (factor structure) of the original version.

7.4   The Use and Translation of the Individualised Care Scale in Different Languages

Individualised nursing care has received great attention in recent years. It serves as a means for providing high standards of nursing care by taking into account the preferences and opinion of patients concerning the nursing care provided by nurses [16, 17]. Through meeting patients' needs and tailoring nursing services based on patients' expectations and preferences, nurses can increase patients' satisfaction from nursing care received and health-care systems in general. It is therefore important to enable both patients and nurses to express their opinion and ideas on the perception of individualised nursing care not only nationally but globally. Through such process, important messages can be derived that may allow all those involved in nursing care (clinical nurses, academics, nurse managers, policy makers) realise what the patients really need and adjust the provision of nursing care accordingly. This is even more important and interesting when the perception of individualised care is measured in an international concept, offering a wider and global look of this aspect.

In order to understand the concept of individualised nursing care but also to facilitate comparisons among different cultural and language settings, the Individualised Care Scale has been extensively used internationally. For this reason, it has been translated, adapted and used in various languages and used in different settings. Appendix presents studies in which the ICS was used and reports the methods used—if applicable—in order to translate and adapt the scale. Internal consistency (Cronbach's alpha) and factor analysis were the principal tests used for validation process. Translation (in those studies that provided description) was reported as forward-back translation. Finally, one study used the Rasch model analysis to test the sensitivity of four translated versions of ICS (patient version).

7.5   Conclusion

The use of the same instrument—for example, the ICS—(either at national or international level) provides the opportunity to researchers, policy makers, nurse managers and clinical nurses to have a more analytic view on individualised nursing care as part of a cross-cultural study of the subject. Data coming from local studies are important; however, their usefulness is limited if they are not compared with international findings. In this way, comparisons are easier to be performed, and conclusions are safer to be made as part of an attempt to implement the concept of individualised nursing care. This fact demonstrates the importance and need to adapt research instruments into different languages and cultures. Only then, a clear, internationally recognised and accepted theory can be developed and implemented as part of the nursing care provision to patients.

Appendix

Examples of the methods used to translate and adapt the Individualised Care Scale into different languages and cultures

Authors	Aim	Methods-tests	Findings
Suhonen et al. [18]	To describe the development of ICS (finish settings) for use among patients (preliminary study)	Literature review to define individual care, items included in first scale draft, expert panel to review draft (including CVI), pilot test among patients (internal consistency), larger study (patients) testing Cronbach's alpha, stability over time (Pearson's correlation coefficient, test-retest), factor analysis	Three-factor solution suggested, useful, quick and easy-to-use scale, stable over time, adequate Cronbach's alpha
Suhonen et al. [19]	To describe the development of ICS, to evaluate its validity and psychometric properties	Data collected from patients being discharged from hospitals. Internal consistency and content validity index of the scale examined. Factor analysis to examine the scale's structure	The reliability and validity properties of ICS (patient version) demonstrated. Three-factor solution confirmed, alpha >0.9 for both parts
Suhonen et al. [20]	To develop the nurse version of ICS and to test its reliability and validity	Items for nurses' version produced from the patients' version. Content validity index evaluated by expert nurses, pilot test (Cronbach's alpha coefficients, inter-item and item-to-total correlations), main testing (internal consistency, construct validity)	Easy to administer, good content validity properties, acceptable internal consistency (Cronbach's alpha >0.72), three-factor structure produced
Suhonen et al. [21]	To investigate the associations between three concepts: professional practic environment, ethical climate and individualised nursing care from the perspective of nurses working in care settings for older people in Finland	Cross-sectional study with the use of three research instruments (including ICS). ANOVA, Pearson's correlations coefficients and stepwise multiple regression analysis were employed	Significant correlations were observed between ethical climate and individualised care and between individualised care and practice environment

(continued)

Authors	Aim	Methods-tests	Findings
Suhonen et al. [22]	To investigate the association between professional nursing caregivers' work satisfaction and individualised care	Three instruments were used (including the ICS, nurse version). ANOVA and multiple regression analyses were conducted. Internal consistency was tested with Cronbach's alpha	Support of patients' individuality from nurses was supported. Significant correlations between aspect of the support of individuality and work satisfaction were observed
Suhonen et al. [23]	To investigate nurses' assessments of individualised care and explore if demographic characteristics affect their opinion on individuality	Exploratory study with the participation of nurses working in long-term care institutions. ANOVA was used to explore any associations, Cronbach's alpha to test the scale's internal consistency and factor analysis to examine its validity	Three-factor structure was supported, and all alphas (for both parts and all subscales) were >0.77. The results indicated that individuality was supported by nurses; however it was not practised on the same level
Charalambous et al. [24]	To explore, from the nurses' point of view, the individualised care and professional practice environment and potential associations between them	Exploratory correlational study in which nurses and nurse managers participated and two scales (including ICS) were used. Mean scores were computed, and Spearman's rho correlations were employed to test for associations between the two concepts. Reliability of the scale was tested with Cronbach's alpha	Internal consistency for both parts and all subscales was satisfactory (alpha ≥0.7). Findings demonstrated association between individualised care and professional practice environment
Suhonen and Leino-Kilpi [25]	To explore and compare the perceptions of older orthopaedic patients and patients of working age regarding individualised care	A descriptive and comparative study. Descriptive and inferential statistics were used	Both support and realisation of individualised care were evaluated as good. Older patients expressed more positive evaluations
Rodríguez-Martín et al. [26]	To explore nurses' possible association between nurses' views and their characteristics and organisational factors in older people health-care settings	A cross-sectional study. Means, percentages and frequencies were computed. Inferential statistics (Spearman's rho correlation and t-tests) were also computed. Internal consistency was evaluated with Cronbach's alpha	The perception of individualised care provided was perceived as positive. Correlations were observed between age and type of organisation on the one hand and assessments of individualised care provided on the other. Internal consistency of the scale was satisfactory

Authors	Aim	Methods-tests	Findings
Köberich et al. [27]	To assess the psychometric properties of the German version of ICS (patient version)	Cross-sectional, methodological study. Analysis included assessment of internal consistency (Cronbach's alpha), confirmatory factor analysis. In addition, concurrent validity was evaluated	German version of the ICS established as a reliable and valid instrument for use
Köberich et al. [28]	To explore factors (individual and organisational) that influence patients' perception of individualisation in their care	Cross-sectional study among German patients (use of ICS and other research instruments)	Several factors extracted as influential. Decision-making process was the only one controlled by nurses. Other factors included self-rated health and educational level
Acaroglu et al. [29]	To assess the psychometric properties of the Turkish version of ICS (patient version)	Cross-sectional study. The English version was used for translation into Turkish (forward-back translation). Expert reviews on the scale's content. Statistical analysis included evaluation of internal consistency (Cronbach's alpha) and factor analysis	German version of the ICS established as a reliable and valid instrument for use
Ceylan and Eser [30]	To explore the perceptions of orthopaedic and trauma patients regarding individualised nursing care	Cross-sectional study among patients. Descriptive statistics were employed, and internal consistency was measured with Cronbach's alpha coefficients	All alphas ≥0.79. Mean scores regarding interventions that support individuality in care were found to be lower than mean scores indicating the practice of individualised care
Gurdogan et al. [31]	To assess the perception of individualised care among internal medicine and surgical patients and also any relationship between individualised care and satisfaction with nursing care	A descriptive, cross-sectional study (ICS was one of the instrument used). Descriptive statistics were computed. Correlations were examined with Pearson's correlation coefficients. Internal consistency was tested with Cronbach's alpha	Positive correlation was observed satisfaction from nursing care and perception of individualised care. Mean score concerning perception of individualised care was higher than realisation of individualised nursing care. Cronbach's alpha for both parts was >0.9

(continued)

Authors	Aim	Methods-tests	Findings
Land and Suhonen [32]	To explore orthopaedic and trauma patients' perceptions of individualised nursing care	A descriptive study, employing both descriptive and inferential statistics. Internal consistency was measured with Cronbach's alpha coefficients. Spearman's rho correlation coefficients, Mann-Witney U-test and Kruskal-Wallis were used to test possible associations between demographics and ICS	Significant associations were observed between demographics and ICS (e.g. duration of stay in hospital). All alpha >0.8
Petroz et al. [33]	To explore the psychometric properties of ICS (patient version, both parts)	A cross-sectional study. Internal consistency (Cronbach's alpha) and factor analysis were employed	Alpha values (both parts) = 0.94. Factor structure of the Canadian version did not support the original one (part B consisted of two factors instead of three)
Amaral et al. [34]	To translate and explore the psychometric properties of the Portuguese version of ICS (patient version)	A cross-sectional survey. Forward and back translation was done to achieve semantic validity. Experts verified the translated version in terms of fluency. Internal consistency was evaluated with Cronbach's alpha coefficients and construct validity via factor analysis	All alphas (except for *subscale clinical situation*—part B) ≥0.77. A three-factor solution was extracted base on factor analysis, supporting the original theoretical model
Rasooli et al. [35]	To examine patients' opinion regarding nurses' support of individualised care (patient version, part A)	A descriptive, cross-sectional study. Mean scores were computed as well as reliability tests	Mean scores were lower than other studies. Cronbach's alpha was adequate
Berg et al. [36]	To explore orthopaedic patients' assessment concerning nurses' support of individuality	A descriptive, cross-sectional study. Descriptive and inferential statistics were used for data analysis. Factor analysis and Cronbach's alpha coefficients were also used to test the scale's reliability and validity	Factor structure of the Swedish version supported the original structure, and internal consistency was demonstrated. Patients assessed support of individuality as an important factor of nursing care

Authors	Aim	Methods-tests	Findings
Papastavrou et al. [37]	To examine the perceptions of individualised care that Cypriot nurses have and any potential associations between individualised care and professional practice environment	A cross-sectional, descriptive, correlational study, using the ICS (among others). Pearson's correlation coefficients were used to examine potential associations. Means were used to measure the perception and Cronbach's alpha coefficients to test internal consistency of the ICS	Nurses in Cyprus support the idea of individuality, which is practised to a lesser degree. Significant associations were observed between individualised care and aspects of professional practice environment
Papastavrou et al. [38]	To study and compare Cypriot nurses' and patients' perception's on individualised care	A cross-sectional, comparative study that use two research instruments (including ICS)	Disagreement between patients and nurses was observed on what is individualised care
Suhonen et al. [23]	To compare nurses' and patients' perceptions of individualised care in five European countries	A cross-sectional and comparative study. Both versions (nurse and patient) administered to 960 patients. Descriptive statistics as well as t-test, chi-square, ANOVA and ANCOVA tests were employed	Differences observed between nurses and patients. Nurses reported that they support patients' individuality more often. Differences between countries in means of ICS were observed
Suhonen et al. [22]	To assess the association between individualised care and patient satisfaction	A cross-sectional study among patients in five European countries. Descriptive statistics and ANOVA and Pearson's correlation coefficients were used	Patients expressed satisfaction with the care received by nurses; however they reported a moderate overall support of their individuality. Difference between countries on the perception of individuality was observed, and positive correlation between patient satisfaction and level of individualised care received was shown
Papastavrou et al. [17]	To explore patients' and nurses' perceptions of patients' decisional control over their care	A cross-sectional and comparative study among 1315 patients and 960 nurses in five European countries. Descriptive and inferential statistics and Cronbach's alpha coefficients for studying the scale's internal consistency were used	Nurses and patients perceived different perceptions on patients' decisional control over their own care. Cronbach's alpha values were adequate

(continued)

Authors	Aim	Methods-tests	Findings
Suhonen et al. [39]	To translate and adapt the ICS (patient version) in different languages	A cross-sectional and comparative study with the participation of 1126 patients from Finland, Greece, Sweden, the United Kingdom and the United States. Internal consistency of ICS was tested with Cronbach's alpha coefficients and its validity through factor analysis. Standard process of forward and back translations was followed	The ICS showed acceptable properties in terms of validity and reliability
Papastavrou et al. [16]	To explore possible associations between nurses' professional practice environment and their perception on the level of care individualisation	A cross-sectional, exploratory study among nurses working in orthopaedic and trauma departments in seven countries. Descriptive statistics and multiple regression analysis were used	Findings demonstrated that aspects of nursing environment could influence individualised care
Idvall et al. [40]	To explore possible associations between nurses' assessments of individualised care and personal characteristics	A cross-sectional, comparative, international study among nurses from seven different countries. Descriptive statistics were used, and general linear model were employed	Personal characteristics of nurses may affect the way they perceive and practice individualised care

References

1. Papastavrou E, Efstathiou G, Charalambous A. Nurses' and patients' perceptions of caring behaviours: quantitative systematic review of comparative studies. J Adv Nurs. 2010;67(6):1191–205.
2. Suhonen R, Papastavrou E, Efstathiou G, et al. Patients satisfaction as an outcome of individualised nursing care. Scand J Caring Sci. 2012;26(2):373–80.
3. Suhonen R, Alikleemola P, Katajisto J, et al. Nurses' assessments of individualised care in long-term institutions. J Clin Nurs. 2012;21(7–8):1178–88.
4. Maneesriwongul W, Dixon JK. Instrument translation process: a methods review. J Adv Nurs. 2004;48(2):175–86.
5. Sousa V, Rojianasrirat W. Translation, adaptation and validation of instruments or scales for use in cross-cultural health care research: a clear and user-friendly guideline. J Eval Clin Pract. 2011;17(2):268–74.
6. Tang ST, Dixon J. Instrument translation and evaluation of equivalence and psychometric properties: the Chinese sense of coherence scale. J Nurs Meas. 2002;10(1):59–76.
7. Brislin RW. Back-translation for cross-cultural research. J Cross Cult Psychol. 1970;1(3):185–216.
8. Brislin RW, Lonner WJ, Throdike RM. Cross cultural research methods. New York: Wiley; 1973.

9. Carlson E. A case study in translation methodology using the health-promotion lifestyle profile II. Public Health Nurs. 2000;17(1):61–70.
10. Gjersing L, Caplehorn J, Clausen T. Cross-cultural adaptation of research instruments: language, setting, time and statistical considerations. BMC Med Res Methodol. 2010;10:13. https://doi.org/10.1186/1471-2288-10-13.
11. Polit D, Beck C. Essentials of nursing research: appraising evidence for nursing practice. 8th ed. Philadelphia: Wolter Kluwer/Lipincott Williams & Wilkins; 2014.
12. Watson R, Thompson DR. Use of factor analysis in journal of advanced nursing: literature review. J Adv Nurs. 2006;55(3):330–41.
13. Bowling A. Research methods in health: investigating health and health services. 4th ed. Berkshire: Open University Press; 2014.
14. Nunnally JC. Psychometric theory. 2nd ed. New York: McGraw-Hill; 1978.
15. Gravetter F, Forzano L. Research methods for the behavioral sciences. 4th ed. Belmont: Wadsworth Cengage Learning; 2012.
16. Papastavrou E, Acaroglu R, Sendir M, et al. The relationship between individualized care and the practice environment: an international study. Int J Nurs Stud. 2015;52(1):121–33.
17. Papastavrou E, Efstathiou G, Tsangari H, et al. Patients' decisional control over care: a cross-national comparison from both the patients' and nurses' points of view. Scand J Caring Sci. 2016;30(1):26–36.
18. Suhonen R, Välimäki M, Katajisto J. Developing and testing an instrument for the measurement of individual care. J Adv Nurs. 2000;32(5):1253–63.
19. Suhonen R, Leino-Kilpi H, Välimäki M. Development and psychometric properties of the individualized care scale. J Eval Clin Pract. 2005;11(1):7–20.
20. Suhonen R, Gustafsson M, Katajisto J, et al. Individualised care scale – nurse version: a Finnish validation study. J Eval Clin Pract. 2010;16(1):145–54.
21. Suhonen R, Schmidt L, Katajisto J, et al. Cross-cultural validity of the individualised care scale – a Rasch model analysis. J Clin Nurs. 2013;22(5–6):648–60.
22. Suhonen R, Charalambous A, Stolt M, et al. Caregivers' work satisfaction and individualised care in care settings for older people. J Clin Nurs. 2012;22(3-4):479–90.
23. Suhonen R, Papastavrou E, Efstathiou G, et al. Nurses' perceptions of individualized care: an international comparison. J Adv Nurs. 2011;67(9):1895–907.
24. Charalambous A, Katajisto J, Välimäki M, et al. Individualised care and the professional practice environment: nurses' perceptions. Int Nurs Rev. 2010;57(4):500–7.
25. Suhonen R, Leino-Kilpi H. Older orthopaedic patients' perceptions of individualised care: a comparative survey. Int J Older People Nursing. 2012;7(2):105–16.
26. Rodríguez-Martín B, Stolt M, Katajisto J, et al. Nurses' characteristics and organisational factors associated with their assessments of individualised care in care institutions for older people. Scand J Caring Sci. 2016;30(2):250–9.
27. Köberich S, Suhonen R, Feuchtinger J, et al. The German version of the individualized care scale – assessing validity and reliability. Patient Prefer Adherence. 2015;9:483–94.
28. Köberich S, Feuchtinger J, Farin E. Factors influencing hospitalized patients' perceptions of individualized nursing care: a cross sectional study. BMC Nurs. 2016;15:14. https://doi.org/10.1186/s12912-016-0137-7.
29. Acaroglu R, Suhonen R, Sendir M, et al. Reliability and validity of Turkish version of the individualised care scale. J Clin Nurs. 2010;20(1–2):136–45.
30. Ceylan B, Eser I. Assessment of individualised nursing care in hospitalized patients in a university hospital in Turkey. J Nurs Manag. 2016;24(7):954–61.
31. Gurdogan E, Findik U, Arslan B. Patients' perceptions of individualized care and satisfaction with nursing care levels in Turkey. Int J Caring Sci. 2015;8(2):369–75.
32. Land L, Suhonen R. Orthopaedic and trauma patients' perceptions of individualized care. Int Nurs Rev. 2009;56(1):131–7.
33. Petroz U, Kennedy D, Webster F, et al. Patients' perceptions of individualised care: evaluating psychometric properties and results of the individualized care scale. Can J Nurs Res. 2011;43(2):80–100.

34. Amaral A, Ferreira P, Suhonen R. Translation and validation of the individualized care scale. Int J Caring Sci. 2014;7(1):90–101.
35. Rasooli AS, Zamanzadeh V, Rahmani A, Shahbazpoor M. Patients' point of view about nurses' support of individualized nursing care in training hospitals affiliated with Tabriz university of medical sciences. J Caring Sci. 2013;2(3):203–9.
36. Berg A, Suhonen R, Idvall E. A survey of orthopaedic patients' assessment of care using the individualised care scale. J Orth Nurs. 2007;11(3–4):185–93.
37. Papastavrou E, Efstathiou G, Suhonen R. The concept of individualized care in nursing [in Greek]. Cyprus Nurs Chron. 2010;11(3):3–19.
38. Papastavrou E, Efstathiou G, Tsangari H. The perception of Cypriot nurses and patients concerning nursing care and individualized nursing care [in Greek]. Cyprus Nurs Chron. 2010;11(2):18–29.
39. Suhonen R, Berg A, Idvall E, et al. Adapting the individualized care scale for cross-cultural comparison. Scand J Caring Sci. 2010;24(2):392–403.
40. Idvall E, Berg A, Katajisto J, et al. Nurses' socio-demographic background and assessment of individualised care. J Nurs Scholarsh. 2012;44(3):284–93.

The Validity and Reliability of the Individualised Care Scale

8

Minna Stolt and Janika Koskenvuori

Abstract

This chapter analyses the psychometric properties of the Individualised Care Scale (ICS). As the scale has been translated into several languages, a wide international perspective to the validity and reliability of the ICS will be provided. The main contents are content, construct, criterion and cross-cultural validity, internal consistency (stability) and item functioning.

Keywords

Individualised Care Scale · Validity · Reliability · Psychometric testing

8.1 Introduction

Validity and reliability are central characteristics of any scale. Validity and reliability are two major concepts including several components. Reliability is seen as a precondition for validity: if a scale fails in measuring, it cannot be used for the intended purpose. Both aspects need to be evaluated each time the scale is used to see if the scale works as planned ([1], p. 25–26). This chapter describes validity and reliability of the Individualised Care Scale (ICS) in the light of international research and ends up with a concise conclusion where some future development suggestions are presented.

M. Stolt (✉) · J. Koskenvuori
Department of Nursing Science, University of Turku, Turku, Finland
e-mail: minna.stolt@utu.fi; janika.j.koskenvuori@utu.fi

© Springer International Publishing AG, part of Springer Nature 2019
R. Suhonen et al. (eds.), *Individualized Care*,
https://doi.org/10.1007/978-3-319-89899-5_8

8.2   Validity

Validity refers to test's ability to measure what was intended to measure [2]. The validity of the ICS has been evaluated in several international research papers. Many kinds of validity types have been under investigation such as face, content, construct and criterion validity.

8.2.1   Face Validity

Face validity is considered as the weakest type of validity, as a subjective evaluation, and refers to whether the scale is measuring the particular construct in focus ([3], p. 458). Face validity of the ICS was ensured during the development process [4] as well as after back and forth translation in cross-cultural research [5, 6] (Table 8.1). Researchers and expert panels evaluated that the items measure the content what it was supposed to measure. Respondents' feedback was requested in all pilot studies (e.g. [4, 22]).

8.2.2   Content Validity

Content validity estimates how much a measure represents every single element of a construct ([3], p. 458, [23]). Content validity can be assessed by an expert panel who critically evaluates the clarity and completeness of the content [24]. The content validity can also be confirmed by comparing the content with the previous literature in the field [24].

Content validity of the ICS was tested in four studies [4, 5, 17, 21] which all supported satisfactory content validity. Content validity was ensured by expert panels [17, 21] with multiple experts (such as nurses, nursing students, nurse teachers [5]) and by analysing different patient data sets with principal component analysis and item analysis [4]. Content validity was also supported in the development phase of the ICS by a comprehensive literature review [4].

Related to content validity, piloting of the ICS with informants outside the health-care system was done to guarantee the clarity and appropriateness of the items [5]. Moreover, adherence to responding indicated by a low number of empty responses in each item [5, 6, 12] can also be seen as supporting the content validity of the ICS.

8.2.3   Construct Validity

Construct validity refers to the extent to which the relationships of the items in a measure are consistent with the theoretical framework behind the content being measured [25]. It is usually assessed with contrasted group approach, hypothesis testing, the multitrait-multimethod approach or/and factor analysis (for more, see, e.g. [25]).

Table 8.1 Validity evidence of the ICS

Country/language version	Validity character													References
	Content validity	Face validity	Principal component analysis	EFA/CFA[a]	Promax rotation	Varimax rotation	Structural equation modelling	Convergent validity	Concurrent validity	Criterion validity	Cultural validity	Known-groups validity	Predictive validity	
Canada (English)			+		+			+						[7]
Finland (Finnish)	+	+	+	+	+		+							[8]
				+	+	+								[4]
							+	+						[9]
							+							[10]
			+				+							[9]
			+			+	+							[11]
			+								+			[12]
											+			[13]
				+				+				+		[14]
			+		+									[15]
												+		[16]
Germany (German)			+						+	+		+		[12]
Greece (Greek)	+		+			+								[17]
Iran (Persian)	+													[18]
Italy (Italian)		+		+		+					+			[5]
Portugal (Portuguese)	+	+	+				+				+			[19]

(continued)

Table 8.1 (continued)

Country/language version	Validity character													References
	Content validity	Face validity	Principal component analysis	EFA/CFA[a] rotation	Promax rotation	Varimax rotation	Structural equation modelling	Convergent validity	Concurrent validity	Criterion validity	Cultural validity	Known-groups validity	Predictive validity	
Sweden (Swedish)	+		+	+		+								[6]
			+											[20]
			+	+		+								[12]
Turkey (Turkish)	+		+	+	+									[21]
UK (English)			+			+								[12]
USA (English)			+			+								[12]

[a]EFA exploratory factor analysis, CFA confirmatory factor analysis

The construct validity of the ICS was tested using a variety of methods. During the development phase of the ICS [4], construct validity was tested with a set of factor analyses, structural equation modelling (LISREL) and using the contrasted group approach [26]. As a result, the three-factor structure was confirmed (correlations ICA 0.48–0.70, ICB 0.39–0.65). This three-factor structure was later confirmed in several studies [12, 14, 20] using principal component analysis and investigating the variance in both scales (ICS-A and ICS-B). Moreover, the hierarchical structure of the ICS was tested with intraclass correlation [27]. In addition, Structural Equation Modelign (SEM) particularly path analysis was used to test the fit of the hypothetical model [28].

The ICS has been developed systematically. The original scale (developed in 2000) has undergone a shortening where some items were removed. The factorial validity of the shorter scale was tested with principal component analysis with Varimax rotation [12] which supported the three-factor solution as well.

Factor analyses have been used to test construct validity using both exploratory [5] and confirmatory [16] factor analysis. In addition, several studies with common factor analysis [6] or principal component analysis (PCA, e.g. [5, 11, 20]) have been reported. In PCA for factor extraction, both orthogonal rotation such as Varimax [5, 11, 20] and oblique rotation (Promax [7, 14, 21]) have been widely used. The ICS has undergone structural equation modelling to test hypothetical causal relationships [8, 9, 11, 19, 21].

Known-group technique, one method to test construct validity, was used in a study of Köberich et al. [16]. They compared ICS-A and ICS-B scores within different groups in the nursing care delivery system (task-oriented nursing, zone nursing and patient-oriented nursing care) and between different patient groups' perceptions of the decision-making process about nursing care (paternalistic, informed, shared). The Individualised Care Scale was able to separate people with different types of admission to hospital, age, gender and education [29]. Younger age, poorer state of health and higher level of education were associated with more critical assessments of individualised care [30]. The results supported the construct validity of the ICS and were also confirmed in studies with patients of different health status [31].

The ICS-A and ICS-B have also been tested using modern test theory, namely, Rasch analysis [32]. Rasch analysis represents modern test theory. It orders persons according to their ability and orders items according to their difficulty. Rasch analysis focuses on indicators which demonstrate how each item fits with the underlying construct ([33], p. 42). The Rasch analysis performed with international data (data from four countries) identified some misfitting items, and some variation in the order of items in different samples was evident. However, the findings supported the use of the ICS in international studies.

8.2.4   Convergent and Discriminant Validity

The multitrait-multimethod matrix method (MTMM) is important while testing the construct validity of a scale [34]. With this method two central concepts of validity, namely, convergence and discriminability, can be tested. Convergence can be achieved by comparing the results obtained with different measurement methods [3], p. 462. Discriminability refers to the scale's ability to differentiate between other similar scales or constructs [3], p. 462.

Convergent validity means the degree to which two expected intercorrelated measures are actually related. This can be analysed with Pearson's correlation or by inspecting item-scale correlations [35]. The convergent validity of the ICS was assessed in three studies [7, 10, 15]. It was tested with Pearson's product-moment correlations between the subscales of the measurement. The analyses from different studies provide somewhat conflicting findings. In the first study where convergent validity was tested [10], the results supported the evidence of convergent validity and positive correlations between subscales measuring individualised care. Similar results were obtained in the study of Petroz et al. [7].

Discriminant validity assesses a scale's capability to differentiate between constructs that are not theoretically the same [2]. The ICS has been tested together with similar scales (such as Schmidt's Perceptions of Nursing Care Survey and Oncology Patients' Perceptions of the Quality of Nursing Care Scale, see [9, 36]), which can be regarded as a potential source of acceptable discriminant validity.

8.2.5   Criterion Validity

Criterion validity reflects the degree to which the scores of the scale correspond with the "gold standard" [23]. Criterion validity in this part is investigated from the perspective of concurrent validity and predictive validity.

8.2.6   Concurrent Validity

Concurrent validity refers to a scale's ability to distinguish between individuals with particular character or behaviour [3], p. 460. Related to ICS, concurrent validity was assessed only in one study [16]. They investigated correlations between the ICS-A/ICS-B and Smoliner Scale subscale where a medium correlation with statistically significant level was found, supporting the concurrent validity of the ICS-A/ICS-B [16].

8.2.7   Predictive Validity

Predictive validity deals with the accuracy of the scale in differentiating between respondent's performance on some certain criterion [3], p. 460. Papastavrou et al. [37] investigated the predictive validity of the ICS-A and ICS-B and the Revised Professional Practice Environment using regression models. They concluded that individualised care was associated with the dimensions of the professional practice environment, thus supporting the predictive validity of the ICS [37].

8.2.8 Cross-cultural Validity

The translated version of the ICS has been used in several studies. As the ICS has been used in many countries and several articles report the results of cross-cultural studies, country comparisons for validity and reliability can be done. The psychometric properties of the ICS are mainly similar indicating high cross-cultural validity (e.g. [12, 13, 18, 32, 37–40]).

8.3 Reliability

The reliability of the ICS has been confirmed in many studies. Internal consistency, stability and item analysis have often been reported while describing the reliability of the ICS.

8.3.1 Internal Consistency

Internal consistency refers to intercorrelation between the items [23]. It can be evaluated with Cronbach's alpha coefficient, Kuder-Richardson formula 20 (targeted to dichotomous scales) and split-half technique [24]. Internal consistency of the ICS has been reported predominantly using Cronbach's alpha coefficient in the majority of the studies with multicultural data (Table 8.2). All Cronbach's alpha values in both ICS-Patient and ICS-Nurse scales were high, above 0.84, indicating good internal consistency. In detail, Cronbach's alpha values in ICS-Patient part A ranged from 0.91 [53] to 0.97 [12, 56] and in part B from 0.90 [12, 51] to 0.97 [12]. In ICS-Nurse scale, Cronbach's alpha values have been slightly lower but still on acceptable level: ICS-A Nurse alpha values ranging from 0.88 [11, 20, 39, 41, 42, 46, 49] to 0.95 [39]. In ICS-B Nurse scale, Cronbach's alpha values were between 0.84 [39] and 0.93 [39]. In addition, several series of factor analyses have also been conducted, all of which support the internal consistency of the ICS [57].

8.3.2 Stability

Stability refers to an instrument's ability to produce similar results on two separate occasions [3], p. 453. Instrument's stability is usually tested with test-retest reliability. In test-retest, the same respondents are administered the same instrument during a certain time period, and their responses are compared and reliability coefficient is calculated [3], p. 453. The ICS has shown acceptable short-term stability when the same informants responded to the ICS scale within a 2-week time period [4, 22, 58].

Table 8.2 Cronbach's alpha coefficients for the ICS

| Country (language) | Cronbach's alpha coefficient | | | | References |
| | ICS-patient | | ICS-nurse | | |
	ICS-A	ICS-B	ICS-A	ICS-B	
Australia (English)	0.94	0.94	0.88	0.90	[41]
Canada (English)	0.94	0.94			[7]
Cyprus (Greek)			0.92	0.92	[39]
	0.93	0.93			[31]
Finland (Finnish)			0.88	0.90	[42]
			0.91	0.91	[15]
	0.94	0.93			[43]
				0.89	[44]
	0.94	0.93			[8]
	0.94	0.93			[4]
	0.94	0.93			[45]
	0.95	0.94			[30]
	0.95	0.94			[36]
	0.95	0.94			[9]
	0.95	0.94			[10]
			0.88	0.90	[11]
			0.88	0.90	[46]
	0.92	0.90			[12]
			0.91	0.92	[47]
			0.88	0.87	[39]
			0.90	0.91	[14]
			0.93	0.92	[48]
	0.96	0.95	0.88	0.90	[49]
				0.89	[50]
	0.95	0.93			[31]
	0.92	0.90			[51]
Germany (German)	0.95	0.93			[16]
Greece (Greek)	0.94	0.94			[31]
	0.97	0.97			[12]
			0.95	0.84	[39]
Iran (Persian)	0.96				[17]
Portugal (Portuguese)			0.91	0.90	[39]
	0.94	0.93			[5]
Sweden (Swedish)	0.94	0.93			[6]
			0.88	0.89	[20]
	0.94	0.92			[52]
	0.91	0.93			[53]
	0.93	0.92			[12]
			0.88	0.88	[39]
	0.94	0.94			[31]

(continued)

Table 8.2 (continued)

| Country (language) | Cronbach's alpha coefficient | | | | |
| | ICS-patient | | ICS-nurse | | |
	ICS-A	ICS-B	ICS-A	ICS-B	References
Turkey (Turkish)	0.92	0.93			[21]
	0.94	0.93			[38]
	0.94	0.95			[54]
	0.95	0.95			[55]
			0.91	0.91	[39]
UK (English)	0.97	0.95			[56]
	0.97	0.95			[12]
USA (English)	0.94	0.93			[12]
			0.95	0.93	[39]

8.3.3   Item Analysis

Item analysis means evaluation of the performance of a single item. An item with high correlation with the underlying construct is ideal but often hard to achieve ([3], p. 486). Item analysis is a well-known method to evaluate internal consistency of the scale, and there are several types to investigate the item functioning, inter-item correlation and item-scale correlation (with uncorrected or corrected approach) being the most popular [59]. Item analysis for ICS has been used several times with different samples (such as [4, 5, 19, 21, 39]). Inter-item correlations were tested particularly during the instrument development process where both ICA and ICB scales showed acceptable (0.30 ≤ r ≤ 0.70, [26]) correlations (0.49–0.62, 0.42–0.59), respectively. This result was supported in later studies [4, 11, 12] and in the study of Amaral et al. [5] where no redundant items were identified. Item-to-total correlations also supported internal consistency of the ICS [4, 9, 11, 16, 36] as well as average inter-item correlations [11] and item-to-total analyses [15].

Conclusions
The process of obtaining information about validity and reliability is an important and ongoing process. Validity and reliability have different levels which can be assessed with different samples. Psychometric testing does not have an endpoint, and whenever an instrument or scale is used, its validity and reliability need to be demonstrated [2, 24].

The ICS has been developed systematically. Its validity and reliability have been confirmed in several national, international and cross-cultural studies. The ICS has excellent internal consistency, which has remained at the same level from study to another. The theoretical structure behind the ICS is strong and has been supported in many studies. Several studies have also demonstrated high construct validity of the ICS. The ICS has undergone a systematic development process, and its psychometric properties have been tested frequently, making it a reliable and valid scale in the context of nursing and health sciences.

References

1. Waltz CF, Strickland OR, Lenz ER. Measurement in nursing and health research. 5th ed. New York: Springer; 2016.
2. DeVon HA, Block ME, Moyle-Wright P, et al. A psychometric toolbox for testing validity and reliability. J Nurs Scholarsh. 2007;39(2):155–64.
3. Polit DF, Beck CT. Nursing research. Generating and assessing evidence for nursing practice. Philadelphia: Lippincott Williams & Wilkins; 2008.
4. Suhonen R, Leino-Kilpi H, Välimäki M. Development and psychometric properties of the individualized care scale. J Eval Clin Pract. 2005;11(1):7–20.
5. Amaral A, Ferreira P, Suhonen R. Translation and validation of the individualized care scale. Int J Caring Sci. 2014;7(1):90–101.
6. Berg A, Suhonen R, Idvall E. A survey of orthopaedic patients' assessment of care using the individualised care scale. J Orthop Nurs. 2007;11(3):185–90.
7. Petroz U, Kennedy D, Webster F, et al. Patients' perceptions of individualized care: evaluating psychometric properties and results of the individualized care scale. Can J Nurs Res. 2011;43(1):80–100.
8. Suhonen R, Välimäki M, Leino-Kilpi H, et al. Testing the individualized care model. Scand J Caring Sci. 2004;18(1):27–36.
9. Suhonen R, Välimäki M, Katajisto J, et al. Provision of individualised care improves hospital patient outcomes: an explanatory model using LISREL. Int J Nurs Stud. 2007;44(2):197–207.
10. Suhonen R, Schmidt LA, Radwin L. Measuring individualized nursing care: assessment of reliability and validity of three scales. J Adv Nurs. 2007;59(1):77–85.
11. Suhonen R, Gustafsson ML, Katajisto J, et al. Individualized care scale - nurse version: a Finnish validation study. J Eval Clin Pract. 2010;16(1):145–54.
12. Suhonen R, Berg A, Idvall E, et al. Adapting the individualized care scale for cross-cultural comparison. Scand J Caring Sci. 2010;24(2):392–403.
13. Suhonen R, Efstathiou G, Tsangari H, et al. Patients' and nurses' perceptions of individualised care: an international comparative study. J Clin Nurs. 2011;21(7–8):1155–67.
14. Suhonen R, Alikleemola P, Katajisto J, et al. Nurses' assessments of individualised care in long-term care institutions. J Clin Nurs. 2012;21(7–8):1178–88.
15. Charalambous A, Chappell NL, Katajisto J, et al. The conceptualization and measurement of individualized care. Geriatr Nurs. 2012;33(1):17–27.
16. Köberich S, Suhonen R, Feuchtinger J, et al. The German version of the individualized care scale - assessing validity and reliability. Patient Prefer Adherence. 2015;23:483–94.
17. Rasooli A, Zamanzadeh V, Rahmani A, et al. Patients' point of view about nurses' support of individualized nursing care in training hospitals affiliated with Tabriz university of medical sciences. J Caring Sci. 2013;2(3):203–9.
18. Rovetta F, Giordano A, Manara DF. The measurement of individualized care: translation and validation semantics of individualized care scale. Prof Inferm. 2012;65:39–45.
19. Amaral A, Ferreira PL, Cardoso ML, et al. Implementation of the nursing role effectiveness model. Int J Caring Sci. 2014;7(7):757–70.
20. Berg A, Idvall E, Katajisto J, et al. A comparison between orthopaedic nurses' and patients' perception of individualised care. Int J Orthop Trauma Nurs. 2012;16(3):136–46.
21. Acaroglu R, Suhonen R, Sendir M, et al. Reliability and validity of Turkish version of the individualised care scale. J Clin Nurs. 2011;20(1):136–45.
22. Suhonen R, Välimäki M, Katajisto J. Developing and testing an instrument for the measurement of individual care. J Adv Nurs. 2000;32(5):1253–63.
23. Mokkink LB, Terwee CB, Patrick DL, et al. The COSMIN study reached international consensus on taxonomy, terminology, and definitions of measurement properties for health-related patient-reported outcomes. J Clin Epidemiol. 2010;63(7):737–45.
24. Bannigan K, Watson R. Reliability and validity in a nutshell. J Clin Nurs. 2009;18(11–12):3237–43.

25. Soeken KL. Validity of measures. In: Waltz CF, Strickland OL, Lenz ER, editors. Measurement in nursing and health research. 5th ed. New York: Springer; 2017. p. 209–60.
26. Davis AE. Instrument development: getting started. J Neurosci Nurs. 1996;28(3):204–7.
27. Köberich S, Feuchtinger J, Farin E. Factors influencing hospitalized patients perception of individualized nursing care - a cross-sectional study. BMC Nurs. 2016;15:14. https://doi.org/10.1186/s12912-016-0137-7.
28. Charalambous A, Radwin L, Berg A, et al. An international study of hospitalized cancer patients' health status, nursing care quality, perceived individuality in care and trust in nurses: a path analysis. Int J Nurs Stud. 2016;61(1):176–86.
29. Suhonen R, Välimäki M, Berg A, et al. The impact of patient characteristics on orthopaedic and trauma patients' perceptions of individualised nursing care. Int J Evid Based Healthc. 2010;8(4):259–67.
30. Suhonen R, Välimäki M, Katajisto J, et al. Patient characteristics in relation to perceptions of how individualized care is delivered-research into the sensitivity of the individualized care scale. J Prof Nurs. 2006;22(4):253–61.
31. Suhonen R, Charalambous A, Berg A, et al. Hospitalised cancer patients' perceptions of individualised nursing care in four European countries. Eur J Cancer Care (Engl). 2018;27(1):1–12. https://doi.org/10.1111/ecc.12525.
32. Suhonen R, Schmidt LA, Katajisto J, et al. Cross-cultural validity of the individualised care scale - a Rasch model analysis. J Clin Nurs. 2013;22(5–6):648–60.
33. Bond TG, Fox CM. Applying the Rasch model. Fundamental measurement in the human sciences. New York: Routledge; 2015.
34. Campbell DT, Fiske DW. Convergent and discriminant validation by the multitrait-multimethod matrix. Pscyhol Bull. 1959;56(1):81–105.
35. Hays RD, Hayashi T. Beyond internal consistency reliability: rationale and user's guide for multitrait scaling analysis program on the microcomputer. Behav Res Methods Instrum Comput. 1990;22(2):167–75.
36. Suhonen R, Välimäki M, Katajisto J, et al. Hospitals' organizational variables and patients' perceptions of individualized nursing care in Finland. J Nurs Manag. 2007;15(2):197–206.
37. Papastavrou E, Acaroglu R, Sendir M, et al. The relationship between individualized care and the practice environment: an international study. Int J Nurs Stud. 2015;52(1):121–33.
38. Gurdogan E, Findik U, Arslan B. Patients' perception of individualized care and satisfaction with nursing care levels in Turkey. Int J Caring Sci. 2015;8(2):369–75.
39. Suhonen R, Papastavrou E, Efstathiou G, et al. Nurses' perceptions of individualized care: an international comparison. J Adv Nurs. 2011;67(9):1895–907.
40. Yang I. Individualized care, satisfaction with nursing care and health-related quality of life-focusing on heart disease. J Women's Health. 2008;9(1):37–56.
41. Rose PM. Individualized care in the radiation oncology setting from the patients' and nurses' perspectives. Cancer Nurs. 2016;39(5):411–22.
42. Charalambous A, Katajisto J, Valimaki M, et al. Individualised care and the professional practice environment: nurses' perceptions. Int Nurs Rev. 2010;57(4):500–7.
43. Makkonen A, Hupli M, Suhonen R. Potilaiden näkemys hoidon yksilöllisyydestä ajanvarauspoliklinikalla. Hoitotiede. 2010;22(2):129–40.
44. Rodríguez-Martín B, Stolt M, Katajisto J, et al. Nurses' characteristics and organisational factors associated with their assessments of individualised care in care institutions for older people. Scand J Caring Sci. 2016;30(2):250–9.
45. Suhonen R, Välimäki M, Leino-Kilpi H. Individualized care, quality of life and satisfaction with nursing care. J Adv Nurs. 2005;50(3):283–92.
46. Suhonen R, Gustafsson ML, Katajisto J, et al. Nurses' perceptions of individualized care. J Adv Nurs. 2010;66(5):1035–46.
47. Suhonen R, Stolt M, Puro M, et al. Individuality in older people's care - challenges for the development of nursing and nursing management. J Nurs Manag. 2011;19(7):883–96.
48. Suhonen R, Charalambous A, Stolt M, et al. Caregivers' work satisfaction and individualised care in care settings for older people. J Clin Nurs. 2013;22(3–4):479–90.

49. Suhonen R, Tsangari H, Leino-Kilpi H, et al. Individualised care - comparison of patients' and nurses' assessments. Hoitotiede. 2013;25(2):80–91.
50. Suhonen R, Stolt M, Gustafsson ML, et al. The associations among the ethical climate, the professional practice environment and individualized care in care settings for older people. J Adv Nurs. 2014;70(6):1356–68.
51. Suhonen R, Leino-Kilpi H. Older orthopaedic patients' perceptions of individualised care: a comparative survey. Int J Older People Nursing. 2012;7(2):105–16.
52. Berg A, Rask M. Patienternas syn på individualiserad vård på en ortopedisk klinik. Collaborative and integrated approaches to health. Kristianstad: Forskningsplattformen för utveckling av närsjukvård; 2008. p. 25.
53. Nygårdh A, Malm D, Wikby K, et al. Empowerment intervention in outpatient care of persons with chronic kidney disease pre-dialysis. Nephrol Nurs J. 2012;39(4):285–93.
54. Tekin F, Findik UY. Level of perception of individualized care and satisfaction with nursing in orthopaedic surgery patients. Orthop Nurs. 2015;34(6):371–4.
55. Ceylan B, Eser I. Assessment of individualized nursing care in hospitalized patients in a university hospital in Turkey. J Nurs Manag. 2016;24(7):954–61.
56. Land L, Suhonen R. Orthopaedic and trauma patients' perceptions of individualized care. Int Nurs Rev. 2009;56(1):131–7.
57. Terwee CB, Bot SD, de Boer MR, et al. Quality criteria were proposed for measurement properties of health status questionnaires. J Clin Epidemiol. 2007;60(1):34–42.
58. Suhonen R, Välimäki M, Katajisto J. Individualized care in a Finnish healthcare organization. J Clin Nurs. 2000;9(2):218–27.
59. Ferketich S. Focus on psychometrics. Aspects of item analysis. Res Nurs Health. 1991;14(2):165–8.

Other Instruments Measuring Individuality and Related Concepts

9

Janika Koskenvuori, Minna Stolt, and Riitta Suhonen

Abstract

This chapter aims to describe the variety of instruments developed for the measurement of individuality and person-centredness in healthcare from patients' and healthcare professionals' perspective. As the topics of individualised care and person-centredness have long been of interest and researchers have defined these concepts in different ways, instruments have also been developed for the measurement of these abstract concepts.

Keywords

Scales · Instruments · Measures · Existing measurement tools

9.1 Introduction

In addition to the Individualised Care Scale, there are many other instruments designed to measure individuality from different points of view, especially from patients' and healthcare professionals' (mainly nurses) perspective. Individuality has been the main target of some of the instruments, but also one of the sub-concepts of other constructs. Furthermore, there are many instruments measuring concepts related to individuality, such as person-centredness (see Table 9.1). Comprehensive definitions for such concepts are presented in Chap. 4.

J. Koskenvuori (✉) · M. Stolt
Department of Nursing Science, University of Turku, Turku, Finland
e-mail: janika.j.koskenvuori@utu.fi; minna.stolt@utu.fi

R. Suhonen
Department of Nursing Science, University of Turku, Turku, Finland

Turku University Hospital, City of Turku, Welfare Division, Turku, Finland
e-mail: riisuh@utu.fi

© Springer International Publishing AG, part of Springer Nature 2019
R. Suhonen et al. (eds.), *Individualized Care*,
https://doi.org/10.1007/978-3-319-89899-5_9

91

Table 9.1 Instruments measuring individuality and related concepts

	Instrument	Main target	Subscale	Respondents	
				Patient/client	Healthcare professionals
Individuality	Schmidt perception of nursing care survey (SPNCS) [1]	Nursing care	Seeing the individual patient	x	
	Oncology patients' perceptions of the quality of nursing care scale (OPPQNCS) [2]	Quality of nursing care	Individualisation	x	
	Individualized care index (ICI) van [3]	Individualised care			x
	Individualized care inventory (ICI) [4]	Individualised care			x
	Assessment of the approach to nursing care [5]	Approach for nursing care	Individualised nursing care		x
Person-centredness	The person-centered inpatient scale [6]	Person-centredness		x	
	Client-centred care questionnaire (CCCQ) [7]	Person-centred care		x	
	Person-centred care climate questionnaire-patient version (PCQ-P) [8]	Person-centred care environment		x	
	The person-centred nursing index (PCNI) [9, 10]	Person-centred nursing care		x	x
	Person-centred climate questionnaire-staff version (PCQ-S) [11]	Person-centred care environment			x
	Person-centered care assessment tool (P-CAT) [12]	Person-centred care			x
	Patient-centred care competency scale (PCC) [13]	Person-centred care competency			x

Twelve different instruments reflecting individuality and related concepts will be briefly described, including their purpose, theoretical basis, and operationalisation and scaling. In the first subchapter, two instruments measuring individuality from the patients' perspective through subscales are presented. In the second subchapter, three instruments focusing on individualised care from healthcare professionals' perspective are presented followed by the third subchapter in which seven instruments measuring person-centredness from both patients' and/or healthcare professionals' perspectives are described. The expressions used in the original papers are used, and no interpretations are made.

9.2   Measuring Individuality from the Patients' Viewpoint

There are a few instruments that can be used to measure individuality from the patients' perspective. In this section two of them are presented: *Schmidt Perception of Nursing Care Survey (SPNCS)* and *Oncology Patients' Perceptions of the Quality of Nursing Care Scale (OPPQNCS)*.

9.2.1   Schmidt Perception of Nursing Care Survey (SPNCS)

Schmidt Perception of Nursing Care Survey (SPNCS), originally designed in the USA, is an empirically derived instrument aimed to measure patients' perceptions of their nursing care [1]. The theoretical basis for the development of the SPNCS is provided by a grounded theory study about medical-surgical patients' perceptions of the nursing care they received while hospitalised. Four categories of patients' perceptions of their nursing care emerged: 'Seeing the Individual Patient', 'Explaining', 'Responding' and 'Watching Over' [14].

The psychometric properties of the initial 37-item measure were tested in a US sample of discharged medical-surgical patients. Acceptable reliability was obtained for the scale, and factor analysis suggested four factors. According to Suhonen et al. [15], also satisfactory inter-item correlations, criterion validity against typical satisfaction surveys and discriminant validity of the SPCNS have been reported. Furthermore, the SPCNS has been further validated using structural equation modelling (SEM), implemented through LISREL in a sample of medical and surgical patients [16], and some evidence for the convergent validity of the 'Seeing the Individual Patient' subscale has been provided among Finnish hospital patients [17]. The SPCNS has been used in the USA among medical-surgical [16], bariatric [18] and critical care [19] patients. One European comparative study was conducted among orthopaedic and trauma patients in Finland, Greece, Sweden and the UK [15].

The SPCNS consists of 15 items that are scored by the patient using a Likert-type scale (from 1, strongly disagree to 5, strongly agree). The SPNCS is divided into four subscales: 'Seeing the Individual Patient' (five items), 'Explaining' (three items), 'Responding' (three items) and 'Watching Over' (four items) [16].

'Seeing the Individual Patient' represents the extent to which patients perceive they were treated as unique individuals by the nursing staff providing care. 'Explaining' represents the extent to which the nursing staff meets the patients' information needs. 'Responding' represents the actions of nursing staff that result from the patient's request or symptom. 'Watching Over' represents patients' knowledge that nursing staff were in close proximity and alert to their needs [14].

9.2.2   Oncology Patients' Perceptions of the Quality of Nursing Care Scale (OPPQNCS)

The Oncology Patients' Perceptions of the Quality of Nursing Care (OPPQNCS), originally designed in the USA, is an instrument that measures the quality of cancer nursing care from the patient's perspective [2]. The development of the OPPQNCS is based on the middle-range theory of high-quality cancer nursing care by Radwin [20]. The theory is comprised of two multidimensional concepts: (1) attributes of high-quality cancer nursing and (2) outcomes of high-quality cancer nursing. The OPPQNCS operationalises the eight attributes: professional knowledge, continuity, attentiveness, coordination, partnership, individualisation, rapport and caring [20, 21]. The conceptual definitions of the eight attributes, theoretical descriptions and verbatim data from the study [20] were used to construct the OPPQNCS subscales and items. One hundred twelve initial items underwent expert consultant evaluation, after which content validity was assessed using an expert panel consisting of patients and healthcare professionals.

The preliminary study leading to the development of the OPPQNCS was performed with a sample of 552 cancer patients. Data from the research supported the reliability ($\alpha = 0.99$) of the scale, and factorial analysis suggested four components. Further research has provided evidence for the convergent validity of the Individualization subscale among Finnish hospital patients [17]. The OPPQNCS has been used only in oncology patient settings in the USA [21] and Turkey [22] as well as in a few international studies conducted in the European countries of Finland, Cyprus, Greece and Sweden [23, 24].

The OPPQNCS includes 40 items (or 18 items in the short form) that are recorded by the patients on a 6-point Likert scale reflecting the frequency of the nursing activity (from 1, never to 6, always). The scale is composed of four subscales: 'Responsiveness', 'Individualization', 'Coordination' and 'Proficiency'. 'Responsiveness' designates the degree to which the nurse demonstrates that he/she is able to meet patient's needs in an attentive and caring manner. 'Individualization' designates the degree to which the nurse personalises care according to the patient's feelings, preferences and desired level of involvement in care. 'Coordination' designates the degree to which the nurse promotes communication among other nurses and the patient, while 'Proficiency' designates the degree to which the nurse provides knowledgeable and skilful nursing care [2].

9.3   Measuring Individuality from the HealthCare Providers' Point of View

The individuality of care can also be measured from the healthcare provider's perspective. In this section, three instruments focusing on this are presented: *Individualized Care Index (ICI)*, *Individualized Care Inventory (ICI)* and *assessment of the approach to nursing care*.

9.3.1   Individualized Care Index (ICI)

The Individualized Care Index (ICI), originally designed in the USA, is aimed to measure the extent to which nurses perceive they are individualising the care they are providing to their patients, and it is addressed specifically at nurses delivering direct patient care in inpatient hospital settings [3]. The theoretical basis for the Individualized Care Index was created by establishing a valid definition of the concept of individualised care through a threefold process. First, a comprehensive review of the literature was conducted. The concept of individualised care, as well as various related phenomena, such as patient-centred care, coordinated-continuous patient care and comprehensive nursing care, was explored, leading to generation of a list of nursing care behaviours. Second, a panel of judges reviewed the list of nursing care behaviours, of which 64 out of 80 were judged to be individualised care actions. Third, an initial pretest was conducted leading to a final selection of action referring to individualised care. The actions included three individualised care factors: patient-centred comprehensive care, patient-centred coordinated care and patient-centred inquiry/assessment [3].

The preliminary study leading to the development and psychometric testing of the Individualized Care Index was conducted among 838 nurses working in medical-surgical settings [3]. Each of the subscales had acceptable alpha values (factor 1, 0.91; factor 2, 0.85; factor 3, 0.91) indicating good reliability of the measurement. Construct validity, inter-item correlations and discriminant validity have been reported [3]. The Individualized Care Index has primarily been used in Canada, for example, among nurses working in cardiology, neurology and orthopaedic units [25] as well as in acute care settings [26, 27].

The Individualized Care Index consists of 45 items that are scored by the nurses on a 5-point rating scale from 1, with none of my patients, to 5, with all of my patients. A total of 29 items elicit the frequency with which nurses perceive themselves as fulfilling each of discrete individualised nursing care actions for their patients. The ICI includes an additional 13 items from the Qualpacs instrument and 3 items addressing indirect aspects of care. These items were used to mask the original intent of the survey, which had a heavy focal point on patient-centred interactions of the nurse-patient dyad [3]. Higher ICI scores indicate higher levels of individualisation of patient care.

9.3.2   Individualized Care Inventory (ICI)

The Individualized Care Inventory (ICI), originally designed in Canada, is aimed to measure individualised care from the staff perspective. It was initially developed to capture staff perceptions of individualised care for persons with dementia in long-term care institutions [4]. The theoretical basis of the ICI was established through a literature review, direct observation of care at long-term care facilities and ongoing consultation with an expert panel. Three domains focusing on staff members and their interactions with each other and with the resident were eventually chosen as appropriate for the development of the Individualized Care Inventory: '(1) the individuality of the resident, i.e. knowing the person/resident, (2) an opportunity for autonomy and choice for the resident, (3) open communication between staff themselves and between staff and residents' [4]. Item generation included development of an item pool for each domain, expert panel assessments, revisions and piloting [4].

Psychometrics of the instrument were assessed using a sample of 58 care aides working in long-term care facilities. The evidence of construct validity demonstrated a three-factor model. Reliability for each of the three subscales was acceptable as the Cronbach's α coefficient ranging from 0.77 to 0.80. Test-retest reliability was also reported [4]. Further support for the psychometric properties of the Individualized Care Inventory was provided in the study by O'Rourke et al. [28]. It has also been adapted and validated for a Chinese population [29], and it has been used in Canadian long-term care settings [4, 28, 30] as well as in nursing home settings in Australia [31] and Sweden [32].

The Individualized Care Inventory consists of three scales, 'IC-KNOW', 'IC-AUTONOMY' and 'IC-COMMUNICATION', measuring long-term aged care staff's perceptions of the individualised care they have recently been providing. The first scale, 'IC-KNOW', refers to how well staff perceives they know the residents they are caring for as persons. The scale includes 13 items that are rated by the staff on a 4-point Likert scale (from 1, strongly disagree, to 4, strongly agree). The second scale, 'IC-AUTONOMY', refers to how much control the staff perceives residents have over their everyday environment and their ability to choose to participate in activities directly related to their care or well-being. The scale includes 15 items reflecting frequency that are recorded on a 5-point Likert scale (from 1, very frequently, to 5, never). Lower scores indicate increased resident autonomy. The third scale, 'IC-COMMUNICATION', consists of 2 subscales that measure both staff-to-resident communication and staff-to-staff communication through 18 items. Responses are given on a four-point scale (from 1, never, to 4, always). Higher scores report better communication [4].

9.3.3   Assessment of the Approach to Nursing Care

Assessment of the approach to nursing care seems to be the first published assessment regarding individualisation in nursing care. The precise name of the scale is unclear, and it has also been named as a questionnaire for determining if nursing care is individualised or functional. It was introduced by Mackay and Ault in 1977 when they presented their plan that could be used to move the approach to nursing care in units from a functional, task-oriented approach to individualised nursing care to meet the physical, psychological and social needs of the patient. This plan included nearly 30 different steps, in one of which nursing units were recommended to assess their current approach to nursing care using a simple 12-question assessment. This questionnaire is divided into two parts: individualised nursing care and functional nursing care. Both parts consist of six dichotomous questions (YES/NO). YES to all answers in part 1 indicates an individualised approach to nursing care within the nursing unit, whereas YES to all answers in part 2 indicates a functional approach. YES answers in both parts indicate that the nursing unit uses both individualised and functional components in the nursing care provided [5].

Very little is known about the use of the assessment of the approach to nursing care in the practical or research field. However, it was probably one of the baseline factors launching the interest in developing more comprehensive measurements targeting individualisation in the healthcare context.

9.4 Measuring Person-Centred Healthcare

There are many instruments available that are designed to measure person-centredness in healthcare from both patients' and healthcare providers' perspectives. In this section, three instruments are presented measuring person-centredness from patients' perspective (*Person-Centered Inpatient Scale*, *Client-Centred Care Questionnaire (CCCQ)* and *Person-Centered care Climate Questionnaire-Patient version (PCQ-P)*) and four instruments measuring the same phenomenon from healthcare providers' perspective (*Person-Centred Nursing Index (PCNI)*, *Person-Centered Care Assessment Tool (P-CAT)*, *Person-Centred Climate Questionnaire-Staff version (PCQ-S)* and *Patient-Centred Care Competency Scale (PCC)*).

9.4.1 The Person-Centred Inpatient Scale

The Person-Centered Inpatient Scale, originally designed in the UK, is an instrument purposed to assess 'Valuing people as individuals' under the term person-centredness in healthcare from patients' perspective [6]. Theoretical basis of the Person-Centered Inpatient Scale is provided by a previous qualitative study examining how people talked about their disappointments with healthcare. The study identified 'personal identity threat' as a key concept explaining how people accounted for their experiences. The categories of 'personal identity threat' included perceptions of being dehumanised, objectified, stereotyped, devalued and disempowered. The first two categories of dehumanisation and objectification referred to the patients feeling that they had been treated as 'non-persons' and with little attention paid to their feelings, unique knowledge and experience. Being stereotyped included having low intelligence and being incompetent, infantile, idle/dishonest and unbalanced. Being disempowered meant having that person little control over one's body, feeling frustrated at being unable to gain access to care or carrying out one's social roles and feeling unable to assert the authentic self. Being devaluated included a feeling of being devalued as a human being [6].

An initial questionnaire consisting of 72 items covering the dimensions of the concept of 'personal identity threat' was developed through a process that included piloting, testing and refinement of the items. The initial questionnaire was used in a sample of Scottish inpatients discharged from a hospital. However, no validity or reliability testing was presented [6] According to the paper of Davis et al. [33], Coyle and Williams presented in their unpublished paper a rigorous process with established criteria for item retention, reducing the questionnaire to a 20-item tool. According to the same paper, the final scale was unidimensional and had good reliability ($\alpha = 0.91$). The utility of the scale was further studied in an Australian sample of older subacute care patients. The study found that the Person-Centered Inpatient Scale has the ability to detect variation in frequency scores. However, no validity or reliability estimates were presented in this study, either [33].

The Person-Centered Inpatient Scale consists of 20 items in 5 dimensions: (1) personalization (four items), (2) empowerment (four items), (3) information (four items), (4) approachability/availability (four items), (5) respectfulness (two items) and (6) miscellaneous (two items). Items are scored on a five-point Likert scale including the categories 'strongly agree', 'agree', 'uncertain', 'disagree' and 'strongly disagree' [33].

9.4.2 Client-Centred Care Questionnaire (CCCQ)

The Client-Centred Care Questionnaire (CCCQ), originally designed in the Netherlands, is purposed to evaluate person-centred care from a client perspective in home-care setting [7]. The CCCQ is based on a framework that emerged during a study on client perspectives of client-centred care and the competencies professionals should have in order to provide it [7]. The study results suggested that care is experienced as client-centred when clients 'feel recognised and respected by the nurse and when they experience autonomy with respect to the way in which care is delivered' [7]. Five central values (autonomy, continuity of life, uniqueness, comprehensiveness and fairness) and three underlying values (equality, partnership and interdependence) were identified as essential to client-centredness and relationships with caregivers [7].

Fifteen items referring to the values and expectations mentioned above were formulated and assessed through discussion with experienced nurses and clients. The initial questionnaire was piloted and, following minor revisions, tested with a sample of clients receiving home care ($n = 107$). Internal consistency using Cronbach's alpha for total questionnaire was 0.94. Factorial analysis suggested that CCCQ has a unidimensional construct [7].

The CCCQ consists of 15 items that are rated by the clients using a five-point Likert scale (from 1, totally disagree, to 5, totally agree) [7]. The questionnaire has been used within home-care settings in the Netherlands [34, 35] and Canada [36]. It has also been subjected to research in long-term care settings in Estonia and among Chinese chronic patients [37].

9.4.3 Person-Centred Climate Questionnaire-Patient Version (PCQ-P)

The Person-Centered Climate Questionnaire-Patient version (PCQ-P), originally designed in Sweden, is an instrument designed to measure the extent to which patients perceive their care environments as person-centred. The PCQ-P is intended to be used with adults receiving somatic care in subacute and acute hospital settings. The theoretical framework for developing the PCQ-P emerged from the authors' qualitative research programme exploring care environments perceived as caring. Patients and their significant others described that physical and psychosocial dimensions of care environments that supported their personhood were important for their well-being. The theoretical framework describes person-centred environments as consisting of three dimensions: a climate of safety, a climate of everydayness and a climate of hospitality. Drawing on this theoretical framework, a preliminary 45-item questionnaire was constructed embracing the 3 climate dimensions and further validated by its content through expert panel and patient assessments [8].

The PCQ-P underwent an initial testing and reduction process with a sample of hospital patients ($n = 544$). The internal consistency coefficient was satisfactory for the total scale when estimated with Cronbach's alpha (0.93), and a three-domain factorial structure was found. The test-retest reliability of the questionnaire was estimated to be satisfactory [8]. The PCQ-P was later translated into English and validated in an Australian hospital patient sample, confirming appropriate psychometric properties [38]. More recently, the PCQ-P was evaluated for its psychometrics in long-term care settings using a sample of older residents in North America. The PCQ-P was demonstrated as a valid and reliable tool that could also be used beyond hospital settings [39].

The PCQ-P includes 17 items that are rated by patients on a 7-point Likert scale (from 1, no, I disagree completely to 7, yes, I agree completely). The scale has the following three dimensions: (1) 'a climate of safety' (ten items), (2) 'a climate of everydayness' (four items) and (3) 'a climate of hospitality' (three items). 'A climate of safety' refers to staff who talk in an understandable lay language; are available, approachable and competent; and respond quickly. Furthermore, a clean and well-organised physical environment symbolises safe care. 'A climate of everydayness' refers to experiences of a 'de-institutionalised' environment that contains the aspects of the familiar and every day and of being home-like. 'A climate of hospitality' refers to the reception and entertainment of people in the environment, conveying both feelings of being welcome and receiving the best treatment and care. Higher scores indicate a climate that is very person-centred [8].

9.4.4 The Person-Centred Nursing Index (PCNI)

The Person-Centred Nursing Index (PCNI) developed by Slater and McCormack in the UK in 2006 is an instrument purposed to measure the processes and outcomes of person-centred nursing care from nursing and patient perspectives [9, 10]. The PCNI measures factors identified in McCormack and McCance's [40] 'Person-centred nursing theoretical framework', which brings together previous empirical research focusing on person-centred practice with older people and the experience of caring in nursing. The framework comprises four constructs: prerequisites, care environment, person-centred processes and outcomes. Prerequisites focus on the attributes of the nurses and include being professionally competent, having developed interpersonal skills, being committed to the job, being able to demonstrate clarity of beliefs and values and knowing self. The care environment focuses on the care context and includes appropriate skill mix, systems facilitating shared decision-making, effective staff relationships, supportive organisational systems, shared power and the potential for innovation and risk-taking. Person-centred processes focus on delivering care through a variety of activities and include working among patient's beliefs and values, engagement, having sympathetic presence, sharing decision-making and providing for physical needs. Outcomes are the results of effective person-centred nursing and include satisfaction with care, involvement in care, feeling of well-being and creation of a therapeutic environment [40].

The PCNI was developed as an integral part of the study described in the paper by McCance et al. [41], and it was generated from an amalgamation of key findings from an extensive literature review, focus groups and a pilot study. The PCNI consists of three parts—the Nursing Context Index (NCI), the Caring Dimensions Inventory (CDI) and the Nursing Dimensions Inventory (NDI). The NCI consist of 89 items covering 19 domains relevant to the nursing work environment. The CDI is an instrument designed to measure perceptions of caring in the nurse-patient relationship. It consists of 35 items that are categorised into 5 labels: technical, intimacy, psychosocial, unnecessary and inappropriate. Items are rated on a five-point Likert scale ranging from 'strongly agree' to 'strongly disagree'. The NDI is an instrument for non-nurses (including patients) to assess non-nursing views of what constitutes caring. It is based on the CDI and replicates the items from a non-nursing perspective [41].

The PCNI has been used in the UK within residential care [41] and hospital [10] settings. Another study within residential care settings was conducted in Australia [42], whereas Deravin et al. [43] used the instrument within medical-surgical settings [42]. The PCNI has also been subjected to research within adult psychiatric hospital settings in Finland [44].

9.4.5 Person-Centred Climate Questionnaire-Staff Version (PCQ-S)

The Person-Centred Climate Questionnaire-Staff version (PCQ-S), originally designed in Sweden, is an instrument aimed at measuring to what extent the climate of healthcare settings is experienced as person-centred by staff. Similar to the PCQ-P introduced previously, the theoretical framework for developing the PCQ-S emerged from the authors' qualitative research programme exploring care environments. The theory describes person-centred environments as consisting of the following three main climate categories: a climate of safety, a climate of everydayness and a climate of hospitality. Based on theory and other research literature, an initial pool of items covering the three main climate categories was formulated and validated by its content through expert panel evaluation [11].

The initial questionnaire consisting of 45 items was subjected to item analysis and reduction using a sample of Swedish hospital staff ($n = 600$). Cronbach's alpha, indicating internal consistency, was 0.88 for the final 14-item questionnaire. Factorial analyses resulted in a three-factor structure. Test-retest reliability confirmed satisfying stability and reliability of the PCQ-S over time [11]. The PCQ-S has been translated into English and validated in an Australian sample of day surgery care staff, supporting the reliability of the scale. However, the scale was found to have a four-component structure, which deviated somewhat from the three-factor structure found earlier [45]. There is also a study validating the PCQ-S in a Norwegian sample of nursing home staff, demonstrating good psychometric properties, which indicates that the scale can be used in such settings as well [46]. Furthermore, the PCQ-S has been used in studies conducted in Sweden in acute care settings [47, 48] and in residential care settings for older people [49] as well as in Korea in long-term care settings [50].

The PCQ-S contains 14 items in 3 subscales: (1) 'a climate of safety' (five items), (2) 'a climate of everydayness' (five items) and (3) 'a climate of community' (four items). Safety relates to experiences of being safe in the environment, everydayness relates to the environment as having an everyday and neat character, while community involves possibilities to maintain previous and establish new social contacts in the environment. Items are rated by the staff members on a six-point Likert scale (from 1, no, I disagree completely, to 6, yes, I agree completely). Higher scores indicate a climate that is very person-centred [11].

9.4.6 Person-Centred Care Assessment Tool (P-CAT)

The Person-Centered Care Assessment Tool (P-CAT), originally designed in Sweden and Australia, is an instrument purposed to measure the extent to which professionals working in residential aged care facilities rate their settings as being person-centred [12]. The theoretical basis for the P-CAT was generated through a process of review of literature, expert panel consultations and interviews. First, a literature review was conducted to summarise the knowledge about person-centred care for people with dementia. Person-centred care was described through four dimensions as 'maintaining personhood in spite of declining cognitive ability, striving to take the standpoint of the patient, acknowledging personal experiences of life and relationships, and including the social environment as a therapeutic agent'. Based on the description, initial items for the P-CAT were formulated and further modified and verified through expert consultations and interviews with staff members, patients and family members [12].

To undergo a systematic process of item reduction and psychometric testing, the preliminary tool was distributed to an Australian sample (n = 220) of aged care staff. Data from the research supported the reliability (α = 0.84) of the scale, and factorial analysis suggested three domains: personalised care, accessibility and organisational support. Furthermore, test-retest reliability of the tool indicated satisfactory estimates [12]. The P-CAT has subsequently been adapted and validated in residential care settings in Sweden [51] and Norway [52]. A version has also been adapted and validated for Chinese [53] and, more recently, Spanish populations [54]. All of this research confirmed the acceptable psychometric properties of this instrument. The P-CAT has been used in research conducted in residential care settings for older people in Australia [55] and Sweden [56] as well as in long-term care settings in Korea [50].

The Person-Centered Care Assessment Tool consists of 13 items reflecting the content of individualised care, environmental accessibility and organisational support. Items are rated by the professionals using a five-point Likert scale (from 1, disagree completely, to 5, agree completely). Higher values indicate a higher degree of person-centredness [12].

9.4.7   Patient-Centred Care Competency Scale (PCC)

The Patient-Centred Care Competency Scale (PCC), developed in South Korea, is an instrument designed to assess hospital nurses' perceptions of their patient-centred care competency. The development of the PCC is based on a definition of patient-centred care competency proposed by the Quality and Safety Education for Nurses (QSEN) faculty. The QSEN defines patient-centred care competency as *knowledge*, *skills* and *attitudes* regarding patient-centred care. Drawing on this definition and a review of previous research, an initial 41-item draft of the questionnaire was composed and validated by its content through an expert panel. The resulting 25 items were pretested among nurse professionals to verify their clarity and comprehensibility, leading to minor modifications of the wording of the questionnaire [13].

For psychometric testing of the PCC scale, the 25-item questionnaire was distributed to a sample of hospital nurses (n = 594). Cronbach's alpha indicating internal consistency coefficient was satisfactory (0.92) for the final 17-item questionnaire. Initial factor analysis revealed a four-factor solution, and multitrait scaling analysis supported satisfying convergent and discriminant validity for the four-subscale structure. There seems to be no other research on the PCC, and further validation of the instrument is suggested [13].

The PPC contains 17 items in four subscales: (1) 'respecting patients' perspectives' (six items), (2) 'promoting patient involvement in care processes' (five items), (3) 'providing for patient comfort' (three items) and (4) 'advocating for patients' (three items). Nurses rate their competencies for each item on a five-point Likert scale (from 1, minimal to 5, excellent). Higher scores indicate nurses' higher competency with respect to patient-centred care [13].

Conclusion

There are a variety of instruments aimed to measure individuality and related concepts both from patients' and healthcare professionals' perspectives. Some of the instruments have been widely used in different countries, also in comparative studies, while others have been used less and in national contexts only. To measure abstract concepts, the definition of the concept has to be operationalised in the instrument. Therefore, it was important to describe the background of each instrument and the purpose for which it was developed. In order to measure concepts such as individuality, individualised care and patient-centredness of care, valid and reliable instruments are needed. The validity and reliability assessment of these instruments has been varying, and it seems that only few instruments have been systematically developed and tested. However, developing an instrument takes years and is not an easy task to undertake.

After describing the different instruments in this chapter, it can be seen that the approaches have been different and the purposes of the instruments have been many. The fact that there are so many instruments lends support to the importance of the topic in clinical practice as well from both patients' and professionals' point of view. All of these instruments are potential choices when measuring individuality and related concepts. In addition, they could be used as criterion instruments when demonstrating criterion validity of another instrument. In all, more research using such instruments is needed in order to verify their relevance in measuring individuality and person-centredness in the healthcare context.

References

1. Schmidt LA. Development and testing of a measure of patient satisfaction with nursing care. Dissertations from ProQuest. 2001. 1756. https://scholarlyrepository.miami.edu/dissertations/1756. Accessed 28 Mar 2018.
2. Radwin L, Alster K, Rubin KM. Developments and testing of the oncology patients' perceptions of the quality of nursing care scale. Oncol Nurs Forum. 2003;30(2):283–90.
3. van Servellen G. The individualized care index. In: Strickland O, Dilor C, editors. Measurement of nursing outcomes: volume 2, client outcomes and quality of care. 2nd ed. New York: Springer; 2003. p. 280–4.
4. Chappell NL, Reid RC, Gish JA. Staff-based measures of individualized care for persons with dementia in long-term care facilities. Dementia. 2007;6(4):527–47.
5. Mackay C, Ault LD. A systematic approach to individualizing nursing care. J Nurs Adm. 1977;7(1):39–48.
6. Coyle J, Williams B. Valuing people as individuals: development of an instrument through a survey of person-centredness in secondary care. J Adv Nurs. 2001;36(3):450–9.
7. de Witte L, Schoot T, Proot I. Development of the client-centred care questionnaire. J Adv Nurs. 2006;56(1):62–8.
8. Edvardsson D, Sandman PO, Rasmussen B. Swedish language person-centred climate questionnaire patient version: construction and psychometric evaluation. J Adv Nurs. 2008;63(3):302–9.
9. Slater P. Person-centred nursing: the development and testing of a valid and reliable nursing outcomes instrument. Unpublished PhD thesis. Jordanstown: University of Ulster; 2006.

10. McCormack B, Dewing J, Breslin L, et al. Developing person-centred practice: nursing outcomes arising from changes to the care environment in residential settings for older people. Int J Older People Nursing. 2010;5(1):93–107.
11. Edvardsson D, Sandman PO, Rasmussen B. Swedish language person-centred climate questionnaire-staff version. J Nurs Manag. 2009;17(7):790–5.
12. Edvardsson D, Fetherstonhaugh D, Nay R, et al. Development and initial testing of the person-centered care assessment tool (P-CAT). Int Psychogeriatr. 2010;22(1):101–8.
13. Hwang JI. Development and testing of a patient-centred care competency scale for hospital nurses. Int J Nurs Pract. 2015;21(1):43–51.
14. Schmidt LA. Patients' perceptions of nursing care in the hospital setting. J Adv Nurs. 2003;44(4):393–9.
15. Suhonen R, Berg A, Idvall E, et al. European orthopaedic and trauma patients' perceptions of nursing care: a comparative study. J Clin Nurs. 2009;18(20):2818–29.
16. Schmidt LA. Patients' perceptions of nurse staffing, nursing care, adverse events, and overall satisfaction with the hospital experience. Nurs Econ. 2004;22(6):295–306.
17. Suhonen R, Schmidt LA, Radwin L. Measuring individualized nursing care: assessment of reliability and validity of three scales. J Adv Nurs. 2007;59(1):77–85.
18. Wolf D, Lehman L, Quinlin R, et al. Can nurses impact patient outcomes using a patient-centered care model? J Nurs Adm. 2008;38(12):532–40.
19. Golembeski S, Willmitch B, Kim SS. Perceptions of the care experience in critical care units enhanced by a Tele-ICU. AACN Adv Crit Care. 2012;23(3):323–9.
20. Radwin L. Oncology patients' perceptions of quality nursing care. Res Nurs Health. 2000;23(3):179–90.
21. Radwin LE. Cancer patients' demographic characteristics and ratings of patient-centered nursing care. J Nurs Scholarsh. 2003;35(4):365–70.
22. Can G, Akinb S, Aydinerc A, et al. Evaluation of the effect of care given by nursing students on oncology patients' satisfaction. Eur J Oncol Nurs. 2008;12(4):387–92.
23. Adam C, Patiraki E, Chryssoula L, et al. Quality of nursing care as perceived by cancer patients: a cross-sectional survey in four European countries. J BUON. 2017;22(3):777–82.
24. Charalambous A, Radwin L, Berg A, et al. An international study of hospitalized cancer patients' health status, nursing care quality, perceived individuality in care and trust in nurses: a path analysis. Int J Nurs Stud. 2016;61(1):176–86.
25. Poochikian-Sarkissian S, Sidani S, Ferguson-Pare M, et al. Examining the relationship between patient-centred care and outcomes. Can J Neurosci Nurs. 2010;32(4):14–21.
26. Sidani S, Doran D, Porter H, et al. Processes of care: comparison between nurse practitioners and physician residents in acute care. Nurs Leadersh. 2006;19(1):69–85.
27. Sidani S, Irvine D, Porter H, et al. Practice patterns of acute care nurse practitioners. Can J Nurs Leadersh. 2000;13(3):6–12.
28. O'Rourke N, Chappell NL, Caspar S. Measurement and analysis of individualized care inventory responses comparing long-term care nurses and care aides. Gerontologist. 2009;49(6):839–46.
29. Chappell NL, Chou KL. Chinese version of staff-based measures of individualized care for institutionalized persons with dementia. Asian J Gerontol Geriatr. 2010;5(1):5–13.
30. Caspar S, O'Rourke N. The influence of care provider access to structural empowerment on individualized care in long-term-care facilities. J Gerontol. 2008;63B(4):S255–65.
31. Davis S, Campbell A. The practice of individualized dementia care in Australian nursing homes. Alzheimers Dement. 2012;8(4S):S753. https://doi.org/10.1016/j.jalz.2013.08.051.
32. Elfstrand Corlin T, Kajonius PJ, Kazemi A. The impact of personality on person-centred care: a study of care staff in Swedish nursing homes. Int J Older People Nursing. 2017;12:e12132.
33. Davis S, Byers S, Walsh F. Measuring person-centred care in a sub-acute health care setting. Aust Health Rev. 2008;32(3):496–504.
34. Bosman R, Boursa GJJW, Engelsc J, et al. Client-centred care perceived by clients of two Dutch homecare agencies: a questionnaire survey. Int J Nurs Stud. 2008;45(4):518–25.

35. Muntinga ME, Mokkink LB, Knol DL, et al. Measurement proprieties of the client-centred care questionnaire (CCCQ): factor structure, reliability and validity of a questionnaire to assess self-reported client-centeredness of home services in a population of frail, older people. Qual Life Res. 2014;23(7):2063–72.
36. Brazil K, Bainbridge D, Ploeg J, et al. Family caregiver views on patient-centred care at the end of life. Scand J Caring Sci. 2012;26(3):513–8.
37. Liu S, Chen Y, Fan F. Reliability and validity of Chinese version of the client-centred care questionnaire. Chin J Pract Nurs. 2015;31(19):1460–3.
38. Edvardsson D, Koch S, Nay R. Psychometric evaluation of the English language person-centered climate questionnaire-patient version. West J Nurs Res. 2009;31(2):235–44.
39. Yoon JY, Roberts T, Grau B, et al. Person-centered climate questionnaire-patient in English: a psychometric evaluation study in long-term care settings. Arch Gerontol Geriatr. 2015;61(1):81–7.
40. McCormack B, McCance TV. Development of a framework for person-centred nursing. J Adv Nurs. 2006;56(5):472–9.
41. McCance T, Slater P, McCormack B. Using the caring dimensions inventory as an indicator of person-centred nursing. J Clin Nurs. 2009;18(3):409–17.
42. White C, Wilson V. A longitudinal study of aspects of a hospital's family centred nursing: changing practice through data translation. J Adv Nurs. 2015;71(1):100–14.
43. Deravin L, Karen F, Nielsen S, et al. Nursing stress and satisfaction outcomes resulting from implementing a team nursing model of care in a rural setting. J Hosp Adm. 2017;6(1):60–6.
44. Kurjenluoma K, Rantanen A, McCormack B, et al. Workplace culture in psychiatric nursing. Scand J Caring Sci. 2017;31(4):1048–58.
45. Edvardsson D, Koch S, Nay R. Psychometric evaluation of the English language person-centred climate questionnaire-staff version. J Nurs Manag. 2010;18(1):54–60.
46. Bergland Å, Kirkevold M, Edvardsson D. Psychometric properties of the Norwegian person-centred climate questionnaire from a nursing home context. Scand J Caring Sci. 2012;26(4):820–8.
47. Lehuluante A, Nilsson A, Edvardsson D. The influence of a person-centred psychosocial unit climate on satisfaction with care and work. J Nurs Manag. 2012;20(3):319–25.
48. Nilsson A, Lindkvist M, Rasmussen BH, et al. Staff attitudes towards older patients with cognitive impairment: need for improvements in acute care. J Nurs Manag. 2012;20(5):640–7.
49. Edvardsson D, Sjogren K, Lindkvist M, et al. Person-centred climate questionnaire (PCQ-S): establishing reliability and cut-off scores in residential aged care. J Nurs Manag. 2015;23(3):315–23.
50. Ha JY, Park SH. Person-centered care and person-centered care climate of long-term care facilities for the elderly. IJIPHM. 2017;4(1):59–66.
51. Sjögren K, Lindkvist M, Sandman P, et al. Psychometric evaluation of the Swedish version of the Person-Centered Care Assessment Tool (P-CAT). Int Psychogeriatr. 2012;24(3):406–15.
52. Rokstad AMM, Engedal K, Edvardsson D, et al. Psychometric evaluation of the Norwegian version of the Person-Centred Care Assessment Tool. Int J Nurs Pract. 2012;18(1):99–105.
53. Zhong XB, Lou VWQ. Person-centered care in Chinese residential care facilities: a preliminary measure. Aging Ment Health. 2013;17(8):952–8.
54. Martínez T, Suárez-Álvarez J, Yanguas J, et al. Spanish validation of the person-centered care assessment tool (P-CAT). Aging Ment Health. 2016;20(5):550–8.
55. Edvardsson D, Fetherstonhaugh D, McAuliffe L, et al. Job satisfaction amongst aged care staff: exploring the influence of person-centered care provision. Int Psychogeriatr. 2011;23(8):1205–12.
56. Edvardsson D, Sandman PO, Borell L. Implementing national guidelines for person-centered care of people with dementia in residential aged care: effects on perceived person-centeredness, staff strain, and stress of conscience. Int Psychogeriatr. 2014;26(7):1171–9.

Part III

Research Evidence: The Delivery of Individualised Care

Individualised Nursing Care of Operative Surgical Patients

10

Helena Leino-Kilpi and Sunna Rannikko

Abstract

The purpose of this chapter is to describe the nature and implementation of individualised nursing care among surgical patients. The nature of this care is operational, the patient-professional contact is short and the emphasis is on supporting recovery and self-management by educational activities. In this chapter, we first describe the nature of individualised surgical nursing care and then move on to the support of this care.

Keywords

Individualised care · Operative care · Surgical nursing care · Surgical patient

10.1 The Nature of Individualised Surgical Nursing Care

In surgical nursing care, there are many challenges for individualised care. These challenges have to do with the short contact times between patients and professionals, the high-level standardisation of the procedures and high technical orientation. All these mean high expectations for the patients' self-management and individual responsibility of their recovery.

Shortening contact times between patients and professionals is mainly due to the increase of ambulatory care and short-stay clinics, leading to shorter hospital stays [1]. This emphasises the importance of preoperative education and patients' individual preparation for the operation, as well as recovery time at home. This requires

H. Leino-Kilpi (✉) · S. Rannikko
Department of Nursing Science, University of Turku,
Turku University Hospital, Turku, Finland
e-mail: heleiki@utu.fi; seeran@utu.fi

© Springer International Publishing AG, part of Springer Nature 2019
R. Suhonen et al. (eds.), *Individualized Care*,
https://doi.org/10.1007/978-3-319-89899-5_10

multidimensional empowering knowledge (e.g. [2])—as well as understanding of the individual patient's own contribution and empowerment.

The aim of high-level standardisation of procedures is to achieve what is best for the patients. This has to do with the definition of surgical protocols and clinical pathways as well as with patient safety guidelines. At the same time, however, these pose challenges for the individual processes of patients and the possibilities to create individual solutions. For example, for the continuity of care in ambulatory surgery, co-ordination flow, time flow, caring relationships flow and information flow all need to be realised at the same time in order to achieve an individual process for patients [3]. In standardised care, the amount of relevant variation of the care is rarely defined, which poses a challenge in terms of responding to each patient's individual needs and expectations. In addition, standardised care emphasises effectiveness and the passive role of the patient instead of the patients taking an active part in their own care [4]. Thus, in certain circumstances, effectiveness may be considered as a threat to individuality [5].

Healthcare technology has brought a lot of advancements in the surgical operational field, from nurses' documentation to the use of surgical robots. However, the use of technology also means some challenges to healthcare professionals in providing individualised care. The time spent on technology is often extensive, and depending on the technological devices, it can also mean time away from the patient's bedside. In addition, it is also a threat to individual care if nurses' skills required in providing individualised care are not valued as highly as their technical skills [6].

Especially, there can be a risk for informational privacy. Sharing patient information with electronic devices may jeopardise information security [7] and thus put patients' privacy at risk. Individual care in the operational surgical field has many dimensions. Patients are mostly physically touched by operations, including procedures such as resections or reconstructions using prosthetic devices. This means that physical privacy and respect of physical dignity have a strong role. Operational care is a process, from the decision of operate to the operation itself and further to the recovery at home. To keep the individual process comprehensive and fluent, there is a need for well-planned, successful patient education and counselling during all the phases of the process. The process also requires individual human understanding and respect of patients' rights as well as tailored patient-oriented solutions. Surgical patients usually have various symptoms, such as pain and fatigue [8]. Pain, for example, can inhibit decision-making and empowerment of a human being. Thus, successful clinical management of pain is part of the respect of individual patients in surgical nursing care [9].

Surgical operational care and treatment require trust: the patient has to trust the professionals, even while under complete anaesthesia during the operation. Correspondingly, this trust requires a high degree of responsibility on the part of the professionals. This reciprocal relationship calls for a deep understanding and respect from both parties. A challenge for individualised care is created if the relationship does not allow enough time to get to know the patients, to listen to their perceptions or to consider individual, exceptional solutions. Thus, there is a clear need to plan and implement individualised surgical nursing care as well as to evaluate the individual outcomes.

10.2   Individualised Surgical Nursing Care in Existing Literature

In the literature, surgical nursing care has been studied using the concepts individualised care, patient-centred care and tailored care. The viewpoint of the studies varies from a general perspective to a very narrow viewpoint of a specific treatment. In this part, we concentrate on the studies using the concept of individualised care from a general perspective. We describe the methods of studying individualised surgical nursing care, its challenges and evaluations for individualisation.

Methodologically, there is a strong tradition of studying individualised surgical nursing care with the Individualised Care Scale (ICS) developed by Suhonen et al. [10]. This scale consists of two subscales, support of individuality in care (ICS-A) and perception of individuality in care (ICS-B), and has versions for both patients [10] and nurses [11]. Qualitative [6] and mixed methods [12] have also been used in this field.

The evaluation of individualised surgical nursing care is methodologically challenging. Patients consider the evaluation difficult as nurses are a heterogeneous group and there can be high variation in the level of individualised care [12]. Nurses have reported experiencing difficulties in individualised care due to the existing resources and emotional demands [6]. Evaluating individualised surgical nursing care is thus somewhat challenging from both patients' and nurses' perspective.

The existing studies from patients' point of view consist of orthopaedic patients [12–14], orthopaedic and trauma patients [15–18], orthopaedic and neurosurgical patients [19] or patients in general surgical wards [20–24]. The literature does not present any clear associations between the surgical patients' background factors and the evaluation of individualised care [12, 14, 15, 18]. Based on the results, it is clear that surgical patients consider it important to be cared for as individuals [13, 16, 17] and they also consider the support for their individuality as rather high [14, 17, 23, 24]. There is, however, variation in the individualisation, ranging from higher [16, 20, 24] to moderate [21]. Surgical patients seem to be satisfied both with the support for [13, 16, 19, 22–24] and the realisation of individuality in clinical situations [16, 19, 21].

Personal life, however, seems to be an area with less received support for individuality [13, 16, 19, 22, 24], and it is not perceived as high in the care, either [13, 16, 19, 21, 23]. Instead, decisional control is highly or well realised in the care of surgical patients [13, 16, 19, 21, 23, 24] except when it comes to deciding when to perform daily hygiene [16]. Individuality in the care realisation is valuable as such, but it is also associated with higher level of patient satisfaction [21, 23] and with health-related quality of life [23].

The study populations in the studies from nurses' point of view consist of nurses working in orthopaedic and trauma wards [25, 26], general surgical wards [20, 22], day surgery or a combination of these [6, 27]. Nurses' support for surgical patients' individuality is connected with their higher level of education, work title and length of working experience [25]. Nurses supporting and providing individualised care is associated with nurses' internal work motivation, cultural sensitivity and staff relationship with physicians. In addition, providing individualised care is connected to nurses' control over practice and teamwork [26]. Nurses consider that they are well able to support surgical patients' individuality [22, 27]. The support is strongest in clinical situations and weakest in the case of personal life situation [22]. Nurses also think that patients' individuality is realised in the care they provide [20, 22, 27]. Individualisation is realised most strongly in decisional control and most weakly in the area of personal life situation [22].

When comparing the viewpoints of patients and nurses, both consider that individuality is supported and realised in the care. Nurses seem to evaluate the individuality as higher than patients [20, 22]. In international comparison, there are some differences in the support and realisation of individuality as evaluated by surgical patients and nurses. However, there is no clear division in the variation on either a North-South or a West-East axis [17, 20, 25, 27]. The variation may be explained by differences in care culture and care arrangements between the countries [17, 20, 27].

The literature on individualised surgical nursing care focuses on the perspectives of patients and nurses. As the surgical field is under fast development and rapid changes in both medical treatment and unit-level nursing, research concerning the requirements for the organisational level is needed. Even though the results of the studies concerning individualised care among surgical patients indicate rather a high level of satisfaction, there is still a need for future studies. In particular, there is a need to find out factors supporting individualised surgical nursing care in different contexts and among different surgical groups of patients, as well as studies testing different interventions to support individualisation. In the next section, we point out some important areas of support of individuality.

10.3 Support of Individualised Surgical Nursing Care

In surgical operational nursing care, there are three main areas of support for the individualisation, i.e. educational, ethical and technological support. The support can include different professional actions, principles and strategies to follow or decisions to be made. In the next paragraphs, all of these will be described, the main emphasis being on educational support.

10.3.1 Educational Support

Educational support for individualisation in surgical nursing care aims to empower individual patients before, during and after the perioperative process. This support can be divided into educational diagnostics, empowering educational discourse, and educational interventions and evaluation of their outcomes.

Educational diagnostics is important for individualised empowering education. Diagnostics means that the professional has to know the existing knowledge base and structure, learning strategies and preferences of the patient. By analysing the patient's existing knowledge, it is possible to construct an individualised educational process for the patient and identify possible gaps in the knowledge. Unfortunately, in healthcare practices, we do not necessarily have systematic educational diagnostic instruments for evaluating the knowledge level of patients or their cognitive structures or ways of processing (e.g. [28, 29]). In the literature, patients' information needs have been one focal topic (e.g. [30]). However, these studies mostly assume that patients' needs can be standardised; subsequently, patient information leaflet material is also created based on that standardisation.

Analysing patients' personal expectations and their evaluations of the received knowledge is fundamental for an individual educational process. This has been done, for example, in the field of orthopaedic care and cancer care. The results indicate that the expectations are multidimensional and have some international correspondence [31]. Especially, the patients expect bio-physiological knowledge, including knowledge about the symptoms and the disease. The results also indicate that, when evaluated postoperatively by the same patients, the expectations are not fully met [31, 32]. In particular, the fulfilment of social, economic and ethical knowledge seems to be a problem. The knowledge received has been shown to be positively connected with patient-centred quality of nursing care [33].

Educational diagnostics can be made using different instruments. A screening instrument for cancer patients ([28]; see also [34]), for example, integrates the critical moments of individual cancer patient education and the knowledge expectation types obtained from patient datasets into assessment of patients' cognitive resources, knowledge expectations and comprehension. Furthermore, knowledge tests can be used for the purpose of identifying individual knowledge gaps [35, 36].

Empowering educational discourse is one method of individualised empowering education (e.g. [37]), but there seem to be problems in the realisation of patient-centred education [38]. Discourse can take different forms, but it can be divided into initiation of the discourse, progress and closing, each having different empowering elements [37]. What is important is shared negotiation and discussion and the content determined by the patient. The individual nature of the discourse allows the identification of knowledge gaps and progress according to the individual situation of each patient.

Different interventions have been tested for supporting individualised education in surgical nursing care (e.g. [39–42]). Most of these interventions have been at least partly effective, eliciting a positive response from patients. For example, Ryhänen et al. [41] were able to show positive outcomes if clinical pathways are used for patient education, while Siekkinen et al. [42] demonstrated the usefulness of knowledge test feedback, as did Kesänen et al. [40]. The positive outcomes included a decrease in preoperative anxiety [40] and an improvement in quality of life [42]. In all of these, the Internet was used in the intervention to give patients more individual opportunities to approach the knowledge available (see [43]). However, there is still a need to develop and test new educational interventions for improving the individual empowerment of surgical patients. A special challenge is the education for ambulatory, short-stay patients. Furthermore, it is clear that educational methods allowing patients to make themselves familiar with new knowledge individually are effective and should be tested. Technological solutions, however, are not the only option: for individual tailoring, it is fundamental to offer patients knowledge in a multidimensional format. The readability and quality of educational materials are also important (e.g. [44]).

10.3.2 Ethical Support

Ethical support in the field of surgical nursing care consists of the support of individual patients' ethical safety, the realisation of patients' rights and the ethical competence of professionals responsible for the care of individual patients. This support has special importance among surgical patients, because they are adults, are willing and capable of making decisions and require rapid recovery, and there are possibilities for surgical errors. Furthermore, especially in surgery, the professionals are allowed to touch the patient physically, even to perform painful actions.

Support for patients' ethical safety aims to improve patients' personal experience of safety, referring to the freedom to express and live according to their own values also in the context of healthcare. This freedom includes freedom for patients to express their own preferences and evaluations of care, as well as to collaborate in an individual way. Safety is a multidimensional concept. According to the WHO, for example, "patient safety is the absence of preventable harm to patient during the process of health care". Thus, ethical safety is the absence of preventable ethical harm, such as non-respect or limited possibilities to decision-making.

The issues in ethical safety are sometimes difficult to identify. Some information can be found in patient complaints (e.g. [45]), satisfaction studies [21] and experience descriptions. Montini et al. [45] have created a classification of patients' complaints; among the "Red flags" they have discrimination, coercion and problems in confidentiality. Ethical safety lists are, however, very rare. As it comes to the individualisation of surgical nursing care, patients have reported [21] that the care they received was only moderately individualised. Individuality was, however, taken into account well in patients' clinical situation and decisional control over care.

The realisation of the ethical rights of patients enacted in legislation and political statements (e.g. [46]) is an individual approach to ethics. The rights are expressed in ethical codes (e.g. [47, 48]), expressions of patients' rights in hospitals or other healthcare organisations (e.g. [49]) and by patients' associations (e.g. [50]). In surgical nursing care, the self-determination [51] and autonomy [52] of patients seem to be on high level, as is also the case with privacy and informed consent [53]. Among professionals, however, there seems to be a lack of knowledge about patients' rights [54].

Ethical competence of professionals is important for the ethical safety of surgical patients. Ethical competence is a multidimensional concept [55], consisting of character strength, ethical awareness, moral judgement skills and willingness to do good. The main part of the competence is moral courage, including seven core attributes, i.e. true presence, moral integrity, responsibility, honesty, advocacy, commitment and perseverance and personal risk ([56]; see also [57]). Although ethical competence is important for professionals to be able to provide ethically oriented individualised care, in the literature, research on ethical competence is scarce.

Based on the literature, nurse leaders have an important role in supporting nurses' ethical competence [58]. Nurse leaders support ethical competence in performance reviews but also, at least on some level, in the recruitment process. In performance reviews, the nurse leaders highlight collegiality and ethical codes, while in the recruitment process, the nurse leaders aim to ensure the nurse's ethical behaviour and knowledge [59]. However, neither nurses nor nurse leaders perceive the support for nurses' ethical competence to be at high level [60]. In addition, the literature points out that nurse leaders' ethical activity is low in many aspects. Nurse leaders are not keen on developing their ethical knowledge or influencing ethical issues. Moreover, they are not enthusiastic about conducting or implementing ethical research [61]. Instead, nurse leaders' ethical activity seems to concentrate on identification of ethical problems [61], and they recognise ethical problems in various areas in the healthcare context [62]. In addition, nurse leaders have many activities aimed to solve the problems although they do not have a systematic model for this ([63]; see also [64]). Thus, in order to support individualised care, we still need evidence about the improvement of the ethical competence of professionals and the role of leaders in that improvement.

The instruments and solutions for ethical support are limited. There are, for example ([65]; see also [66]), clinical ethics consultations, ethics committees, ethics rounds, discussion groups and reflection groups. The first perspective emphasises the importance of ethics consultation, the second one the importance of clinical ethics committees. From the third point of view, professionals' experiences of everyday ethical issues are important, as are also the ethical rounds in different units. The evidence is limited, and individually tailored interventions have not even been tested. It is clear, however, that there is an increased worldwide interest in clinical ethics support.

10.3.3 Technological Support

The use of different technological solutions and devices in everyday life has increased in the last few decades. The technological development gives also healthcare environment possibilities to utilise different kinds of solutions in patient care, including individualised care, and the use of technology has become trivialised in the healthcare context. However, the use of technology in healthcare tends to focus on computer programs and surgical devices used by health professionals, while less attention is given to technological support in individualised patient care used by the patients.

The care of surgical patients may be divided to preoperative, intraoperative and postoperative phases [67]. The literature proposes technological solutions for the preoperative [68, 69] and postoperative phases [70], which may not only ease the patient's care process but also provide possibilities for individualised solutions. These solutions aim to gather, transfer and exchange information [67].

In the preoperative phase, patients' information is usually gathered face-to-face with health professionals. In an alternative solution, patients give information about themselves preoperatively by using technological devices [67], for example, a computer or a tablet. By this, patients are not only able to give information about themselves wherever they want to but also whenever they want to. Thus, patients may provide the information at the time that is most suitable for them. Technological support may also be used in giving information to the patients. In the literature, this has been studied by using a multimedia book with tablets [68] and a preoperative instructional digital video disc [69]. Both these devices are considered applicable in information giving and well received by the patients [68, 69]. By these solutions, patients are able to gather the information when most convenient for them and on repeated occasions, if they wish. However, these solutions provide information selected by the developers of the programmes. In individual preoperative care, patients should also be given the possibility to ask questions and discuss their personal issues.

Patients' knowledge may be supported by technological devices also in the postoperative phase. As in preoperative nursing care, the device may be used in gathering information from the patient and providing information to the patient [67]. The information from the patient may be gathered, for example, in the form of text messages by mobile phone [70]. By gathering postoperative information in real time, the quality of care may be enhanced and the effectiveness of care ensured, thanks to earlier detection of symptoms. In providing tailored information to the patient, the information may consider issues such as side effects and the recovery process. In addition, information may be provided about different kind of services available based on the patient's location, as well as when and who to contact if needed [67]. The technological solutions provide a useful tool in individualised care, especially in ambulatory surgery where the postoperative care time in hospital is minimal.

Less attention has been given to the technological support in the intraoperative phase. As many of the operations are conducted while the patient is asleep, it is fairly obvious that the technological aspect focuses on the devices used by the health professionals. However, there are a number of patients whose operation is done under local anaesthesia. Thus, depending on the selected anaesthesia, there is room for technological innovations that are used by the patients in intraoperative care.

In implementing technological support for the individualisation of surgical nursing care, certain aspects should be taken into consideration. Especially among the ageing population, individuals may not be familiar with the use of devices. In addition, disabilities, e.g. those affecting the senses, may limit the use of technology or at least set some additional requirements to the devices. Despite the high technological orientation of the modern society, there are relatively few studies of the technological support in the surgical field used by the patients. However, this area provides an environment to innovate and implement various technological solutions for individualising nursing care.

Conclusion

Surgical nursing care will increase in the future due to the development of anaesthesia and operative techniques, the growing needs of an older population, especially in orthopaedics, and development of new biomaterials. The patient is always in need of multidimensional knowledge and understanding of the procedures, as well as individual pain management. The quality of surgical nursing care cannot be high without individually tailored solutions. This individual tailoring also means a deep respect for patients as human beings requiring ethical and educational support. The technological changes are substantial and come at high speed, but they are always secondary to the realisation of the value of human beings in surgical nursing care. Research in the field of individualisation calls for a combination of complex interventions, using tested instruments, and a deep narrative approach. In addition to researchers as well as biobanks, registers of surgical patients could be an important data source.

References

1. Eurostat. In-patient average length of stay (days). 2017. http://appsso.eurostat.ec.europa.eu/nui/show.do?dataset=hlth_co_inpst&lang=en. Accessed 15 Jan 2018.
2. Klemetti S, Leino-Kilpi H, Cabrera E, et al. Difference between received and expected knowledge of patients undergoing knee or hip replacement in seven European countries. Clin Nurs Res. 2015;24(6):624–43.
3. Renholm M, Suominen T, Turtiainen A-M, et al. Continuity of care in day surgical care - perspective of patients. Scand J Caring Sci. 2014;28(4):706–15.
4. Hunter B, Segrott J. Re-mapping client journeys and professional identities: a review of the literature on clinical pathways. Int J Nurs Stud. 2007;45(4):608–25.
5. Rogers W, Degeling C, Townley C. Equity under the knife: justice and evidence in surgery. Bioethics. 2014;28(1):119–26.
6. Wigens L. The conflict between 'new nursing' and 'scientific management' as perceived by surgical nurses. J Adv Nurs. 1997;25(6):1116–22.
7. Koivunen M, Niemi A, Hupli M. The use of electronic devices for communication with colleagues and other healthcare professionals – nursing professionals' perspectives. J Adv Nurs. 2015;71(3):620–31.
8. Heikkinen K, Leino-Kilpi H, Vahlberg T, et al. Ambulatory orthopaedic surgery patients' symptoms with two different patient education methods. Int J Orthop Trauma Nurs. 2012;16(1):13–20.
9. Eriksson K, Wikström L, Fridlund B, et al. Patients' experiences and actions when describing pain after surgery – a critical incident technique analysis. Int J Nurs Stud. 2016;56(1):27–36.
10. Suhonen R, Leino-Kilpi H, Välimäki M. Development and psychometric properties of the Individualized Care Scale. J Eval Clin Pract. 2005;11(1):7–20.
11. Suhonen R, Gustafsson ML, Katajisto J, et al. Individualized care scale - nurse version: a Finnish validation study. J Eval Clin Pract. 2010;16(1):145–54.
12. Petroz U, Kennedy D, Webster F, et al. Patients' perceptions of individualized care: evaluating psychometric properties and results of the individualized care scale. Can J Nurs Res. 2011;43(1):80–100.
13. Berg A, Suhonen R, Idvall E. A survey of orthopaedic patients' assessment of care using the Individualised Care Scale. J Orthop Nurs. 2007;11(2):185–93.
14. Tekin F, Findik UY. Level of perception of individualized care and satisfaction with nursing in orthopaedic surgery patients. Orthop Nurs. 2015;34(6):371–4.

15. Ceylan B, Eser I. Assessment of individualized nursing care in hospitalized patients in a university hospital in Turkey. J Nurs Manag. 2016;24(7):954–61.
16. Land L, Suhonen R. Orthopaedic and trauma patients' perceptions of individualized care. Int Nurs Rev. 2009;56(1):131–7.
17. Suhonen R, Berg A, Idvall E, et al. Individualised care from the orthopaedic and trauma patients' perspective: an international comparative survey. Int J Nurs Stud. 2008;45(11):1586–97.
18. Suhonen R, Land L, Välimäki M, et al. Impact of patient characteristics on orthopaedic and trauma patients' perceptions of individualised nursing care. Int J Evid Based Healthc. 2010;8(4):259–67.
19. Acaroglu R, Suhonen R, Sendir M, et al. Reliability and validity of Turkish version of the Individualised Care Scale. J Clin Nurs. 2011;20(1):136–45.
20. Suhonen R, Efstathiou G, Tsangari H, et al. Patients' and nurses' perceptions of individualised care: an international comparative study. J Clin Nurs. 2012;21(7-8):1155–567.
21. Suhonen R, Papastavrou E, Efstathiou G, et al. Patient satisfaction as an outcome of individualised nursing care. Scand J Caring Sci. 2012;26(2):372–80.
22. Suhonen R, Tsangari H, Leino-Kilpi H et al. Individualised care—comparison of patients' and nurses' assessments. Hoitotiede. 2013;25(2):80–91 (Article in Finnish, including English abstract).
23. Suhonen R, Välimäki M, Leino-Kilpi H. Individualized care, quality of life and satisfaction with nursing care. J Adv Nurs. 2005;50(3):283–92.
24. Suhonen R, Välimäki M, Leino-Kilpi H, et al. Testing the individualized care model. Scand J Caring Sci. 2004;18(1):27–36.
25. Idvall E, Berg A, Katajisto J, et al. Nurses' sociodemographic background and assessments of individualized care. J Nurs Scholarsh. 2012;44(3):284–93.
26. Papastavrou E, Acaroglu R, Sendir M, et al. The relationship between individualized care and the practice environment: an international study. Int J Nurs Stud. 2015;52(1):121–33.
27. Suhonen R, Papastavrou E, Efstathiou G, et al. Nurses' perceptions of individualized care: an international comparison. J Adv Nurs. 2011;67(9):1895–907.
28. Vaartio-Rajalin H, Huumonen T, Iire L, et al. Development of an inter-professional screening instrument for cancer patients' education process. Appl Nurs Res. 2016;29:248–53.
29. Vaartio-Rajalin H, Huumonen T, Iire L, et al. Patient education process in oncologic context: what, why, and by whom? Nurs Res. 2015;64(5):381–90.
30. Mavridou P, Manataki A, Arnaoutoglou E, et al. Survey of patients' preoperative need for information about postoperative pain-effect of previous surgery experience. J Perianesth Nurs. 2017;32(5):438–44.
31. Klemetti S, Leino-Kilpi H, Charalambous A, et al. Information and control preferences and their relationship with the knowledge received among European joint arthroplasty patients. Orthop Nurs. 2016;35(3):174–82.
32. Ingadottir B, Johansson Stark A, Leino-Kilpi H, et al. The fulfilment of knowledge expectations during the perioperative period of patients undergoing knee arthroplasty—a Nordic perspective. J Clin Nurs. 2014;23(19-20):2896–908.
33. Leino-Kilpi H, Gröndahl W, Pekonen A, et al. Knowledge received by hospital patients—a factor connected with the patient-centred quality of nursing care. Int J Nurs Pract. 2015;21(6):689–98.
34. Tian C, Champlin S, Mackert M, et al. Readability, suitability, and health content assessment of web-based patient education materials on colorectal cancer screening. Gastrointest Endosc. 2014;80(2):284–90.
35. Kesänen J, Leino-Kilpi H, Arifulla D, et al. Knowledge tests in patient education: a systematic review. Nurs Health Sci. 2014;16(2):262–73.
36. Siekkinen M, Leino-Kilpi H. Developing a patient education method - the e-Knowledge Test with feedback. Stud Health Technol Inform. 2012;180:1096–8.
37. Virtanen H, Leino-Kilpi H, Salanterä S. Empowering discourse in patient education. Patient Educ Couns. 2007;66(2):140–6.

38. Eloranta S, Katajisto J, Leino-Kilpi H. Does the empowerment patient education realize from the perspective of the nurses? Hoitotiede. 2014;26(1):63–73.

39. Johansson K, Nuutila L, Virtanen H, et al. Preoperative education for orthopaedic patients: systematic review. J Adv Nurs. 2005;50(2):212–23.

40. Kesänen J, Leino-Kilpi H, Lund T, et al. Increased preoperative knowledge reduces surgery-related anxiety: a randomised clinical trial in 100 spinal stenosis patients. Eur Spine J. 2017;26(10):2520–8.

41. Ryhänen AM, Rankinen S, Siekkinen M, et al. The impact of an empowering Internet-based Breast Cancer Patient Pathway programme on breast cancer patients' knowledge: a randomised control trial. Patient Educ Couns. 2012;88(2):224–31.

42. Siekkinen M, Pyrhönen S, Ryhänen A, et al. Psychosocial outcomes of e-feedback of radiotherapy for breast cancer patients: a randomized controlled trial. Psycho-Oncology. 2015;24(5):515–22.

43. Salonen A, Ryhänen A, Leino-Kilpi H. Educational benefits of Internet and computer-based programmes for prostate cancer patients: a systematic review. Patient Educ Couns. 2014;94(1):10–9.

44. Cassidy J, Baker J. Orthopaedic patient information on the World Wide Web: an essential review. J Bone Joint Surg Am. 2016;98(4):325–38.

45. Montini T, Noble AA, Stelfox HT. Content analysis of patient complaints. Int J Qual Health Care. 2008;20(6):412–20.

46. UN. United Nations: Universal Declaration of Human Rights. 1948. http://www.un.org/en/universal-declaration-human-rights/. Accessed 10 Jan 2018.

47. International Confederation of Midwives (ICM). International code of ethics for midwives. 2014. http://internationalmidwives.org/who-we-are/policy-and-practice/code-of-ethics-philosophy-model-midwifery-care/. Accessed 6 Oct 2017.

48. International Council of Nurses (ICN). The ICN code of ethics for nurses. 2012. http://www.icn.ch/who-we-are/code-of-ethics-for-nurses/. Accessed 6 Oct 2017.

49. BJC HealthCare. Patient rights and responsibilities. https://www.bjc.org/For-Patients-Visitors/Patient-Rights-Responsibilities. Accessed 15 Jan 2018.

50. Højgaard L, Löwenberg B, Selby P, et al. The European Cancer Patient's Bill of Rights, update and implementation 2016. ESMO Open. 2016;1(6):e000127. https://doi.org/10.1136/esmoopen-2016-000127.

51. Välimäki M, Leino-Kilpi H, Grönroos M, et al. Self-determination in surgical patients in five European countries. J Nurs Scholarsh. 2004;36(4):305–11.

52. Suhonen R, Välimäki M, Dassen T, et al. Patients' autonomy in surgical care: a comparison of nurses' perceptions in five European countries. Int Nurs Rev. 2003;50(1):85–94.

53. Scott PA, Taylor A, Välimäki M, et al. Autonomy, privacy and informed consent 4: surgical perspective. Br J Nurs. 2003;12(5):311–20.

54. Iltanen S, Leino-Kilpi H, Puukka P, et al. Knowledge about patients' rights among professionals in public health care in Finland. Scand J Caring Sci. 2012;26(3):436–48.

55. Kulju K, Stolt M, Suhonen R, et al. Ethical competence: a concept analysis. Nurs Ethics. 2016;23(4):401–12.

56. Numminen O, Repo H, Leino-Kilpi H. Moral courage in nursing: a concept analysis. Nurs Ethics. 2017;24(8):878–91.

57. Lindh I, da Silva B, Berg A, et al. Courage and nursing practice: a theoretical analysis. Nurs Ethics. 2010;17(5):551–65.

58. Poikkeus T, Leino-Kilpi H, Katajisto J. Supporting ethical competence of nurses during recruitment and performance reviews - the role of the nurse leader. J Nurs Manag. 2014;22(6):792–802.

59. Poikkeus T, Numminen O, Suhonen R, et al. A mixed-method systematic review: support for ethical competence of nurses. J Adv Nurs. 2014;70(2):256–71.

60. Poikkeus T, Suhonen R, Katajisto J, et al. Organisational and individual support for nurses' ethical competence: a cross-sectional survey. Nurs Ethics. 2016. https://doi.org/10.1177/0969733016642627.

61. Laukkanen L, Leino-Kilpi H, Suhonen R. Ethical activity profile of nurse managers. J Nurs Manag. 2016;24(4):483–91.
62. Aitamaa E, Leino-Kilpi H, Iltanen S, et al. Ethical problems in nursing management: the views of nurse managers. Nurs Ethics. 2016;23(6):646–58.
63. Laukkanen L, Suhonen R, Leino-Kilpi H. Solving work-related ethical problems. Nurs Ethics. 2016;23(8):838–50.
64. Aitamaa E, Leino-Kilpi H, Puukka P, et al. Ethical problems in nursing management: the role of codes of ethics. Nurs Ethics. 2010;17(4):469–82.
65. Rasoal D, Skovdahl K, Gifford M, et al. Clinical ethics support for healthcare personnel: an integrative literature review. HEC Forum. 2017;29(4):313–46.
66. Stolt M, Leino-Kilpi H, Ruokonen M, et al. Ethics interventions for healthcare professionals and students: a systematic review. Nurs Ethics. 2018;25(2):133–52.
67. Waller A, Forshaw K, Carey M, et al. Optimizing patient preparation and surgical experience using eHealth technology. JMIR Med Inform. 2015;3(3):e29. https://doi.org/10.2196/medinform.4286.
68. Briggs M, Wilkinson C, Golash A. Digital multimedia books produced using iBooks Author for pre-operative surgical patient information. J Vis Commun Med. 2014;37(1):59–64.
69. Ong J, Miller PS, Appleby R, et al. Effect of a preoperative instructional digital video disc on patient knowledge and preparedness for engaging in postoperative care activities. Nurs Clin North Am. 2009;44(1):103–15.
70. Stomberg MW, Platon B, Widén A, et al. Health information: what can mobile phone assessments add? Perspect Health Inf Manag. 2012;9(1):1–10.

Individualised Nursing Care in Older People Care

Beatriz Rodríguez-Martín

Abstract

Individualised care improves the health outcomes of the older patient, particularly their functional ability, and is an essential component of ensuring high-quality care for older people. However, certain problems have been described regarding providing individualised care in facilities for older people. The aims of this chapter are to synthesise and analyse current evidence regarding the delivery of individualised care in care facilities for older people. We undertook a review of studies published in English analysing the delivery of individualised care in facilities for older people. Nurses reported that they largely supported the individualisation of care and considered the older people's clinical situation and their decisional control during their professional practice. The factors associated with the nursing staff's ability to provide individualised care were the following: the access to structural empowerment, the increased age of nurses, the care environment, nurses' work satisfaction, a greater work experience and the implementation of the Facility Specific Social Models of Care. The main barriers were the lack of knowledge and training opportunities, along with rewards and recognition for a job well done. These findings provide key information for the design of plans and programmes dedicated to improving the quality of care in care settings for older people.

Keywords

Aged · Individualised care · Long-term care · Nursing care

B. Rodríguez-Martín
University of Castilla-La Mancha, Faculty of Occupational Therapy, Logopedia and Nursing, Talavera de la Reina, Toledo, Spain
e-mail: Beatriz.RMartin@uclm.es

© Springer International Publishing AG, part of Springer Nature 2019
R. Suhonen et al. (eds.), *Individualized Care*,
https://doi.org/10.1007/978-3-319-89899-5_11

11.1   Introduction

The growing global population currently represents one of the greatest health challenges [1, 2]. The direct effects of this include an increasing prevalence of multi-morbidity and a greater demand for long-term care (LTC) services for older people [3]. Long-term care comprises assisted living, skilled nursing homes, sheltered housing and other residential institutions [4]. In these facilities, the direct care of patients is provided by nursing staff, such as registered nurses (RNs) with 2 to 5 years postsecondary educational training; licenced practical nurses (LPNs) with 1 year of nursing education and who provide basis care; and care aides, who are unlicenced health staff working under the supervision of LPNs or RNs [5].

The number of older people worldwide living in LTC facilities is growing. Factors such as the increased prevalence of chronic diseases and disabilities and changes in both family structure and social dynamics encourage this phenomenon [6]. It is well known that older people living in LTC facilities have a high degree of fragility and dependence [7]. In this regard, previous studies have reported that residents have a lower quality of life and poorer health outcomes than community-dwelling older people [8, 9]. Conversely, older people are not a homogenous group and usually require complex care.

The increase in the number of older people living in LTC facilities and the changes in their needs and demands suggest the need to review the policies with regard to LTC care [10]. The organisational culture involves norms, values, assumptions, behaviours and attitudes [11] adopted at healthcare settings which can affect interpersonal relationships between staff and their patients, as well as the delivery and outcome of care [12, 13]. Accordingly, ethically complicated situations appear when there is no congruence between the individual needs of patients and the organisational culture [14, 15].

A historical review on this subject shows that the dominant institutional model of the care provided at aged care facilities has followed the biomedical model, based on hierarchical decision-making, care provider routines, a disease-oriented focus and the principles of consistency and efficiency [16–18]. In recent years, we have seen a profound culture change in LTC facilities for older people, where institutions are more concerned about the quality of care and the residents' quality of life rather than curing diseases [18, 19]. This movement towards more social models of care has promoted the implementation of different management initiatives, grouped together under the term culture change models (CCMs), Green House Program, the Eden Alternative, Gentle Care, Facility Specific Social Models of Care (FSSMOC), Person-Centred Care, Pioneer Network, Wellspring etc., all of which are aimed at improving individualised care provision [20]. Different terms have been used to express the same concept underlying the new care approach: consumer-directed care, individualised care, person-centred care, self-directed care, resident-centred care, etc. [18]. The principles of CCMs are a person-centred philosophy, the promotion of 'home-like' care environments, the consideration that the 'resident comes first' and the individualisation of care [4].

Within the new paradigm in the care of older people, person-centred care (PCC) was the initial approach to move forward in the provision of individualised care in LTC. The person-centred philosophy of care has been considered a core concept and a standard of practice in LTC and has been widely studied and included in many national care policies [16]. Although focusing on the older person as a whole person is a key element of the PCC approach [21, 22], a wide range of interventions and models of PCC exist [4]. Currently, there are 12 tools that measure person-centred care in older people, including eight tools specifically aimed at nursing homes [22]. Despite the above, more tools have been used in research rather than in practice [22], and PCC is still considered to be a philosophy, rather than a practical approach.

Individualised care is a very important part of nursing practice and is closely connected to the rights of individuals as human beings [23]. This approach considers the following factors: the patient's personal characteristics, clinical condition and personal life circumstances and preferences [13, 24, 25]. Thus, care is based on the specific needs of each individual patient, ensuring that they are treated as an autonomous adult [26, 27]. Moreover, this approach promotes the inclusion of older people and their relatives in the planning of care [20] and encourages professionals to understand situations from the patient's perspective [27].

Individualised care has been widely promoted in nursing care and has been studied from both the nurses' and patients' point of view [28]. Moreover, this concept is judged to be important by patients and nurses in both acute care and LTC [13]. Several studies have clearly shown the benefits of delivering individualised care to improve patient outcomes, their quality of live, autonomy and satisfaction with the care delivered [13, 29]. On the other hand, individualised care can avoid mistakes and improve nurses' work satisfaction and motivation [28, 30, 31].

In the case of the care of older people, it is known that individualised care ensures the well-being of both institutionalised and community-dwelling older people [20]. In aged care facilities, the individualised care approach helps to consider the older person's unique needs and preferences with the goal of guiding caregivers, safe-guarding the older person's identity and relationship and promoting their decision-making and participation in care [20, 32]. Moreover, individualised care is a reflection of older people's individuality, promoting the decision-making about their care process, with the potential to improve residents' quality of life and help-ing to offset their impairments [18, 33, 34]. In addition, individualised care has important benefits for institutionalised older people, such as reducing stress and anxiety, maintaining the person's independence during daily life activities, increas-ing physical activity, decreasing the use of physical restraints and improving staff and family satisfaction, all of which is cost-effective [20]. There is also evidence concerning the benefits of this concept for frail elders [20, 35].

On the other hand, we know that there are differences in patients' and nurses' perceptions about quality of care and good nursing care [36, 37]. Moreover, the needs and demands of older people regarding their care have changed in recent years. Previous studies have shown that older people wish to exercise their control over where they live and the care they receive [16]. Moreover, they consider it important to maintain their autonomy and make their own decisions regarding their care [3].

Although the principles of individualised care are broadly accepted, this concept is not yet part of care plans or implemented in daily practice at older people care facilities [38, 39]. Moreover, although previous studies mention certain barriers for considering the individuality of residents and the ability to provide individualised care in LTC [39], few studies have analysed the factors associated with the provision of individualised care in facilities for older people and the differences in the provision of the same depending on the type of facility. The aims of this chapter are to synthesise and to analyse current evidence regarding the delivery of individualised care in care facilities for older people.

11.2 Studies on Individualised Care in Older People

A narrative review of studies, published in English or Spanish until April 2017, analysed the individualised care provided at care facilities for older people, was carried out in the following databases: Cochrane Plus, PubMed (MEDLINE), Scopus, Web of Science (WoS), CINAHL, Cuiden, ProQuest and PsycINFO. Moreover, the reference lists of all studies found were checked in a secondary search of relevant articles.

The search procedure was based on a combination of the following keywords, depending on the different databases used: individuality, individualised care, nursing science, nursing practice, person-centeredness, person-centred, person-centred resident-centred care, resident-centred care, nursing care, older people, long-term care, nursing homes and residential age-care facilities. During the study selection, the following inclusion and exclusion criteria were used. Inclusion criteria were (1) qualitative studies analysing individualised care in facilities for older people, (2) studies using validated instruments, (3) studies whose target population were older people, (4) studies in which individualised care was provided by nursing staff (ward/nurse manager, registered nurse, licenced practical nurse or care aid), (5) studies published in English or Spanish and (6) studies conducted in any field of older people care. The exclusion criteria were (1) studies in which the intervention was aimed at family members and (2) studies aimed at the development of an assessment instrument.

The methodological quality of the included studies was appraised using the NIH Quality Assessment Tool for Observational Cohort and Cross-Sectional Studies [40]. Seven studies met the inclusion criteria and were reviewed. All were cross-sectional studies [5, 33, 41, 42]. Four studies were conducted in Finland [23, 41–43] and three studies in Canada [5, 33, 34]. The study samples included nursing staff (RN, LPNs and care aides), and the sample size ranged from 96 to 1513 participants. The total sample included in this review was 3790 participants. None of the studies analysed ward/nurse manager's perceptions.

Regarding the settings, the studies included different types of LTC facilities for older people: institutional care (sheltered housing and nursing homes) [5, 23, 33, 34, 43], home healthcare [23], inpatient wards of the municipal health centre hospitals [23, 41–43] and inpatient wards of specialised acute medical care hospitals [43].

The main instruments used for data collection were the following: Conditions of Work Effectiveness Questionnaire (CWEQ) [5, 33, 34], the Job Activities Scale (JAS) [5, 33, 34], the Organizational Relationship Scale (ORS) [5, 33, 34], the Individualised Care Instrument (ICI) [5, 23, 33, 34], the Individualised Care Scale-Nurse (ICS-Nurse) [23, 41–43] and the Index of Work Satisfaction (IWS) [23]. Moreover, the studies gathered participants' demographic variables and organisational variables.

All studies were aimed at exploring the relationships between individualised care provision and the outcomes measured by the abovementioned data collection instruments. In general, nurses working at older people care facilities largely supported the individualisation of care and took into account the older people's clinical situation and their decisional control during their professional practice. However, the ability to consider the residents' personal life situation received the lowest scores [23, 41–43]. One of the studies analysed individualised care provision in facilities that had implemented different types of culture change models (CCMs), concluding that the type of CCMs implemented at each facility affects LPNs' and care aides' access to empowerment and their ability to provide individualised care, although this was not the case with RNs [33].

Access to structural empowerment [5, 33, 34], the increase in the age of nurses [41, 43], the care environment (type of organisation) [23, 42, 43], nurses' work satisfaction [23] and greater work experience [41] all had a positive association with the ability of RNs, LPNS and care aides to provide individualised care in facilities for older people. Moreover, the implementation of a culture change model (CCM) and, in particular, the Facility Specific Social Models of Care (FSSMC) improves the staff's ability to provide individualised care and access to structural empowerment [34]. The main barriers for the implementation of individualised care related to empowerment structures perceived by participant caregivers were the lack of knowledge and training opportunities and providing rewards and recognition for a job well done [33].

Regarding the management strategies for improving individualised care provision in LTC, the result of the studies analysed noted that supervisors should ensure they can motivate and empower staff by actively respecting, valuing and utilising staff's knowledge and skills. This is especially important in the case of front-line care staff (care aides) [33]. Moreover, it is necessary to improve interpersonal staff relationships [5].

11.3   Strategies to Improve Individualised Care in Care Facilities for Older People

This chapter synthesises the current studies analysing factors associated with the provision of individualised care at long-term care facilities for older people. The factors associated with the nursing staff's ability to provide individualised care at LTC facilities for older people are the access to structural empowerment [5, 33, 34], the increased age of nurses [41, 43], the care environment (type of organisation)

[23, 42, 43], nurses' work satisfaction [23], greater work experience [41] and the implementation of the Facility Specific Social Models of Care (FSSMC) [34]. Only a few studies are aimed at analysing factors associated with the provision of individualised care in facilities for older people, and none of these analyse the point of view of older people or their relatives. In this sense, the research findings highlight the need for analysing both patients' and nurses' perceptions regarding individualised care in LTC facilities for older people [41].

Previous studies show that nurses working in LTC (inpatient wards) have the lowest perceptions concerning their ability to provide individualised care [13]. In contrast to this idea, according to other studies conducted in acute care settings [13, 28], the findings of this review show that, in general, nursing staff at LTC facilities for older people perceive that they are able to support patient individuality in their professional practice [23, 41–43]. Regarding the type of facility, the results show that nurses' perceptions about their ability to provide individualised care are higher in nurses working in acute care settings than in nurses working in primary health centre hospitals or in nursing homes [23, 43]. This finding contradicts earlier studies reporting a positive association between knowing patients well and improvements in individualised care provision [13, 44]. This may be because the dependency level is higher in institutionalised older people or due to other factors, such as the organisational culture of care, the working environment or the role of leaders and managers, or staffing levels, all of which need to be examined in more depth in future studies [23, 43].

The role of the patient has changed in healthcare and in long-term care. In this sense, respecting the person's right to self-determination and their active participation in decision-making are several effects of this shift [45]. Although the importance of knowing the previous life history of older people in order to understand their current situation and help to maintain their autonomy and independence has been underlined in several studies [20, 33, 41], the findings of this review show that older people's personal life situations are not always taken into account in the care provided at LTC facilities. As certain studies have noted, one possible solution could be to promote the active participation of older people and their relatives in the care provided [26, 41, 46].

Individualised care is considered a key principle in the nursing care of older people [47]. This chapter confirms that individualised care is perceived as a high-quality approach in nursing care and particularly in the care of older people. In line with previous studies aimed at achieving a culture change in LTC [48, 49], the results of the studies analysed show that the implementation of an individualised care approach requires improving staff training and skills, considering that older people are at the centre of care, promoting resident autonomy and the inclusion of residents and their relatives in care planning (e.g. [5, 41]). Moreover, this chapter provides additional factors affecting individualised care provision in LTC facilities for older people, such as staff's empowerment structures and their job recognition.

As reported by previous studies aimed at person-centred care, the context where care is provided can be a barrier or facilitator for individualised care practice [45,

50, 51]. In this sense, we know that when the quality of the caregivers' care environment improves, staff is more open to improve residents' quality of life [52]. Therefore, managers have an important role for the implementation of individualised care [33, 34]. Moreover, the type of culture change model implemented at each facility can affect LPNs' and care aides' access to empowerment and their ability to provide individualised care, although not in the case of RNs [34]. This may be because LPNs and care aides spend more time with the resident and provide basic care.

As earlier studies have noted, the organisational culture at each institution can affect the outcomes and delivery of individualised care [12, 13]. Moreover, the lack of congruence between the organisational culture and individual patients' needs can cause ethically difficult situations [13, 15]. In line with previous research, the findings of this review show that changes in environmental care are needed to achieve individualised care. Future research should analyse the role of nurse leaders and managers in the development of individualised care in settings for older people [5, 42].

The need to improve staff's training and knowledge has been discussed in previous research [4]. In support of this, the main barrier to the implementation of individualised care perceived by care aides of included studies was the lack of knowledge and training in alternative approaches [33].

As other studies have noted, the implementation of individualised care in long-term care facilities requires an important cultural and institutional change that leaves behind physical task-oriented care and the biomedical approach, focusing more on promoting older people's independence, autonomy and quality of life [4, 20]. Furthermore, the culture change should include institutional policies and philosophy of care, the care environment and staff training [20].

All studies included in this chapter followed a cross-sectional design. Therefore, it is not possible to make causal conclusions. Furthermore, it is important to consider the gender effects of the sample included in the analysed studies (less than 8% of total sample was male). This may be because women are the main LTC force. Additionally, none of studies analysed this phenomena in nurse managers. Thus, future studies should consider these issues. Finally, all included studies analysed individualised care from the professionals' point of view; therefore, future studies should explore the perceptions of older people and family members.

Conclusions

There are few studies aimed at analysing factors associated with individualised care provision in LTC facilities for older people. Although none of these are strong enough for empirical evidence, the findings of this review may help to improve the care of older people. Nursing staff at long-term care facilities for older people consider that they provide individualised care. The factors associated with the nursing staff's ability to provide individualised care are the access to structural empowerment, the increased age of nurses, the type of organisation, nurses work satisfaction, a greater work experience and the implementation of the Facility Specific Social Models of Care (FSSMC).

References

1. Francesca C, Ana LN, Jérôme M et al. OECD health policy studies help wanted? Providing and paying for long-term care: providing and paying for long-term care. OECD; 2011.
2. World Health Organization. World report on ageing and health. Geneva: World Health Organization; 2015.
3. Wilberforce M, Challis D, Davies L, et al. Person-centredness in the care of older adults: a systematic review of questionnaire-based scales and their measurement properties. BMC Geriatr. 2016;16(1):63.
4. Li J, Porock D. Resident outcomes of person-centered care in long-term care: a narrative review of interventional research. Int J Nurs Stud. 2014;51(10):1395–415.
5. Caspar S, Cooke HA, O'Rourke N, et al. Influence of individual and contextual characteristics on the provision of individualized care in long-term care facilities. Gerontologist. 2013;53(5):790–800.
6. Saltman R, Dubois H, Chawla M. The impact of aging on long-term care in Europe and some potential policy responses. Int J Health Serv. 2006;36(4):719–46.
7. Hutchinson A, Rawson H, O'Connell B, et al. Tri-focal model of care implementation: perspectives of residents and family. J Nurs Scholarsh. 2017;49(1):33–43.
8. Hill N, Kolanowski A, Milone-Nuzzo P, et al. Culture change models and resident health outcomes in long-term care. J Nurs Scholarsh. 2011;43(1):30–40.
9. Karakaya M, Bilgin S, Ekici G, et al. Functional mobility, depressive symptoms, level of independence, and quality of life of the elderly living at home and in the nursing home. J Am Med Dir Assoc. 2009;10(9):662–6.
10. Powell JS. The power of global ageing. Ageing Int. 2010;35(1):1–14.
11. Seren S, Baykal U. Relationships between change and organizational culture in hospitals. J Nurs Scholarsh. 2007;39(2):191–7.
12. Hall L, Doran D. Nurse staffing, care delivery model, and patient care quality. J Nurs Care Qual. 2004;19(1):27–33.
13. Suhonen R, Gustafsson M, Katajisto J, et al. Nurses' perceptions of individualized care. J Adv Nurs. 2010;66(5):1035–46.
14. Hart S. Hospital ethical climates and registered nurses' turnover intentions. J Nurs Scholarsh. 2005;37(2):173–7.
15. Wlody G. Nursing management and organizational ethics in the intensive care unit. Crit Care Med. 2007;35(2):S29–35.
16. Brownie S, Nancarrow S. Effects of person-centered care on residents and staff in aged-care facilities: a systematic review. Clin Interv Aging. 2013;8(1):1–10.
17. Rosher R, Robinson S. Impact of the Eden Alternative on family satisfaction. J Am Med Dir Assoc. 2005;6(3):189–93.
18. Sawamura K, Nakashima T, Nakanishi M. Provision of individualized care and built environment of nursing homes in Japan. Arch Gerontol Geriatr. 2013;56(3):416–24.
19. Verbeek H, van Rossum E, Zwakhalen S, et al. Small, homelike care environments for older people with dementia: a literature review. Int Psychogeriatr. 2009;21(2):252–64.
20. Happ M, Williams C, Strumpf N, et al. Individualized care for frail elders: theory and practice. J Gerontol Nurs. 1996;22(3):6–9.
21. Koren M. Person-centered care for nursing home residents: the culture-change movement. Health Aff. 2010;29(2):312–7.
22. Van Haitsma KK, Crespy SS, Humes SS, et al. New toolkit to measure quality of person-centered care: development and pilot evaluation with nursing home communities. J Am Med Dir Assoc. 2014;15(9):671–80.
23. Suhonen R, Charalambous A, Stolt M, et al. Caregivers' work satisfaction and individualised care in care settings for older people. J Clin Nurs. 2013;22(3-4):479–90.
24. Suhonen R, Välimäki M, Katajisto J. Developing and testing an instrument for measurement of individual care. J Adv Nurs. 2000;32(5):1253–63.

25. Suhonen R, Leino-Kilpi H, Välimäki M. Development and psychometric properties of the Individualized Care Scale. J Eval Clin Pract. 2005;11(1):7–20.
26. Chappell L, Colin Reid R, Gish J, et al. Staff-based measures of individualized care for persons with dementia in long-term care facilities. Dementia. 2007;5(4):5227–547.
27. Walker L, Porter M, Grumen C, et al. Developing individualized care in nursing homes: integrating the views of nurses and certified nurse aides. J Gerontol Nurs. 1999;25(3):30–5.
28. Suhonen R, Efstathiou G, Tsangari H, et al. Patients' and nurses' perceptions of individualised care: an international comparative study. J Clin Nurs. 2012;21(7-8):1155–67.
29. Suhonen R, Välimäki M, Leino-Kilpi H. A review of outcomes of individualised nursing interventions on adult patients. J Clin Nurs. 2008;17(12):843–60.
30. Lake E, Friese C. Variations in nursing practice environments: relation to staffing and hospital characteristics. Nurs Res. 2006;55(1):1–9.
31. Suhonen R, Papastavrou E, Efstathiou G, et al. Nurse's perceptions of individualized care: an international comparison. J Adv Nurs. 2011a;67(9):1895–907.
32. Kruijshaar ME, Essink-Bot M-L, Donkers B, et al. A labelled discrete choice experiment adds realism to the choices presented: preferences for surveillance tests for Barrett esophagus. BMC Med Res Methodol. 2009;9:31.
33. Caspar S, O'Rourke N. The influence of care provider access to structural empowerment on individualized care in long-term-care facilities. J Gerontol B Psychol Sci Soc Sci. 2008;63(4):S255–65.
34. Caspar S, O'Rourke N, Gutman GM, et al. The differential influence of culture change models on long-term care staff empowerment and provision of individualized care. Can J Aging. 2009;28(2):165–75.
35. Happ M. Individualized care for frail older adults: challenges for health care reform in acute and critical care. Geriatr Nurs. 2010;31(1):63–5.
36. Rodríguez-Martín B, Martínez-Andrés M, Cervera-Monteagudo B, et al. Perception of quality of care among residents of public nursing-homes in Spain: a grounded theory study. BMC Geriatr. 2013;13:65.
37. Zhao S, Akkadechanunt T, Xue X. Quality nursing care as perceived by nurses and patients in a Chinese hospital. J Clin Nurs. 2009;18(12):1722–8.
38. Rahman A, Schnelle J. The nursing home culture-change movement: recent past, present, and future directions for research. Gerontologist. 2008;48(2):142–8.
39. Wilson D, Neville S. Nursing their way not our way: working with vulnerable and marginalised populations. Contemp Nurse. 2008;27(2):165–76.
40. NHLBI. Quality assessment tool for observational cohort and cross-sectional studies. 2018. Available vía NHLBI https://www.nhlbi.nih.gov/health-pro/guidelines/in-develop/cardiovas-cular-risk-reduction/tools/cohort. Accessed 3 Jan 2018.
41. Suhonen R, Alikleemola P, Katajisto J, et al. Nurses' assessments of individualised care in long-term care institutions. J Clin Nurs. 2011b;21(7-8):1178–788.
42. Suhonen R, Stolt M, Puro M, et al. Individuality in older people's care - challenges for the development of nursing and nursing management. J Nurs Manag. 2011c;19(7):883–96.
43. Rodríguez-Martín B, Stolt M, Katajisto J, et al. Nurses' characteristics and organisational factors associated with their assessments of individualised care in care institutions for older people. Scand J Caring Sci. 2016;30(2):250–9.
44. Gaugler JE, Duval S, Anderson KA, et al. Predicting nursing home admission in the U.S: a meta-analysis. BMC Geriatr. 2007;19:7–13.
45. McCormack B. A conceptual framework for person-centred practice with older people. Int J Nurs Pract. 2003;9:202–9.
46. Reid RC, Chappell NL, Gish JA. Measuring family perceived involvement in individualized long-term care. Dementia. 2007;6(1):89–104.
47. International Council of Nursing. Nursing care of the older person. Genova: International Council of Nursing; 2006.
48. Boise L, White D. The family's role in person-centered care: practice considerations. J Psychosoc Nurs Ment Health Serv. 2004;42(5):1–20.

49. Gnaedinger N. Changes in long-term care for elderly people with dementia: a report from the front lines in British Columbia, Canada. J Soc Work Long Term Care. 2003;2(3-4):355–71.
50. Charalambous A, Kajajisto J, Välimäki M, et al. Individualised care and the professional practice environment: nurses' perceptions. Int Nurs Rev. 2010;57(4):500–7.
51. Suhonen R, Stolt M, Gustafsson M, et al. The associations between the ethical climate, the professional practice environment and individualised care in care settings for older people: a cross-sectional survey. J Adv Nurs. 2014;70:1356–68.
52. Tellis-Nayak V. A person-centered workplace: the foundation for person-centered caregiving in long-term care. J Am Med Dir Assoc. 2007;8(1):46–54.

Individualised Nursing Care in Cancer Care

12

Andreas Charalambous

Abstract

An ideal patient-centred care (or individualised care) environment is necessary within the cancer care context and across the cancer continuum. Persons diagnosed with and living with cancer are facing many varying challenges that can threaten their human dimensions in their totality. Cancer as a disease is typified by emotional, social, spiritual and physical challenges that can be strengthened further by complex treatments, treatment-induced toxicities and uncertain outcomes. These overall effects of cancer and its treatments can negatively influence the perceived quality of nursing care, the patient's quality of life (health status) and trust towards the healthcare professionals. The impact of cancer on the person can be significant but can never be uniformly across different persons. As each person is unique, it is expected that cancer's touch will differ in terms of how the patient is affected and to what extent. By definition this will result in triggering different needs and expectations for the persons affected by cancer. The aim of this chapter is to introduce the reader to the unique conditions induced by cancer and its treatment within the cancer context with reference to the individuality of the person. The way that individualised care can mitigate the impact of cancer on the person by placing the person at the centre of the care will be presented. Finally, the associations between concepts such as quality of oncology care and perceived quality of life with individuality will be lay down to emphasise on the complexity of cancer's impact on the person.

Keywords

Cancer context · Care · Model · Communication · Trust

A. Charalambous
Cyprus University of Technology, Limassol, Cyprus

University of Turku, Turku, Finland
e-mail: andreas.charalambous@cut.ac.cy

© Springer International Publishing AG, part of Springer Nature 2019
R. Suhonen et al. (eds.), *Individualized Care*,
https://doi.org/10.1007/978-3-319-89899-5_12

12.1   Introduction

As a patient I feel that having cancer is the most horrible experience which impacted all aspects of my life [...]. Being diagnosed and living with cancer was a life-changing experience, one I came in as one person and become another [...]. When I was hospitalized (the many times I were) I expect the nurse to be understanding and supportive in my individual and unique cancer journey.

This quotation was retrieved by a patient as part of a study to explore their perspectives along with those of patients' advocates and nurses on what constitutes quality nursing care [1]. Reflecting on this quotation, there are four distinctive words that one should pay attention to. This patient stressed the following words in her description, "individualised", "unique", "understanding" and finally "supportive". On their own, these words have limited meaning in relation to the topic of this chapter. However, if one adds the context, which in this case are cancer and the person diagnosed with and living with cancer, then the essence of the hidden meaning becomes visible. The contextual description is important in order to understand what actually being diagnosed with and living with cancer entails. Cancer is not a rare disease and has in the recent decades become a major cause of morbidity and mortality in many countries with the current statistics showing that it affects approximately one in four of the population. Future projections are more pessimistic, raising the percentage of those that will be affected by cancer to 50% [2, 3].

12.2   The "Case" of Cancer

Cancer is a disease that does not affect solely the person but more likely it affects the person's family and significant others, and here lays the reason for being called a "disease with a social dimension" [4]. The way that cancer can affect the family and the person's significant others can vary on many differing factors (e.g. these can be patient-related and family-related). For example, alongside, the nature of cancer has changed dramatically in recent years, including shorter in-patients' stays, an increasing older cancer population, the growing population of survivors and significant improvements in treatments which however become more complex and demanding (e.g. oral chemotherapy and immunotherapy). Often family and the person's significant others find themselves acquiring the role of informal caregiver [5], a role that calls them to undertake the care of their relative with little or no preparation in complex conditions such as polypharmacy, symptoms clusters and poor professional support [6, 7]. The fact that cancer is a unique disease that is typified by emotional, social, spiritual and physical challenges can have a negative effect on the person living with cancer but also making the provision of informal caregiving more complex and demanding [8]. Informal caregiving comes with a high price, when the demands placed on caregivers exceed their resources, caregivers can feel overwhelmed and experience a deterioration in their physical and psychological well-being [9].

The cancer care context can become further challenging as a result of the complexity of the treatments, the treatment-induced toxicities, the persistency of the side-effects, the likelihood of enduring physical impairment and the uncertainty of the outcomes to report a few. The person diagnosed and living with cancer is often faced with varying needs deriving either from cancer itself or its treatments that can have a depilating effect on the person's life often inflicting devastating changes to his or her view of life (e.g. social withdrawal, stigma, body image changes) and living well (e.g. weakness in performing activities of daily living).

A study by Charalambous [10] on the impact of treatment-induced toxicities on patients with head and neck cancers revealed that even non-life-threatening side effects such as xerostomia can generate severe alterations in one's life including social and psychological manifestations with a negative impact on the person's overall well-being. On this topic, a female patient stated that "I gave it up. I didn't feel and I was not willing to do anything, I didn't recognize myself anymore, this thing had left a shell of my previous self, a self that I despised [...]". Similarly another patient described the impact of living with radiotherapy-induced xerostomia as "[...] I was afraid to talk to anyone, not from a close distance at least, I was afraid of their reaction to my bad breath, they were going to be as sick of it as I was. I didn't know if I could handle this kind of rejection. It seemed better to be alone and silent and keep my dignity. Perhaps the only thing that the treatment hadn't take away from me, yet [...]". The study revealed the diverse ways that patients can experience the impact of cancer and its treatment on their lives highlighting the importance of individuality as a central aspect on the cancer care continuum.

12.3 Individuality in the Cancer Care Context

No matter how great the impact is and no matter how extensive the changes are in a person's life, the person remains unique as it was before becoming diagnosed. Cancer actually strengthens and highlights the uniqueness of the person as it identifies it as the pathway to provide comprehensive and quality care based on the patient's needs, preferences and limitations. Since the 1990s, the Institute of Medicine (IOM) in two reports, namely, *Ensuring Quality Cancer Care* [11] and *Delivering High-Quality Cancer Care: Charting a New Course for a System in Crisis* [12], has directed attention to quality issues including the provision of care that is informed by the patient's perspective and preferences. Put in simple words, whether the issue is developing a quality framework or taking a personalised clinical decision for a patient, the essence in both cases is what Balint back in the late 1960s called taking into consideration the "unique human being" [13]. This is the point where the word *unique* gains significance in relation to the above quotation.

Within the healthcare context, the uniqueness of the person becomes the point of reference for individualised care, which takes into account a person's own values, preferences and beliefs related to health in personally meaningful ways [14] and one that can have a positive impact on patient related outcomes [15–17]. Therefore, it becomes of paramount importance to acknowledge the uniqueness of the person throughout the cancer care continuum and to address it as part of a model for providing quality care within the cancer care context [18]. Let's take, for example, the conceptual framework of quality of oncology nursing care developed by Charalambous et al. [1, 18] as a means to understand the importance of individualised care in providing quality care as this is perceived by the patients, nurses and patients advocates. The authors proposed a six-dimensional framework that comprises nursing care quality: *being valued*, *being respected*, *being confirmed*, *being cared for religiously and spiritually*, *sense of belonging*, and *being cared for by communicative and supportive nurses*. Reflecting on the study's data and the factors description, individualised care plays a decisive role in how the perceptions of the patients are defined in relation to receiving care that meets their needs and expectations. All the six dimensions have an inherent aspect of patient centredness built into them. For example, the dimension of *being respected* entails that the patient's uniqueness is acknowledged and respected throughout the care. The person expects the nurse to elicit his or her needs as part of the care and address them throughout the care delivery. Being unique from the patient's perspective is not only about meeting the needs that the cancer and its treatment induce. It also involves the nurse's behaviour towards the person. This should be done within the results of advanced assessment of the situation, respecting, for example, a patient's agitation when pain is present and persistent, respecting his or her preferences, facilitating the patient's need to express his or her feeling on bad news that have been just delivered to him or her or simply sharing an honest conversation with the nurse on what the future lies ahead.

The theme *being cared for religiously and spiritually* is another dimension of the nursing care quality framework that has individuality as its cornerstone. Equally patients and nurses raised the personalised meanings that they attributed to these concepts as well as the importance these concepts can have on providing holistic care [18]. What has been emphasised is that spirituality is realized as an essential aspect to be included in order to achieve the "whole" in holistic care. To highlight this assertion, a female cancer patient narrated "Praying, reading the Holy Bible took my mind off the constant thought of death [...] but it was through the nurse's caring I saw what the true meaning of life is [....]".

Essentially, this quotation reveals the complementary nature of the two concepts that of holistic caring and individualised care within the cancer care context. Holistic care lays on the philosophy of holism that emphasises that the human being, composed of a mind, body and soul integrated into an inseparable whole that is greater than the sum of the parts, is in constant interaction with the universe and all that it contains [19]. Within this philosophical approach in order to providing holistic care, the person is acknowledged as a whole where there is interdependence among one's biological, social, psychological and spiritual aspects. With individualised nursing care being defined as patient perceptions of nurses' activities and being cared for as an individual [20, 21], there is an apparent connection between the concept of individuality and holistic care. Whereas holistic care provides a macro perspective to the person as a whole, individualised care provides a micro perspective. Therefore, whilst holistic care calls for the person to be cared for as a whole, individuality calls for the person to be cared for based on his or her individual needs according to the circumstances at hand and how these circumstances might alter a person's preferences and expectations.

Whilst the biological, social, psychological and spiritual dimensions of the person remain equally important, specific conditions necessitate that there is a prioritisation of the needs that need to be addressed based on which of the person's dimensions are mostly affected. This approach is based on the fact that cancer does not affect all the persons in the same way and most definitely its impact on the person fluctuates and changes over time. In order to address these variations in the level and the type of care needed in each situation, each patient needs to be assessed and cared for based on his or her individual perspectives where an approach "one size fits for all" is inappropriate and likely to fail. For example, patients with highly developed supportive networks might not require extensive emotional support during the diagnosis phase. This phase is accompanied with distress, such as unwanted intrusive thoughts about cancer for patients, and it may lead to emotional reactions and psychological challenges, such as anxiety, despair, fear of dying, sense of aloneness and sexual and body image problems. These patients can often rely on internal and external resources such as family and significant others to overcome the stressing effects of receiving a cancer diagnosis [22, 23].

The individualised approach inherent in this six-dimensional framework is further warranted by the fact that in the study, the patients reported that it was only when the incorporation of all the six dimensions (without any hierarchical order) within their caring was achieved that they truly experienced a sense of emotional and physical well-being [1].

Within the complex cancer care context, individualised care is not a concept that occurs in isolation. It has been related to several other concepts such as the overall quality of oncology nursing care and one that can influence patient outcomes [24] and healthcare quality [25]. On a European level, the latter was partly the result of various patient lobbying groups such as the European Cancer Patient Coalition (ECPC) placing pressure on policymakers, healthcare providers and other relevant stakeholders to increase their involvement as service users in the development of healthcare and healthcare policy [26]. The rise of empowered patients is highly reflected in ECPC's motto: "Nothing about us, without us". This motto demonstrates also an acceptance that, to be appropriate and efficient, patients as a group need a variety of approaches to care highlighting the need for patient centredness [27, 28]. Equally strategically, taking into account of individuals' own values, preferences and beliefs about their health issues in personally meaningful ways may prevent and undermine the illness process or may simplify the management of complex healthcare.

There has been increasing evidence in the literature that adopting a more patient-centred model of care, one that promotes active participation of patient in planning their care and decision-making, improves healthcare outcomes and patient safety [29, 30]. In the cancer care context, a correlational survey of hospitalised surgical cancer patients found a positive correlation between the level of individuality in care delivered and health status scores [21]. Radwin et al. [31] found that individualisation of nursing interventions was positively related to cancer patients' sense of well-being. Within the individualised care context, the provision of patient-centred communication promotes patient's participation in decision-making and increases patient-healthcare professional trust, respecting the uniqueness of the patient, navigating patients to the appropriate care in a timely manner and facilitating the decision-making process based on the evidence and consistent with patients values [32].

Patient-centred communication has been adopted as an indicator of quality healthcare and a contributor (direct or indirect) to improved clinical outcomes and health-related quality of life. For example, Arora et al. [33] evaluated pathways linking physicians' decision-making style with cancer survivors' health-related quality of life (HRQOL). They found that a participatory physician style that abided to the principles of patient-centred communication and individuality may improve survivors' mental health by a complex two-step mechanism of improving survivors' proximal communication and intermediate cognitive outcomes. These studies demonstrated that patients perceive cancer care to be of high quality when it is practised within a person-centred approach that fosters the individualised caring of the patient. However, it also demonstrates the fact that individualised care is associated with other concepts such as the nursing care quality, trust and patient's health status. Charalambous et al. [34] in a cross-sectional, exploratory and correlational study in Cyprus, Finland, Greece and Sweden tested a hypothesised model linking hospitalised cancer patients' health status, nursing care quality, perceived individuality in care and trust in nurses. The aim was to test the various hypothetical associations between these four variables. According to the model, nursing care quality and perceived individuality on care mediated the effects of the health status factor on patients' reports of trust in nurses (Fig. 12.1) [34].

The strongest relationship in all the studied factors was found in the direct effect of health status scores on nursing care quality followed by individualised care which was the second strongest factor influenced by health status. These associations were consistent to the findings of earlies studies suggesting that there was an association between the provision of individualised care and health status. For example, Suhonen et al. [24] in a cross-sectional correlational survey with a sample of 861 predischarged hospitalised adult patients highlighted the contribution of individualised nursing care to positive patient outcomes, such as patient satisfaction, patient autonomy and perceived health-related quality of life. Jones [35], using a classical grounded theory methodology, demonstrated the positive correlation between individualised nursing response to patients' needs and the improvement of the patients'

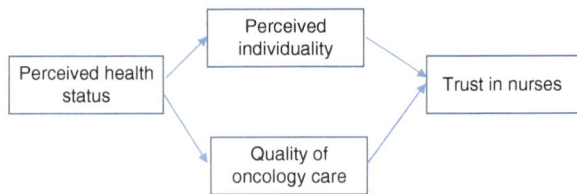

Fig. 12.1 Model of trust

perceived health status. The model also warrants that trust in nurses is influenced by perceived individuality.

Caring for the person diagnosed with and living with cancer is complex and demanding and one that requires nurses to engage in a therapeutic relationship with their patients that fosters trust between the two parties as the pathway to providing quality care [1, 36]. The onset of such successful relationships lays on patient-centred communication which promotes the development of trust between the patient and the healthcare professional. Cancer is a chronic disease that requires long-term and genuine commitment on behalf of the two parties as to maintain these trusting relationships. Additionally, for nurses working in cancer care, it is important to develop ways that would allow them to recognise, understand and use the factors which influence the generating, maintaining and regaining of trust between nurses and patients. Overall the model championed the complexity of caring for patients diagnosed and living with cancer highlighting the many factors involved. Adopting a caring philosophy inspired by the principles of patient centredness is demanding but essential in achieving patient-nurse trust and in turn accomplishing the provision of nursing care quality. These are the ideal conditions that can promote the patients' health status within the cancer care context.

Conclusion

Reflecting back to the initial patient quotation, the four words used convey the idea that the care provided should take place into a context that it is informed by the individuals' needs, desires, experiences, preferences, behaviours, feelings, perceptions and understandings. In other words, this quotation encapsulates what patients cherish the most when they face a life-threatening disease, not only maintaining their unique identity when being cared for but also being respected as a unique human being by those involved in the care. It is not surprising that often patients referred to being identified by their disease status. This is an essential concern on behalf of the patients diagnosed with and living with cancer that can generate significant anxiety and depression and lead to a deterioration in the perceived quality of life. The extent to which one's life can be negatively influenced by the feeling of identity loss under conditions of illness was captured by Taylor [37]: "The notion of identity refers to us certain evaluations which are essential because they are the indispensable horizon or foundation out of which we evaluate as persons. To lose this horizon, or not to have found it, is indeed a terrifying experience of disaggregation and loss (p. 125)". The philosophical underpinnings of individualised caring adhere to the principle of maintaining one's unique identity throughout the disease journey and attributing the necessary attention to those specific needs experienced by the person. By attributing attention to individualised care, positive effects can also be recorded on the patient's health status, the provision of quality nursing care and promoting trust between patients-healthcare professionals.

References

1. Charalambous A, Papadopoulos R, Beadsmoore A. Listening to the voices of patients with cancer their advocates and their nurses: a hermeneutic-phenomenological study of quality nursing care. Eur J Oncol Nurs. 2008;12(5):436–42.
2. Ferlay J, Soerjomataram I, Dikshit R, et al. Cancer incidence and mortality worldwide: sources, methods and major patterns in GLOBOCAN 2012. Int J Cancer. 2015;136(5):E359–86.
3. Rahib L, Smith BD, Aizenberg R, et al. Projecting cancer incidence and deaths to 2030: the unexpected burden of thyroid, liver, and pancreas cancers in the United States. Cancer Res. 2014;74(11):2913–21.
4. Cordella M, Poiani A. The social dimension of cancer. In: Behavioural oncology. New York: Springer; 2014.
5. Papastavrou E, Charalambous A, Tsangari H, et al. The cost of caring: the relative with schizophrenia. Scand J Caring Sci. 2010;24(4):817–23.
6. Given B, Given C, Kozachik S. Family support in advanced cancer. CA Cancer J Clin. 2001;51(4):213–31.
7. Kitrungrote LCM. Quality of life of family caregivers of patients with cancer: a literature review. Oncol Nurs Forum. 2006;33(3):625–32.
8. Kent EE, Rowland JH, Northouse L, et al. Caring for caregivers and patients: research and clinical priorities for informal cancer caregiving. Cancer. 2016;122(13):1987–95.
9. Northouse LL, Katapodi MC, Schafenacker AM, et al. The impact of caregiving on the psychological well-being of family caregivers and cancer patients. Semin Oncol Nurs. 2012;28(4):236–45.
10. Charalambous A. Hermeneutic phenomenological interpretations of patients with head and neck neoplasm experiences living with radiation-induced xerostomia: the price to pay? Eur J Oncol Nurs. 2014;18(5):512–20.
11. Hewitt M, Simone JV. Ensuring quality cancer care. Washington: National Academy Press; 1999.
12. Institute of Medicine. Delivering high-quality cancer care: charting a new course for a system in crisis. Washington, DC: National Academies Press; 2013. https://doi.org/10.17226/18359.
13. Balint E. The possibilities of patient-centered medicine. J R Coll Gen Pract. 1969;17(82):269–76.
14. Suhonen R, Valimaki M, Leino-Kilpi H, et al. Testing the individualised care model. Scand J Caring Sci. 2004;18(1):27–36.
15. Qamar N, Pappalardo AA, Arora VM, et al. Patient-centered care and its effect on outcomes in the treatment of asthma. Patient Relat Outcome Meas. 2011;2:81–109.
16. Sidani S. Effects of patient-centered care on patient outcomes: an evaluation. Res Theory Nurs Pract. 2008;22(1):24–37.
17. Suhonen R, Valimaki M, Leino-Kilpi H. A review of outcomes of individualised nursing interventions on adult patients. J Clin Nurs. 2008;17(7):843–60.
18. Charalambous A, Papadopoulos IR, Beadsmoore A. Towards a theory of quality nursing care for patients with cancer through hermeneutic phenomenology. Eur J Oncol Nurs. 2009;13(5):350–60.
19. Erickson HL. Philosophy and theory of holism. Nurs Clin North Am. 2007;42(2):139–63.
20. Radwin L, Alster K, Rubin K. The development and psychometric testing of the Oncology Patients' Perceptions of the Quality of Nursing Care Scale (OPPQNCS). Oncol Nurs Forum. 2003;30(2):283–90.
21. Suhonen R, Leino-Kilpi H, Valimaki M. Development and psychometric properties of the Individualised Care Scale. J Eval Clin Pract. 2005;11(1):7–20.
22. Mehrabi E, Hajian S, Simbar M, et al. Coping response following a diagnosis of breast cancer: a systematic review. Electron Physician. 2015;7(8):1575–83.

23. Silva SM, Crespo C, Canavarro MC. Pathways for psychological adjustment in breast cancer: a longitudinal study on coping strategies and posttraumatic growth. Psychol Health. 2012;27(11):1323–41.
24. Suhonen R, Välimäki M, Katajisto J, et al. Provision of individualised care improves hospital patient outcomes: an explanatory model using LISREL. Int J Nurs Stud. 2007;44(2):197–207.
25. OECD. Towards high-performing health systems. OECD health project. Paris: Organisation for Economic Co-operation and Development (OECD); 2004.
26. deBronkart D. From patient centred to people powered: autonomy on the rise. BMJ 2015;350. doi: https://doi.org/10.1136/bmj.h148.
27. ECPC. Challenges in cancer policy at EU level: the role of patients and future challenges. Paper presented at the CanCon Final Conference, Malta, 17th February 2017. 2017.
28. Wessels H, de Graeff A, Wynia K, et al. Gender-related needs and preferences in cancer care indicate the need for an individualized approach to cancer patients. Oncologist. 2010;15(6):648–55.
29. Hansson E, Ekman I, Swedberg K, et al. Person-centred care for patients with chronic heart failure - a cost-utility analysis. Eur J Cardiovasc Nurs. 2015;15(4):276–84.
30. Mazurenko O, Bock S, Prato C, et al. Considering shared power and responsibility: diabetic patients' experience with the PCMH care model. Patient Exp J. 2015;2(1):61–7.
31. Radwin LE, Cabral HJ, Wilkes G. Relationships between patient-centered cancer nursing interventions and desired health outcomes in the context of the health care system. Res Nurs Health. 2009;32:4–17.
32. Street RL, Mazor KM, Arora NK. Assessing patient-centered communication in cancer care: measures for surveillance of communication outcomes. J Oncol Pract. 2016;12(12):1198–202.
33. Arora NK, Weaver KE, Clayman ML, et al. Physicians' decision-making style and psychosocial outcomes among cancer survivors. Patient Educ Couns. 2009;77(3):404–12.
34. Charalambous A, Radwin L, Berg A, Sjovall K, Patiraki E, Lemonidou C, Katajisto J, Suhonen R. An international study of hospitalized cancer patients' health status, nursing care quality, perceived individuality in care and trust in nurses: a path analysis. Int J Nurs Stud. 2016;61:176–86.
35. Jones SM. Making me feel comfortable: developing trust in the nurse for Mexican Americans. West J Nurs Res. 2015;37(11):1423–40.
36. Rchaidia L, Dierckx de Casterle´ B, De Blaeser L, et al. Cancer patients' perceptions of the good nurse: a literature review. Nurs Ethics. 2009;16(5):528–42.
37. Taylor C. Sources of the self: the making of the modern identity. Cambridge: Harvard University Press; 1989.

13

Maritta Anneli Välimäki and Tella Jemina Lantta

Abstract

Individualised care has been part of international discussion in mental health services and psychiatric care since 1990s. The discussion is originally based on a wide movement in psychiatry towards community care away from institutionalised and less human approaches in mental health services. However, a connotation of the concept of 'individualised care' varies in the literature. There is also a great variation on how the concept of individualised care has been used in different mental healthcare services or in psychiatric care regarding guidelines, strategies, research or educational purposes. In addition, different methods have been used to describe a realisation in individualised care in different target population. In this book chapter, we will first overview how individualised care in mental health and psychiatric care has been defined in different context. Second, we will list the measures and outcomes, which have been used to assess the realisation of individualised care in daily practices. Third, the interventions or programmes used to support individualised care in special target groups will be described. Fourth, the realisation and impact of individualised care will be described.

Keywords

Individualised care · Primary nursing · Psychiatric care · Mental health · Mental illness

M. A. Välimäki (✉)
School of Nursing, The Hong Kong Polytechnic University, Hong Kong, China SAR

Department of Nursing Science, University of Turku, Turku, Finland
e-mail: mavalim@polyu.edu.hk; mava@utu.fi

T. J. Lantta
Department of Nursing Science, University of Turku, Turku, Finland
e-mail: tejela@utu.fi

13.1 Introduction

Since 1990s, individualised care has been discussed in mental health services and psychiatric care. The discussion is originally based on a wide movement in psychiatry towards community care away from institutionalised and less human approaches in mental health services. However, a connotation of the concept of 'individualised care' may still be vague, and its meaning is unclear in the literature. There is also a great variation on how the concept of individualised care has been used in different mental healthcare services or in psychiatric care regarding guidelines, strategies, research or educational purposes. In addition, different methods have been used to describe a realisation in individualised care in different target population.

In this chapter, we will first overview how individualised care in mental health and psychiatric care has been defined in different context. Second, we will list the measures and outcomes, which have been used to assess the realisation of individualised care in daily practices. Third, the interventions or programmes used to support individualised care in special target groups will be overviewed. Fourth, the realisation and impact of individualised care will be described.

13.2 Definitions and Context of Individualised Care in Mental Health and Psychiatric Care

In the literature and empirical studies, a concept of individualised care has been described using a high number of different connotations and definitions. Already in early 1990s, Burchard and Clarke [1] used the concept of individualised care related to children who had severe maladjusted behaviour. The authors described individualised care from the point of view of the service environment and called it as 'a total system'. This means that the care is tailored to fit the needs of each individual child. For example, the services to be tailored are 'unconditional, flexible, child and family focused and interagency coordinated'. The services follow the child until he or she is adjusting in a normalised, mainstream environment. Based on the description, individualised care can be seen as a feature, which should be included in the healthcare services and the process of care. On the other hand, individualised care has also been used as a separate entity. In that case, 'individualised' is something to be developed and late to be integrated into an existing system of care [2].

Jones [3] explored perceptions of individualised care in mental health services. Jones's qualitative findings indicated two major themes in description individualised care: 'knowing the patient' and 'developing a relationship'. Indeed, a relationship between a patient and a nurse is a fundamental issue in psychiatric care [4]. On the other hand, pitfall of individualised care was recognised. Values of the professionals may have an influence to what kind of treatment is provided to a patient; a patient may be subjected to professionals' individual styles and decisions about what is important for the patient [3].

As manifestation of individualised care in mental health area, individualised care can be seen as a method of delivering nursing care or responsibilities of nurses, such as 'named nursing' or 'primary nursing.' 'Named nurse' includes critical elements with specific concepts. First, a single nurse has responsibility over decision-making for a patient. Second, a single nurse is responsible of patients' daily care. Third, a single nurse is responsible for direct communication to patient's network. And fourth, a single nurse is responsible for the quality of patient care administered for a patient on 24-h basis. [5]. Primary nursing also means delivering patient-centred and individualised treatment for a patient and makes patient management less fragmented and aims to fulfil patient's wishes and needs [6]. More recently, the emphasis of 'named nurses' has been moved towards multidisciplinary teams, which are comprised of staff who vary in their educational and professional experiences and bring together diverse perspectives, expertise and skills [7].

The studies have been conducted to find out different technical tools to support individualised care from the point of view of risk factors or predictors. Gowin et al. [8] used neuroimaging to predict patient relapses. The goal was to find out whether this advanced neuroimaging tool can use to make decisions about individualised treatment of substance use disorders. Zilcha-Mano et al. [9] also aimed to find out predictors for patient dropout to be used in individualised treatment recommendations. Further, Cannon et al. [10] used an individualised, web-based risk calculator tool to predict the risk for psychosis. They found based on the calculator that the 2-year probability of conversion to psychosis was 16%, which was predicted by higher levels of unusual thought content and suspiciousness, greater decline in social functioning, lower verbal learning and memory performance, slower speed of processing and younger age at baseline which contributed to individual risk for psychosis. Individualisation has also been used for diagnosis purposes for patients with schizophrenia and mood disorders [11].

13.3 The Measures and Outcomes Used to Assess the Realisation of Individualised Care in Daily Practices

Individualised care has been described to be something 'mystical' and specific in psychiatric care [3]. Some nurses has thought that it is impossible to make any structured assessment about patients' status or outcome because each individual nurse can make their own judgement based on their experiences and intuition. Indeed, standardisation of care has been resisted due to this unique nature of psychiatric practice [3]. Different instruments have still been developed to measure individualised care, its process or outcomes in mental health and psychiatric nursing. The instrument has been used from patients' and nurses' viewpoints.

13.3.1 Instrument to Be Used by Patients

Pesola et al. [12] have developed Individualized Outcome Measure (IOM). The final version of IOM has two components: goal attainment (GA) and personalised primary outcome (PPO). For goal attainment, patients will identify first one relevant goal for his or her treatment. The same goal will be rated again from the point of view of the goal attainment at follow-up. For personalised primary outcome (PPO), patient will choose an outcome domain related to their goal from a predefined list at baseline and complete a standardised questionnaire assessing the chosen outcome domain at baseline and follow-up. There are ten outcome domains from which a patient can choose from. All of these ten outcome domains are patient-rated, pre-existing measures. These include (1) the Empowerment Scale (ES) which has 28 items that are rated on a 4-point Likert scale [13], (2) the Herth Hope Index (HHI) which has 12 items that are rated on a 4-point Likert scale [14], (3) the Rosenberg Self-esteem Scale (RSES) which consists of 10 items that are rated on a 4-point Likert scale [15], (4) the Stigma Scale (SS) which has 28 items rated on a 5-point Likert scale [16], (5) the Meaning of Life Questionnaire (MLQ) which has 10 items rated on a 7-point Likert scale [17], (6) The MOS Social Support Survey (MOS) scale which consists of 21 items that are rated on a 5-point Likert scale [18], (7) the Community Integration Measure (CIM) which consists of 10 items rated on a 5-point Likert scale [19], (8) the Warwick–Edinburgh Mental Well-Being Scale (WEMWBS) which has 14 items rated on a 5-point Likert scale [20], (9) the Service User Perception of Functioning Scale (PPFS) which consists of 5 items that are rated on a 5-point Likert scale [21] and (10) the Manchester Short Assessment of Quality of Life (MANSA) which has 12 items rated on a 7-point Likert scale [22]. The authors recommend that the instrument can be used as a patient-specific outcome measure in RCTs of complex interventions, but further assessment of the psychometric properties of the instrument should be conducted. However, the PPO has been found to be feasible instrument approach? in ways that patients with mental illness are able to use the instrument properly.

The realisation of individualised care has been measured by assessing treatment outcomes: cognition level (The Brief Assessment of Cognition in Schizophrenia—Japanese version (BACS-J), [23]), psychiatric symptoms (Positive and Negative Syndrome Scale (PANSS), [23]) and physical health status [24]. Patients' individualised treatment as means of realisation of primary nursing in care has also been evaluated by asking patients' feedback with survey instrument whether patients were aware of a name of their primary nurse [25]. Further, realisation of individualised care has been assessed by identifying changes in care restrictions in primary nursing care by assessing the use of seclusion and restraints [25].

13.3.2 Instruments to Be Used by Nurses

The realisation of individualised care in psychiatric hospital has been measured by using Individualised Care Scale—Nurse—instrument [26]. This instrument is used to assess nurses' views about delivery of individualised care. The measurement scale guides nurses to rate in 5-point Likert-type scale how they support patients' individuality in clinical situations, in patients' personal life situation and in decisional control over care with a total of 34 items [26].

Impact of realisation of primary nursing care has been assessed by measuring work satisfaction [25] with the Index of Work Satisfaction Questionnaire (IWS, [27]). The instrument contains 44 items with six components: pay, autonomy, task requirements, professional status, interaction and organisational policies [28]. Further, the impact of primary nursing has been evaluated related to ward environment from nurses' perspectives [29] by using Ward Atmosphere Scale (WAS, [30]). This instrument with 100 statements has been used to capture various aspects of ward environment.

Moreover, as an outcome of providing more individualised care in primary nursing, nurses' burnout and job turnover have been measured [31]. As a burnout measure, the Maslach Burnout Inventory (MBI) has been used. The MBI contains 22 items that are assessed with 7-point Likert scale divided to dimensions of emotional exhaustion, depersonalisation and personal accomplishment subscales that are parts of the 22-item MBI [32].

13.4 Examples of the Interventions and Programmes to Support Individualised Care in Special Target Groups

A high variety of interventions and programmes have been developed to support individualised care. Burchard and Clarke [1] described two programmes for children. The Alaska Youth Initiative programme was established in which individualised care was used to return children from out-of-state, residential programmes. The other is Project Wraparound where it was used to prevent children from being removed from their families. Further, Curtis et al. [33] used a 12-week individualised intervention targeted to 14–25 years people with first-episode psychosis (FEP). The lifestyle and life skills intervention was delivered by specialist clinical staff (nurse, dietician and exercise physiologist) and youth peer wellness coaches. The importance of the intervention lies on the fact that antipsychotic medication frequently induces clinically significant weight gain.

Individualised care has been connected with a care pathway programme for mental health residential services. Care pathway programme emphasises individualised care for people with serious mental illnesses. In this programme, the strengths and individual goals of service users were assessed. Individual goals will be set together with healthcare professional, and these goals are written on a personal plan. Personal plan are used to decide what kinds of interventions are suitable to help the service user reach their goal [34].

Schneider et al. [35] planned to investigate the efficacy of an individualised metacognitive therapy programme (MCT+) for psychosis. The individualised version of the intervention was developed to allow for more detailed targeting of patient-specific problems, and therefore it should be used for individual persons only. Although the programme is highly structured and fully manualised, the therapist can select the therapy units that fit best to the patient's current difficulties and cognitive biases [35].

Further, Velligan et al. [36] examined the short-term efficacy of two treatments using environmental support to improve behaviours in individuals with schizophrenia. In this study, environmental support meant signs, alarms, pill containers or checklists. In the study, a group of patients participated in the treatment called 'cognitive adaptation training' (CAT). The training is a manual-driven set of environmental supports, which are customised based on individual's cognitive impairments and behaviours. They are further established and maintained in participants' homes on weekly visits. In the second group, 'Generic Environmental Supports' (GES) offered a generic set of supports given to patients at a routine clinic visit and replaced on a monthly basis. After 3 months, patients in both CAT and GES groups had better global function than those participants who continued in usual care. Further, patients in 'cognitive adaptation training' group were more likely to improve on, for example, orientation, hygiene and medication adherence.

Individual Placement and Support (IPS) is an approach used in the United States of America to improve employment rates for persons facing significant barriers. The IPS is an evidence-based programme, which includes a set of core principles, such as small caseloads, integrating treatment teams into vocational plans, no exclusion criteria, rapid job search and services provided in the community. The core components support the implementation of the principles: job exploration, individualised planning, job development and job carving, job coaching and natural supports. The programme has successfully used for persons with serious mental illness [37, 38]. More recently, IPS has been found to be more beneficial than a job club in working with individuals with severe mental illness who have legal convictions, misdemeanours or felonies [39].

13.5 Realisation and Impact of Individualised Care

It has been evaluated that patients with schizophrenia who have received individualised care interventions may have improvements in cognition and reduction in psychiatric symptoms [23] compared to treatment groups without individualised components. Health promotion of patients with severe mental illnesses seems also to benefit from individualised care planning: positive outcomes may be seen in actual physical health of individuals and in mental status as in patients' own satisfaction with their physical health [24]. In care of depression, realisation of individualised care has been showed to increased commitment to treatment and lead to reduced dropout from treatment [9].

In psychiatric inpatient settings, reduction in use of seclusion and restrains has been detected as a result of primary nursing care model. This has been estimated to be an outcome that nurses spend more time with patients and that nurses are able to recognise developing patient crisis earlier and they are more familiar how these crises would be managed when they know the patients in more individual level. Patients' has been also more aware who their primary nurse is after more individualised practices had been introduced [25].

Dechamps et al. [40] used the cognition-action (CA) intervention for severely deconditioned institutionalised old adults to reduce their behavioural disturbances. Patients received short bouts of 5–15 min and accumulated 50 min of interaction per week. Intervention included five standardised exercises as tools to enhance communication and social interactions between staff and old adults. The study showed that for institutionalised old adults, the combination of tailored guidance and simple standardised exercises can be an effective behavioural management approach for behavioural disturbances reduction and functional autonomy improvement.

For nurses, the introduction of primary nursing has had positive impact on nurses work satisfaction [25] and led to reduction in job turnover [31]. Mental health nurses, for example, have assessed how individualised care has realised in their daily practice. In generally, mental health nurses' assessments have been positive. They have perceived that nurses support well patients' individuality through nursing activities in clinical situations. For example, nurses talk with patients about their needs that require specific attention. Nurses also take into account the meaning of the illness to the patient personally [26].

On the other hand, opposite results have also been found when outcomes of primary nursing have been evaluated by asking nurses' thoughts about ward environment [29]. Like any other approach, individualised care may also include practical and ethical issues, which should be taken into collaboration in care environment. For example, the change towards more individualised care practices may cause resistance in psychiatric care, which was seen, for instance, when nurses assessed that ward atmosphere weakened as a result of introducing a working method, primary nursing, which they did not consider themselves as superior working style [29]. Individualised care of patients may also lead to incoherent treatment practices [3]. If 'individuality' means totally unstructured and invisible approaches, it cannot be measured or subjected to audit. For instance, it has been stated that nurses assess patients' needs and mental status in very different ways and using different concept areas [41]. This may result that professionals hide behind concept of 'individualised care' and are reluctant to open treatment practices to others or write them down [3].

13.6   Discussion

Individualised care in mental health and psychiatric services seems to be an integral element of care provision. Psychiatric care has traditionally been based on interaction between a professional and a patient [42], which provides a good starting point for creating individualised care. In its basic form, manifestation of individualised care in mental health area can be seen to lie on practice of primary nursing, where every patient is met as an individual with unique needs, problems and goals [6].

Besides nursing care practices, individualised care realises in different psychological and psychosocial interventions, which are structured, but able to be tailored based on individual needs. Instead of providing all patients the same therapy treatment, individual patients' preferences can be taken into account when there exist two or more treatment options which have been shown to be equally effective [43].

Besides, providing an opportunity to make individual care decisions has been evaluated to lead to higher patient satisfaction, increased treatment engagement and better treatment outcomes as well [9, 23, 24, 43], and individualised care for patients with mental illnesses is rewarding also to a professional [25]. As its best, it empowers professionals who know the patient best to coordinate the care based on individual needs and creates an environment where mental health professionals feel they make a difference [44].

However, there is still a lack of evidence-based and robust studies of individualised care in mental health area [45, 46]. For example, primary nursing care model has been launched decades ago, but still its realisation possesses challenges [25, 47]. There may also be doubts about the quality of care: patients may not have individualised treatment plans [47], or they are not aware who is responsible of planning, implementing and assessing their care based on their needs [48].

The future of individualised care in mental health and psychiatric care may lie on advances of personalised medicine. We may be able to predict disease vulnerability based on, for example, individuals' genetic information, other biomarkers and environmental exposures [49]. Thus, preventive mental health work could be targeted for individuals in risk of developing a mental illness. In future, especially pharmacology treatments could be optimised based on the individual patients' biological characteristics [49]. Although some promising results in this field have been achieved, personalised medicine is in its early development stages in psychiatric care [50]. While waiting for scientific breakthroughs in more enhanced prevention of mental illnesses and optimised drug therapies, clinical practice and mental health professionals need to ensure that each patient receives well-planned care of uniform quality with full respect, taking into account individual's needs and preferences.

Conclusions

A connotation of the concept of 'individualised care' may be vague, and its meaning is unclear in the literature. There is also a great variation how the concept of individualised care has been used in different mental healthcare and psychiatric services. In addition, different interventions and programmes have been developed and implemented to support a realisation in individualised care in different target populations. Although positive impacts have been described in patient and nurse population, the effectiveness of individualised care has not been evaluated with rigour and robust research methods.

References

1. Burchard JD, Clarke RT. The role of individualized care in a service delivery system for children and adolescents with severely maladjusted behavior. J Ment Health Adm. 1990;17(1):48–60.
2. VanDenBerg JE. Integration of individualized mental health services into the system of care for children and adolescents. Admin Pol Ment Health. 1993;20(4):247–57.
3. Jones A. Perceptions on individualized approaches to mental health care. J Psychiatr Ment Health Nurs. 2005;12(4):396–404.

4. Peplau HE. Psychiatric nursing: role of nurses and psychiatric nurses. Int Nurs Rev. 1978;25(2):41–7.
5. Manthey M. The practice of primary nursing. Boston: Blackwell Scientific; 1980.
6. Rose D. Users' voices: the perspectives of mental health service users on community and hospital care. London: Sainsbury Centre for Mental Health; 2001.
7. Kozlowski SWJ, Ilgen DR. Enhancing the effectiveness of work groups and teams. Psychol Sci Public Interest. 2006;7(3):77–124.
8. Gowin JL, Ball TM, Wittmann M, et al. Individualized relapse prediction: personality measures and striatal and insular activity during reward-processing robustly predict relapse. Drug Alcohol Depend. 2015;152:93–101.
9. Zilcha-Mano S, Keefe JR, Chui H, et al. Reducing dropout in treatment for depression: translating dropout predictors into individualized treatment recommendations. J Clin Psychiatry. 2016;77(12):e1584–90.
10. Cannon TD, Yu C, Addington J, et al. An individualized risk calculator for research in prodromal psychosis. Am J Psychiatry. 2016;173(10):980–8.
11. Koutsouleris N, Meisenzahl EM, Borgwardt S, et al. Individualized differential diagnosis of schizophrenia and mood disorders using neuroanatomical biomarkers. Brain. 2015;138(7):2059–73.
12. Pesola F, Williams J, Bird V. Development and evaluation of an Individualized Outcome Measure (IOM) for randomized controlled trials in mental health. Int J Methods Psychiatr Res. 2015;24(4):257–65.
13. Rogers E, Chamberlin J, Ellison M. A consumer-constructed scale to measure empowerment among users of mental health services. Psychiatr Serv. 1997;48(8):1042–7.
14. Herth K. Abbreviated instrument to measure hope: development and psychiatric evaluation. J Adv Nurs. 1992;17(10):1251–9.
15. Rosenberg M. Society and the adolescent self-image. Princeton: Princeton University Press; 1965.
16. King M, Dinos S, Shaw J. The Stigma Scale: development of a standardized measure of the stigma of mental illness. Br J Psychiatry. 2007;190(3):248–54.
17. Steger MF, Frazier P, Oishi S, et al. The meaning in life questionnaire: assessing the presence of and search for meaning in life. J Couns Psychol. 2006;53(1):80–93.
18. Sherbourne C, Stewart A. The MOS social support survey. Soc Sci Med. 1991;32(6):8.
19. McColl MA, Davies D, Carlson P. The community integration measure: development and preliminary validation. Arch Phys Med Rehabil. 2001;82(4):429–34.
20. Tennant R, Hiller L, Fishwick R, et al. The Warwick–Edinburgh Mental Well-being Scale (WEMWBS), development and UK validation. Health Qual Life Outcomes. 2007. https://doi.org/10.1186/1477-7525-5-63.
21. Horn KK, Jennings S, Richardson G, et al. The patient-specific functional scale: psychometrics, clinimetrics, and application as a clinical outcome measure. J Orthop Sports Phys Ther. 2012;42(1):30–42.
22. Priebe S, Huxley P, Knight S. Application and results of the Manchester Short Assessment of Quality of Life (MANSA). Int J Soc Psychiatry. 1999;45(1):7–12.
23. Shimada T, Nishi A, Yoshida T, et al. Development of an individualized occupational therapy programme and its effects on the neurocognition, symptoms and social functioning of patients with schizophrenia. Occup Ther Int. 2016;23(4):425–35.
24. Bressington D, Chien WT, Mui J, et al. Chinese Health Improvement Profile for people with severe mental illness: a cluster-randomized, controlled trial. Int J Ment Health Nurs. 2018;27(2):841–55.
25. Allen DE, Bockenhauer B, Egan C, et al. Relating outcomes to excellent nursing practice. J Nurs Adm. 2006;36(3):140–7.
26. Suhonen R, Gustafsson ML, Katajisto J, et al. Nurses' perceptions of individualized care. J Adv Nurs. 2010;66(5):1035–46.
27. Stamps P. Nurses and work satisfaction: an index of measurement. Chicago: Health Administration Press; 1997.

28. Ahmad N, Oranye NO, Danilov A. Rasch analysis of Stamps's Index of Work Satisfaction in nursing population. Nurs Open. 2016;4(1):32–40.
29. Rigby A, Leach C, Greasley P. Primary nursing: staff perception of changes in ward atmosphere and role. J Psychiatr Ment Health Nurs. 2001;8(6):525–32.
30. Moos RH. Ward atmosphere scale manual. Palo Alto: Consulting Psychologists; 1989.
31. Melchior ME, Philipsen H, Abu-Saad HH. The effectiveness of primary nursing on burnout among psychiatric nurses in long-stay settings. J Adv Nurs. 1996;24(4):694–702.
32. Maslach C, Jackson SE. Maslach burnout inventory. 2nd ed. Palo Alto: Consulting Psychologists; 1981.
33. Curtis J, Watkins A, Rosenbaum S, et al. Evaluating an individualized lifestyle and life skills intervention to prevent antipsychotic-induced weight gain in first-episode psychosis. Early Interv Psychiatry. 2016;10(3):267–76.
34. Rayner L. Language, therapeutic relationships and individualized care: addressing these issues in mental health care pathways. J Psychiatr Ment Health Nurs. 2005;12(4):481–7.
35. Schneider BC, Brüne M, Bohn F. Investigating the efficacy of an individualized metacognitive therapy program (MCT+) for psychosis: study protocol of a multi-center randomized controlled trial. BMC Psychiatry. 2016;16:51. https://doi.org/10.1186/s12888-016-0756-2.
36. Velligan DI, Diamond P, Mueller J, et al. The short-term impact of generic versus individualized environmental supports on functional outcomes and target behaviors in schizophrenia. Psychiatry Res. 2009;168(2):94–101.
37. Becker DR, Drake RE. Supported employment interventions are effective for people with severe mental illness. Evid Based Ment Health. 2006;9(1):22.
38. Tsang HW, Chan A, Wong A, et al. Vocational outcomes of an integrated supported employment program for individuals with persistent and severe mental illness. J Behav Ther Exp Psychiatry. 2009;40(2):292–305.
39. Bond GR, Kim SJ, Becker DR, et al. A controlled trial of supported employment for people with severe mental illness and justice involvement. Psychiatr Serv. 2015;66(10):1027–34.
40. Dechamps A, Alban R, Jen J, et al. Individualized Cognition-Action intervention to prevent behavioral disturbances and functional decline in institutionalized older adults: a randomized pilot trial. Int J Geriatr Psychiatry. 2010;25(8):850–60.
41. Coombs T, Crookes P, Curtis J. A comprehensive mental health nursing assessment: variability of content in practice. J Psychiatr Ment Health Nurs. 2013;20(2):150–5.
42. Peplau HE. Peplau's theory of interpersonal relations. Nurs Sci Q. 1997;10(4):162–7.
43. Lindhiem O, Bennett CB, Trentacosta CJ. Client preferences affect treatment satisfaction, completion, and clinical outcome: a meta-analysis. Clin Psychol Rev. 2014;34(6):506–17.
44. Allen DE, Vitale-Nolen RA. Patient care delivery model improves nurse job satisfaction. J Contin Educ Nurs. 2005;36(6):277–82.
45. Butler M, Collins R, Drennan J, et al. Hospital nurse staffing models and patient and staff-related outcomes. Cochrane Database Syst Rev. 2011;7:CD007019. https://doi.org/10.1002/14651858.CD007019.pub2.
46. Farrelly S, Brown GE, Flach C, et al. User-held personalised information for routine care of people with severe mental illness. Cochrane Database Syst Rev. 2013;10:CD001711. https://doi.org/10.1002/14651858.CD001711.pub2.
47. Payne R, Steakley B. Establishing a primary nursing model of care. Nurs Manag. 2015;46(12):11–3.
48. Shebini N, Aggarwal R, Gandhi A. Improved patient awareness of named nursing through audit. Nurs Times. 2008;104(21):30–1. https://www.nursingtimes.net/roles/mental-health-nurses/improved-patient-awareness-of-named-nursing-through-audit/1425602.article. Accessed 20 Dec 2017.
49. Alhajji L, Nemeroff CB. Personalized medicine and mood disorders. Psychiatr Clin North Am. 2015;38(3):395–403.
50. Costa e Silva JA. Personalized medicine in psychiatry: new technologies and approaches. Metabolism. 2013;62(Suppl 1):S40–4.

Individualised Care and Rehabilitation

Lena von Koch

Abstract

In this chapter individualised rehabilitation is referring to the process of returning to, or maintaining, a meaningful everyday life, valued activities and roles in the context of an illness or a health condition. Rehabilitation usually involves at least two perspectives, i.e. that of the individual person who has a health condition or an illness and that of the enablers, e.g. health service workers. In individualised rehabilitation, the medical diagnosis itself is not enough for the understanding of the individual person's situation nor for his/her needs of rehabilitation. Instead, a wider framework is useful such as the biopsychosocial model in which the state of health is seen as an interaction between biological, psychological, and social factors as outlined in WHO's *International Classification of Functioning, Disability and Health* (ICF). Health can be promoted by creating environments where people in need of rehabilitation are active participating actors, who are supported to identify their internal and external resources and learn how to use and reuse them to reach vital goals in their everyday lives. Individualised rehabilitation entails a problem-solving process of interrelated phases performed by the individual in partnership with health professionals in a rehabilitation team. The process entails to establish a shared understanding; identify, negotiate and agree on short-term and long-term goals; together plan interventions required to reach the goals; put the plan into action; and evaluate and reflect on goal attainment.

Keywords

Activities · Everyday life · Functioning · Goals · Health promotion · Participation · Shared decision-making

L. von Koch
Karolinska Institutet, Solna, Sweden
e-mail: Lena.Von.Koch@ki.se

14.1   Rehabilitation: A Process

Rehabilitation is the process of returning to, or the process of enabling a person to return to, a meaningful everyday life, valued activities, participation and roles in the context of an illness or a health condition. This entails that rehabilitation can have several end points as we usually have several different roles, e.g. roles in the family, at work, etc. Furthermore, in the situation of a chronic or a long-term health condition, rehabilitation includes the process of maintaining or the process of enabling someone to maintain a meaningful everyday life, valued roles and activities. Hence, rehabilitation is a process in which an individual with or without the support of health services personnel and other support regains and/or maintains a meaningful life, valued roles and activities. Rehabilitation for a limited health condition may require input from one profession only and for a limited time. For rehabilitation of more complex health conditions, a team approach is more common with several professions involved.

14.2   Perspectives

As revealed in the description of the rehabilitation process, there can be at least two parties involved, and consequently more than one perspective might be at hand, that of the individual person, who has a health condition or an illness, and that of the enablers, e.g. health service workers. There are empirical studies that show that these two perspectives are not always well aligned and in agreement [1, 2]. Additional perspectives of importance are those of significant others. Significant others include people who are close to the person who has the illness, and they can be family, friends, etc. In healthcare, there is a growing contemporary trend not only to include the person with an illness but also significant others, in particular the family in the individualised rehabilitation process. Hence, in individualised rehabilitation significant others may have dual roles and perspectives. They may both be enablers in the rehabilitation process but also themselves recipients of support in order to maintain their own valued roles and activities in everyday life. Even though the text hereafter will be phrased in relation to the person who has an illness, it might as well include the family, even if this is not explicitly stated.

From the perspective of the enabler, i.e. the healthcare professionals, an overarching goal of individualised rehabilitation could be stated as to support or enable the individual's role fulfilment and her/his functioning in her/his environment/context within the limitations imposed by a health condition or an illness. If there are gaps between roles achieved and roles desired, individualised rehabilitation includes to support the individual to live with these differences [3]. An aspect that is not included in this statement is the relation to the availability of health services resources, an aspect of utmost importance considering the need for equality in access to healthcare, both on a national and a global level. Albeit the issue of equity and equality in healthcare has extensive ethical underpinnings, which by no means should be neglected, it will not be further considered in this chapter.

14.3 International Classification of Functioning, Disability and Health (ICF): A Framework

The terminology used in this chapter stems to a large extent from the framework of the WHO's international classification of functioning, disability and health (ICF) [4]. The framework is based upon the biopsychosocial model proposed by Engel in 1977 [5] in response to the dominating biomedical model of illness, which still remains the dominant healthcare model, in particular in acute healthcare. In contrast, in rehabilitation, the medical diagnosis itself is rarely useful for the understanding of the individual person's situation nor for which are his/her needs of rehabilitation. Instead by applying the biopsychosocial model in which the state of health is seen as an interaction between biological, psychological, and social factors [6], a better guide for the understanding of the individual person's situation is at hand and which issues should be considered and addressed in the rehabilitation process.

The ICF framework, depicted in Fig. 14.1, integrates two major models of disability—the medical model and the social model. The framework states that an individual's health condition is dependent on the interplay between an individual's functioning (function, activity and participation), personal factors and environmental factors. In ICF, functioning is conceptualised as a 'dynamic interaction between a person's health condition, environmental factors and personal factors' [4].

There are two overarching terms in the ICF—functioning and disability—denoting the positive and the negative aspects of functioning from the individual, biological and social perspectives [7]. Hence, functioning is the umbrella term for function, activity and participation, where function refers to body function and structure, activities denotes the execution of tasks or actions and participation refers to the involvement in life situations. Disability then is the umbrella term for impairments in body function or body structures, and activity limitations denoting difficulties encountered when executing tasks or actions and restrictions in participation are problems experienced by the individual in the involvement in life situations.

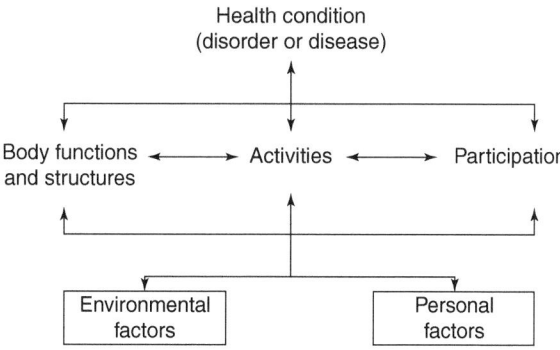

Fig. 14.1 The ICF Model: Interaction between ICF components (Reproduced from: WHO A Practical Manual for using the International Classification of Functioning, Disability and Health (ICF) [7])

14.4   Environmental and Personal Factors

The ICF framework also includes and puts emphasis on environmental factors, which are external to the individual and constitutes the physical, societal and attitudinal context in which a person lives. Environmental factors are considered both at the micro level, e.g. access to and access in the own home but also include the neighbourhood, the workplace, etc. At the meso or macro levels, environmental factors refer to the access to health services, prevailing policies and laws that impact on a person's life and health. Hence, environmental factors are to be considered from the perspective of the individual whose situation is to be described and in need of rehabilitation. An environmental factor that increases the level of functioning or decreases the level of disability is a facilitator, whereas the opposite constitutes an environmental barrier. Thus, in the ICF model disability is not just a health problem but a complex phenomenon, reflecting the interaction between a person and the society in which he or she lives. Lastly the model includes personal factors, which are the more internal aspects of the individual that may impact on functioning, e.g. age, gender, coping style, previous experiences, etc. The personal factors have not been well developed in the framework, and further work is needed. The ICF framework has rightfully been criticised for not including dimensions of individual meanings, own will and choice and for not recognising that there may be several perspectives involved [8]. Despite the shortcomings of the ICF, it can still be considered to supply a neutral nonprofession-specific common language that can be used to describe the individual's situation when in need of rehabilitation or health services as well as in rehabilitation research and scientific communication.

14.5   To Promote Health

As health is the focus of individualised rehabilitation as well as the ICF framework, Antonovsky's theory of salutogenesis, which focuses on resources for health and health-promoting processes rather than on disease as in pathogenesis [9], can be useful. A core construct in salutogenesis is a person's sense of coherence, which comprises comprehensibility, manageability and meaningfulness. In salutogenesis experiences of health and wellbeing are hypothesised to depend on general resistance resources (GRR), which are postulated to be personal factors but GRR also include assets available in people's environments. The key factor for health is to have the knowledge and be able to use and reuse the GRR. Health promotion is identified as the process of enabling individuals to increase control over the determinants of health and thereby improve health to live an active and a productive life [10]. Thus, health can be promoted by creating environments where people are the active participating actors, who are supported to identify their internal and external resources, learning how to use and reuse them to reach vital goals in their everyday lives [11]. In rehabilitation, there is a growing emphasis on health promotion and self-management, which entails to include key features such as problem-solving, decision-making and the formation of a partnership [12].

14.6   The Individualised Rehabilitation Process

Schematically individualised rehabilitation can be seen as a process made up of a set of interrelated phases, which might be reiterative, performed by the individual himself/herself in close collaboration, in partnership, with a rehabilitation team [13]. The process entails to identify, negotiate and agree on short-term and long-term goals, together plan interventions required to reach the goals, put the plan into action, evaluate and reflect on goal attainment, set new goals and so on. The phases can be seen as problem-solving processes in which the person in partnership is coached by the rehabilitation team. The individual practises a problem-solving process in order to be able to apply the process over and over again on her/his own when new challenges in everyday life appear. Monitoring of the process and progress is attained by reflecting on own performance and improvements made [14]. Hence, the individualised rehabilitation includes a learning process aimed to boost and support self-efficacy and self-management and trust in self as a competent person with resources, i.e. GRRs, to meet the challenges in the future and to avoid and not foster dependence on health services.

14.7   Shared Perspectives

It is imperative for the rehabilitation team to initially strive for an empathetic understanding of the individual person in need of rehabilitation. An agreement in perspectives will enable the individual's partaking, learning and shared responsibility in the rehabilitation process. The empathetic perspective was proposed as one of the core elements of client-centred practice by Carl Rogers [15]. It is a trust in that the individual person has a strong drive and to rely on that force and not only on the therapists' own powers [15]. Hence, in the initial phase of individualised rehabilitation, ways to reach an empathetic understanding and common shared perspectives are in focus. In order for a rehabilitation team to obtain such an understanding of the individual person and of his/her account of the own functioning and the situation, a partnership relation based on mutual trust needs to be established. This can be obtained by dialogues, narratives and diaries and by means of other expressions, e.g. art and photography as in photovoice [16]. Applying the ICF framework and the salutogenic perspective, the person shares experiences of internal and external resources available and functioning as well as impairments, activity limitations and participation restrictions encountered. In addition, the person shares descriptions of what it is that is valued and give meaning to his or her everyday life and what might be the desired goals for the rehabilitation. In order to reach a common and shared understanding, the individual person together with the rehabilitation team shares these accounts as a team, i.e. the individual is not external to, but an included partner, a member of the team. Likewise, documents and assessments should be shared by the team in which the individual is included throughout the rehabilitation process.

14.8 Awareness

For the individual to describe and reflect on the own situation and to be supported in identifying the resources available rather than to just focus on the problems is likely to increase the awareness of the own situation both regarding the resources and the limitations at hand. Awareness could also enhance motivation and self-efficacy. How the individual understands the own situation is likely to be revealed in the individual's own description, which will guide the rehabilitation team. Specific instruments developed with the aim to reflect the subjective perspective could as well be used to capture what is of importance to the individual. However, awareness of a disability might not always be present and might be dependent on a discovery process to take place first as it might be hard for a person to fully assess the consequences, in particular if the onset of disability was sudden. This has been reported by Tham et al. [17] to be the experience of people with hemi-neglect after a stroke. It is likely that other disabilities with sudden onsets might require a discovery process as well. Such discovery processes might be supported by a familiar context such as in the home environment where the individual's own functioning is familiar and known. Hence, when the awareness is low, gaps in functioning, i.e. disability, might be more easily uncovered by the individual in a familiar context [18]. In contrast the unfamiliar hospital environment in which an individual's functioning before a sudden onset of disability is not known and therefore difficult to use for comparisons and discovery of discrepancies in ability. Empirical studies support the suggested advantages of using the context of the home environment [14, 19] and to include home visits during hospital stays to increase awareness and motivation as this have been found feasible and beneficial [20]. Thus in the initial phase when the rehabilitation team establishes an empathetic understanding by sharing the individual's account and the team needs to pay specific attention to the individual's awareness of disability and if not present gently guide the person in the discovery process as awareness appears to be a prerequisite for motivation for rehabilitation [17].

14.9 Shared Decisions and Individual Goals

In the next phase of the rehabilitation process, shared decision-making and goal-setting are two cornerstones in individualised rehabilitation. These are constructs of increasing importance in legislation and policy documents in the health service sector. A transition can be detected from a view of the patient as the passive recipient of health services to a respected competent partner and user of health services, informed and updated on knowledge regarding alternative interventions. Studies on shared decision-making have shown that involvement in decisions on care and treatment was associated with the experience of having the own needs of health services met to a larger extent [21].

Goal-setting is widely recognised as a vital part of rehabilitation. Most behaviour is goal-directed and people usually have a reason for their doings. Thus, in individualised rehabilitation, goal-setting performed in partnership based on an empathetic understanding of the individual's situation is thought to increase the person's motivation and to ascertain that the goals are relevant and reachable. This is supported by theories of goal-setting indicating that the goal-performance relationship is strongest when people are committed to the goals [22]. Furthermore, satisfaction with services received appears to increase when people experience that they have been actively taking part in the goal-setting.

The goal-setting in partnership may in addition assist the rehabilitation team to achieve a common understanding and to act together as a team in the interventions. It will furthermore assist in how the monitoring of progresses should be made and how goals or outcomes of interventions could be captured. In line with the overarching goal of rehabilitation presented initially in this chapter reaching a goal will either involve a change or an improvement, or the maintenance or the slowing down of a deterioration of the current situation. A goal should not be a forecast but should be the intended outcome of an intervention performed in the partnership between the person and the rehabilitation team.

To invite and support the individual to take part in the goal-setting might require training and change in behaviour. This was the experience of team members in an individualised rehabilitation intervention in the home environment [14]. Similarly, an empirical study in which occupational therapists were trained to enhance an individualised client-centred rehabilitation approach revealed that indeed the trained therapists did include the individuals in the goal-setting, planning, actions to reach the goals and in the evaluation of goal attainment to a larger extent than therapists who had not received such training [23]. However, there was no difference in outcome between individuals who had received rehabilitation from the trained therapists compared to those who had received training from therapists without such training neither in the short term [24] nor in the long term [25]. Though, family members to the former group unexpectedly had beneficial long-term development of caregiver burden compared to family members in the latter group [26]. A qualitative longitudinal study of the experiences of the family members to individuals who had received rehabilitation from the trained therapists revealed that their partners were self-regulating and in charge of their own rehabilitation process while also supporting their spouses to engage in their own activities [27]. Similar results have been reported in systematic reviews of goal pursuit in rehabilitation where some evidence appear to suggest that goal-setting may improve psychosocial outcomes for adults receiving rehabilitation for acquired disability [28].

There are different ways in which goals can be set. There are at least two components that should be present. The first is that there should be an agreed way to tell if the goals—the intended outcomes—are reached by all members of the rehabilitation team. The second is that it should not be a forecast but a goal that is meaningful to the individual, feasible and attainable given the individual's functioning. Here the expertise of the health professionals can assist the individual in the negotiation of feasible goals and the time needed to achieve them. The use of so called SMART goals has been advocated in rehabilitation, that is specific, measurable, achievable, realistic/relevant and timed goals [29].

14.10 Measures to Capture Individualised Goals and Goal Attainment

There are several established measures that can be used to capture goals and outcomes related to the ICF domains function, activity and participation. In rehabilitation, until recently such measures presented the perspective of the health professionals in the rehabilitation team only. Though, in the last decades, measures presenting outcomes or experiences as perceived by the individual (Patient reported experience measures PREM and Patient reported outcome measures PROM) have been developed and have received much interest. Now PROMs and PREMs are increasingly used and recommended in rehabilitation and research [30].

In addition there are measures that capture and monitor progress in the context of individualised goals [31]. Goal attainment scaling was originally developed for community mental health programmes [32] and then for clinical and healthcare programmes [33]. Goal attainment scaling has been used for the assessment of individualised goal attainment in rehabilitation of people with complex health conditions and found feasible [31, 34]. The Canadian Occupational Performance Measure [35], which was developed for occupational therapy to monitor individualised occupation based goals has also been found to be feasible for monitoring progress and the attainment of individualised goals [31, 36], also for the use by the entire rehabilitation team [37]. A third measure that can capture and monitor individualised goals is the Patient Goal Priority Questionnaire [38], which in comparison is less investigated than the two measures before mentioned.

14.11 How to Meet the Individualised Goals

When goals have been set, the next phase involves planning and implementing interventions to meet the goals that have been agreed upon. Together the individual and the health professionals in the rehabilitation team plan actions to take. Interventions can target one or several of the domains in the ICF framework and can involve regular training sessions together with a therapist, e.g. to improve strength or oxygen uptake, learning activities to increase the individual's own knowledge base, techniques for behavioural changes and self-management related to, e.g. lifestyle, coping with pain, etc. Additionally, in the case of environmental barriers when the environmental demands exceed the individual's capacity, environmental adjustments might be part of the solution, e.g. adaptation of the home or the work environment. Similarly, tools, assistive devices, can be prescribed to improve functioning. These are just a few examples of the actions that might be taken. Moreover, the organisation of how the actions are implemented can vary, e.g. self-directed training can be performed in a dedicated training area but as well in the home environment. It should be emphasised that interventions in individualised rehabilitation are tailored to the individual's needs but not restricted to individual interventions. Indeed, a group intervention, which supported individuals with neck pain to work on own goals, rendered sustainable reductions in disability [39]. Furthermore, there is an increasing use of information and communication technology in rehabilitation services and there are indications that outcomes can be as good as face-to face sessions with a therapist [40]. This opens up new avenues where rehabilitation can be individualised even further as interventions can be tailored both to individual goals and needs and delivered in accordance to individual preferences.

Contemporary information and communication technology calls for an increased awareness of e-health literacy and health literacy [41]. In order to make informed health decisions it is vital for the individual to be able to obtain, understand and use health information, which is defined as health literacy and to be able to seek, find, understand, and appraise health information from electronic sources and apply the knowledge gained to address or solve a health problem, known as eHealth literacy. Some health conditions may render the use of electronic sources particularly difficult and decrease e-health literacy yet the opposite may also be the case, i.e. the use of electronic sources may offer new opportunities and means to perform the desired activities.

14.12   Individualised Rehabilitation and Self

It is not uncommon that people with disabilities refer to their state of health in the light of how life was before the disability was present. In comparison with the state before the disability occurred, it might be hard for the person to see any progress made after the onset of disability. As a consequence, a deterioration of motivation and signs of a depressed mood might appear. Hence it might be useful to apply and support a more flexible approach to self. Theories of psychological flexibility, acceptance and commitment [42] have been shown to be useful in the context of rehabilitation. Supporting psychological flexibility by acceptance and commitment in people with chronic pain was shown to improve their functioning [43]. This approach entails to coach the individual not only to reflect on own behaviour and self in relation to self before the disability but rather to reflect on self and improvements made after the disability.

Another theory that has been shown useful in rehabilitation in regard to behavioural changes and self-management is self-efficacy, which is rooted in social cognitive theory by Bandura [44, 45]. Self-efficacy refers to the individuals' belief in his/her capability to perform a course of action to attain a desired outcome. The theory of self-efficacy suggests that the stronger the individuals' efficacy expectations the more likely they will initiate and persist with a given activity. Hence actions that supply tools for self-management and that boosts self-efficacy are likely to contribute to sustainability of gains made during the rehabilitation and that behavioural changes are maintained over time.

14.13   The Individualised Rehabilitation Process and Transitions in the Care Trajectory

In the contemporary fragmented healthcare, a major challenge for individualised rehabilitation is the threat to the continuity of the rehabilitation process. To develop respect and trust takes time and to start fresh in new contexts is demanding and information may be lost in the transition between caregivers. Effective team work requires openness and mutual respect and the sharing of information and documents between all involved. This calls for the development of strategies to strengthen the individual through the transitions in the continuum between caregivers in the rehabilitation process, and it emphasises the importance of rendering support and coaching of the individual in assuming responsibility for the own rehabilitation process.

References

1. Coran JJ, Koropeckyj-Cox T, Arnold CL. Are physicians and patients in agreement? Exploring dyadic concordance. Health Educ Behav. 2013;40(5):603–11.
2. Tistad M, Ytterberg C, Tham K, et al. Poor concurrence between disabilities as described by patients and established assessment tools three months after stroke: a mixed methods approach. J Neurol Sci. 2012;313(1-2):160–6.
3. Wade DT. Stroke: rehabilitation and long-term care. Lancet. 1992;339(8796):791–3.
4. World Health Organisation. Towards a common language for functioning, disability and health. International classification of functioning, disability and health (ICF). Geneva: WHO; 2001 http://www.who.int/classifications/. Accessed 3 Oct 2017.
5. Engel GL. The need for a new medical model: a challenge for biomedicine. Science. 1977;196(4286):129–36.
6. Wade DT, Halligan PW. The biopsychosocial model of illness: a model whose time has come. Clin Rehabil. 2017;31(8):995–1004.
7. World Health Oragnization. How to use the ICF. A practical manual for using the international classification of functioning, Disability and Health (ICF); 2013. http://www.who.int/classifications/drafticfpracticalmanual.pdf. Accessed 3 Jan 2018.
8. Wade DT, Halligan PW. Do biomedical models of illness make for good healthcare systems? BMJ. 2004;329(7479):1398–401.
9. Antonovsky A. Unraveling the mystery of health: how people manage stress and stay well. San Francisco: Jossey-Bass; 1987.
10. WHO. Milestones in health promotion statements from global conferences, Geneva; 2009. http://www.who.int/healthpromotion/. Accessed 3 Oct 2017.
11. Eriksson M, Lindström B. A salutogenic interpretation of the Ottawa Charter. Health Promot Int. 2008;23(2):190–9.
12. Lorig K, Holman H. Self-management education: history, definition, outcomes, and mechanisms. Ann Behav Med. 2003;26(1):1–7.
13. Wade DT, Smeets RJ, Verbunt JA. Research in rehabilitation medicine: methodological challenges. J Clin Epidemiol. 2010;63(7):699–704.
14. von Koch L, Holmqvist LW, Wottrich AW, et al. Rehabilitation at home after stroke: a descriptive study of an individualized intervention. Clin Rehabil. 2000;14(6):574–83.
15. Rogers C. Significant aspects of client-centered therapy. Class Hist Psychol. 1946;1:415–22.
16. Wang C, Burris M. Photovoice: concept, methodology, and use for participatory needs assessment. Health Educ Behav. 1997;3(3):369–87.
17. Tham K, Borell L, Gustavsson A. The discovery of disability: a phenomenological study of unilateral neglect. Am J Occup Ther. 2000;54(4):398–406.
18. von Koch L, Wottrich AW, Holmqvist LW. Rehabilitation in the home versus the hospital: the importance of context. Disabil Rehabil. 1998;20(10):367–72.
19. Turner B, Fleming J, Ownsworth T, et al. Perceptions of recovery during the early transition phase from hospital to home following acquired brain injury: a journey of discovery. Neuropsychol Rehabil. 2011;21(1):64–91.

20. Rasmussen RS, Ostergaard A, Kjaer P, et al. Stroke rehabilitation at home before and after discharge reduced disability and improved quality of life: a randomised controlled trial. Clin Rehabil. 2016;30(3):225–36.

21. Kristensen HK, Tistad M, von Koch L, et al. The importance of patient involvement in stroke rehabilitation. PLoS One. 2016;11(6):e0157149.

22. Locke EA, Latham GP. Building a practically useful theory of goal setting and task motivation. A 35-year odyssey. Am Psychol. 2002;57(9):705–17.

23. Flink M, Bertilsson AS, Johansson U, et al. Training in client-centeredness enhances occupational therapist documentation on goal setting and client participation in goal setting in the medical records of people with stroke. Clin Rehabil. 2016;30(12):1200–10.

24. Bertilsson AS, Ranner M, von Koch L, et al. A client-centred ADL intervention: three-month follow-up of a randomized controlled trial. Scand J Occup Ther. 2014;21(5):377–91.

25. Guidetti S, Ranner M, Tham K, et al. A "client-centred activities of daily living" intervention for persons with stroke: one-year follow-up of a randomized controlled trial. J Rehabil Med. 2015;47:605–11.

26. Bertilsson AS, Eriksson G, Ekstam L, et al. A cluster randomized controlled trial of a client-centred, activities of daily living intervention for people with stroke: one year follow-up of caregivers. Clin Rehabil. 2016;30(8):765–75.

27. Bertilsson AS, von Koch L, Tham K, Johansson U, et al. Client-centred ADL intervention after stroke: significant others' experiences. Scand J Occup Ther. 2015;22(5):377–86.

28. Levack WM, Weatherall M, Hay-Smith EJ, et al. Goal setting and strategies to enhance goal pursuit for adults with acquired disability participating in rehabilitation. Cochrane Database Syst Rev. 2015;7:CD009727.

29. Bovend'Eerdt TJ, Botell RE, Wade DT. Writing SMART rehabilitation goals and achieving goal attainment scaling: a practical guide. Clin Rehabil. 2009;23(4):352–61.

30. Nelson EC, Eftimovska E, Lind C, et al. Patient reported outcome measures in practice. BMJ. 2015;350:g7818.

31. Doig E, Fleming J, Kuipers P, et al. Clinical utility of the combined use of the Canadian Occupational Performance Measure and Goal Attainment Scaling. Am J Occup Ther. 2010;64(6):904–14.

32. Kiresuk TJ, Sherman RE. Goal attainment scaling: a general method for evaluating comprehensive community mental health programs. Community Ment Health J. 1968;4(6):443–53.

33. Kiresuk TJ, Lund SH, Larsen NE. Measurement of goal attainment in clinical and health care programs. Drug Intell Clin Pharm. 1982;16(2):145–53.

34. Moorhouse P, Theou O, Fay S, et al. Treatment in a Geriatric Day Hospital improve individualized outcome measures using Goal Attainment Scaling. BMC Geriatr. 2017;17(1):9.

35. Law M, Baptiste S, McColl M, et al. The Canadian occupational performance measure: an outcome measure for occupational therapy. Can J Occup Ther. 1990;57(2):82–7.

36. Law M, Polatajko H, Pollock N, et al. Pilot testing of the Canadian Occupational Performance Measure: clinical and measurement issues. Can J Occup Ther. 1994;61(4):191–7.

37. Yang SY, Lin CY, Lee YC, et al. The Canadian occupational performance measure for patients with stroke: a systematic review. J Phys Ther Sci. 2017;29(3):548–55.

38. Asenlof P, Siljeback K. The Patient Goal Priority Questionnaire is moderately reproducible in people with persistent musculoskeletal pain. Phys Ther. 2009;89(11):1226–34.

39. Gustavsson C, von Koch L. A 9-year follow-up of a self-management group intervention for persistent neck pain in primary health care: a randomized controlled trial. J Pain Res. 2017;10:53–64.

40. Bring A, Asenlof P, Soderlund A. What is the comparative effectiveness of current standard treatment, against an individually tailored behavioural programme delivered either on the Internet or face-to-face for people with acute whiplash associated disorder? A randomized controlled trial. Clin Rehabil. 2016;30(5):441–53.

41. Kim H, Xie B. Health literacy in the eHealth era: a systematic review of the literature. Patient Educ Couns. 2017;100(6):1073–82.
42. Hayes SC, Strosahl KD, Wilson KG. Acceptance and commitment therapy: an experiential approach to behavior change. New York: Guilford Press; 1999.
43. Yu L, Norton S, McCracken LM. Change in "Self-as-Context" ("Perspective-Taking") occurs in acceptance and commitment therapy for people with chronic pain and is associated with improved functioning. J Pain. 2017;18(6):664–72.
44. Bandura A. Self-efficacy: toward a unifying theory of behavioural change. Psychol Rev. 1977;84:191–215.
45. Bandura A, Adams NE, Beyer J. Cognitive processes mediating behavioral change. J Pers Soc Psychol. 1977;35(3):125–39.

Individual's Foot Health

15

Minna Stolt

Abstract

Feet are a part of the human body that allows daily movement and functioning. Feet are considered intimate, and ethical aspects related to them are rarely investigated. This chapter describes ethical issues from the perspective of the individual in the context of foot health care. The foot-related ethical issues are approached from the perspectives of individuality and availability of services. This chapter will also highlight the meanings and values how individuals experience their own foot health. Some long-term health problems, such as rheumatoid arthritis or diabetes mellitus, cause foot disorders that change normal foot structure. Therefore individual's body image and aesthetic perspective are discussed.

Keywords

Foot health · Individuality · Ethical issues

15.1 Introduction

Healthy feet make walking and living an active life possible. The main features of healthy feet are straight toes, neutral heel position, good condition of the skin and nails, and the absence of foot pain. Despite the fundamental importance of feet, they are often taken for granted, and their care remains on poor or at most satisfactory level. Related to foot self-care and professional care, there are several ethical issues that are rarely in the focus of interest. Issues such as individuality, access to care,

M. Stolt

Department of Nursing Science, University of Turku, Turku, Finland

e-mail: minna.stolt@utu.fi

coping with decreasing foot health and body image are common ethical issues identified from recent foot-related literature and research. Ethical issues in foot care do not differ from other health-care sectors or areas. However, these issues are seldom studied and infrequently brought up in discussion.

15.2 Individuality

All humans have individual footprints and their own kind of way of walking [1]. The footprints can change, however, due to reasons such as self-care habits, occupational circumstances, and physical loadings and long-term diseases. Long-term diseases such as rheumatoid arthritis [2, 3], diabetes mellitus [4] and psoriasis [5] affect the foot, causing significant visible changes. Foot self-care is one method to prevent and promote foot health. However, individuals have different kinds of resources to care for their own feet. One may need help with putting on socks, while another needs support in cutting the nails or creaming the skin of the foot. In all, individual resources need to be taken into account while educating patients in foot self-care.

15.2.1 Foot Problems Have Individual Effects on One's Life

Foot problems affect each person individually. Firth et al. [6] investigated how foot ulceration impacted on patients' daily life. They found that patients' health-related quality of life in three domains (physical, social and psychological) was decreased. In addition, as the ulcer was in the foot, it caused pain and walking disability. Together, both pain and walking disability led to limitations to take care of household tasks and independent personal hygiene and care. Related to ulcer care itself, the patients found it very problematic to keep the ulcer dry during daily activities and personal hygiene. Due to foot ulceration, they needed to change their footwear and clothing style, which directly affected their self-esteem and body image. Decreased walking activities and footwear restrictions led to changes in social participation. Psychologically, foot ulceration caused low mood, depression and frustration. In addition, more concerns were caused by the financial costs related to ulcer care and footwear alterations or modifications [6].

As an example, the aforementioned patient experience gives an extensive overview of how a problem in the foot can have a comprehensive effect on a person's physical, psychological and social interactions. When caring for people with foot problems, it is essential to identify and support their needs on a large scale. A partnership model where a professional has an equal position towards the patient has been observed to be the most appropriate, leading to desired outcomes ([7], p. 319). During the patient contact or appointment, sufficient time to discuss with the patient is needed. There is some evidence that patients with foot problems tend to suffer with their foot problems, failing to report them or identify them as medical problems that may be cared for by health-care professionals [8, 9]. Patients might thus benefit from an individual approach during nurse/physician/podiatrist appointments where the focus is on foot health. Professionals could use validated instruments to identify their patients' foot problems (e.g. foot health assessment instrument [10]) and their impact on daily life (Foot Health Status Questionnaire [11]).

15.3   Body Image

Body image refers to internal understanding of individual's appearance comprising attitudes, perceptions and behaviours [12, 13]. A long-term health condition, such as rheumatoid arthritis, changes the body in many ways. These changes are often visible. Related to feet, rheumatoid arthritis causes toe deformities, overlapping toes and changes in the foot arch shape and position of the heel, leading to a situation where the appearance of the feet is different compared to the normal feet. These changes in the feet cause negative feelings in the patient, such as shame, despair and embarrassment [9]. These feelings are related to individual's body image. Individuals have a certain perception of a healthy or normal body and its parts. However, among patients with long-term diseases, their body image does not often correspond with the reality [14, 15]. This causes negative feelings for them and feelings of being visibly different from healthy individuals. For example, persons with lower limb amputations have lower body image and quality of life [14].

15.3.1 Footwear as Part of Body Image

In the same way as clothing or accessories, footwear is part of body image and demonstrates social status [16]. Proper footwear produces happy feelings and has a positive impact on self-esteem [17]. However, rheumatoid arthritis causes significant disorders in the feet, leading to a situation where normal retail footwear is no longer suitable. In addition, finding suitable footwear is often hard for patients [18]. Therefore, therapeutic footwear is often recommended to support safe and painless mobility and to prevent new foot problems from occurring [19]. Despite the benefits of therapeutic footwear, only a minority of patients wear them on a regular basis.

Finding appropriate footwear can cause significant problems for patients with foot problems in terms of suitability, look (body image) and availability. The reasons for non-adherence to wearing therapeutic footwear can be several. One major factor is the limited selection and the appearance of therapeutic footwear [6]. Patients with foot problems are usually knowledgeable as to what kind of properties of footwear should have to fit their feet. This knowledge relates to their understanding of their own body and body image. However, these properties are not often met. Footwear that does not comply with aesthetic values and fashion can easily limit patients' clothing choices [20]. Unaesthetic footwear can change their body image and, especially among females, change their femininity [21]. Females feel that unattractive footwear decreases the enjoyment of wearing different clothes which match their individual look [20]. Footwear is something that everyone can see; when using therapeutic footwear, people feel that it is a symbol of health problems [22]. For example, despite the bodily changes caused by rheumatoid arthritis and the benefits of proper footwear, some patients choose to wear footwear that follows current fashion trends. With footwear, they show their social status, which improves their self-image and self-presentation [16].

Therapeutic footwear is beneficial only when used regularly. However, patients often find the therapeutic footwear unattractive, giving rise to negative feelings like sadness, shame and anger [21, 23] and a feeling of being stigmatised [24]. Silvester et al. [18] reported that only 5% of patients with rheumatoid arthritis used the prescribed footwear, while the majority preferred to comply with fashion [18]. Therapeutic footwear is often larger in size than normal footwear (due to modifications made for foot/toe disorders), and the colour selection is limited [21]. Moreover, the price of therapeutic footwear is high [19, 25]. Footwear is part of individuality and body image, especially for females [21, 23]. Outfit choice is the most important factor for female patients when they select a new pair of footwear [16, 17]. These aspects need to be taken into account when designing and recommending therapeutic footwear to patients with foot problems. Some long-term health conditions, such as rheumatoid arthritis and diabetes mellitus, change the shape of the foot continuously [22]; a patient might thus need many pairs of therapeutic footwear within a short time period. Discussion about the manufacturing costs and finding potential funders is needed to support patients to comply with the footwear.

15.4   Availability of Services

Patients with long-term health conditions often consider that they have inadequate care for their health problems. This might be partly explained by the complex nature and bodily consequences of long-term health conditions. From professionals' perspective, the problems that the patients consider the most disabling might be the ones requiring the least care, and vice versa. To overcome these discrepancies, it is essential to give and share information about long-term health conditions and educate patients to take care of themselves according to their own abilities and resources. Individualised foot care education, tailored for patients' foot health needs and adjusted by their resources, led to significant changes in foot care knowledge, foot self-care activities and confidence to care for own feet among home care patients with diabetes [26].

Access to care for people with foot problems is diverse. Current foot care services have predominantly focused on caring for foot problems in people with rheumatoid arthritis and diabetes. Although the importance of foot care services for patients is widely acknowledged, there are difficulties worldwide to organise timely care for people with foot problems [25, 27]. Patients often feel that health-care professionals ignore their foot problems [28, 29], and only a minority of patients feel that they have access to appropriate foot care specialist [27]. This lack of interest towards foot care may have several reasons:

1. Lack of knowledge to identify foot problems [28]
2. Lack of a suitable foot health-care provider to refer the patient to, such as a podiatrist [25, 29]
3. Prioritisation of patient's other health concerns before foot problems [25]

All these potential reasons for ignoring patient's foot health problems are manageable. Providing the best possible care and responding to patients' foot health needs call for a patient-centred and foot-oriented approach where the patient with foot problems is in the focus, and tailored care is provided to manage often multifaceted foot health problems. For patients with rheumatoid arthritis, Blake et al. [8] have suggested a three-way model where patients, members of the rheumatology team and podiatrists all identify the foot problems of the patient to support their early care and functional ability.

Individual foot care education interventions, as described above, are needed to support patients' knowledge and activities in foot self-care. Adequate foot self-care can alleviate existing foot problems and prevent new ones from occurring. This could lead to a reduction in health-care costs [30] and improvement in patients' quality of life [31] when they feel that they can promote their own foot health.

15.5 Fear of Coping with Decreasing Foot Health

Foot health is not a stable status. It can change along with ageing, foot self-care, way of life and health status. Especially older persons are worried about how they will cope when their foot health decreases. When foot problems are related to certain long-term health conditions such as diabetes mellitus or rheumatoid arthritis, all other health issues are discussed more frequently than foot problems during physical appointments. Despite this, foot problems cause significant deficiencies and trouble in patients' daily lives. Because of foot problems, the patients must modify their daily activities and coping strategies to be able to live as active a life as possible. Due to these modifications, they are afraid of how they can cope in the future with decreasing foot health [9].

Despite these strong concerns, patients rarely report their foot problems [8]. They find the look of their feet irritating and sometimes ugly [23] and are not willing to show their feet. They are also unsure who to contact [25]. They only mention the problems when they consider that the situation is unbearable. Foot health status is not stable, it changes; when having a physician's appointment, the foot problems may not be evident and thus remain unassessed. Instead, the patients try to do everything they can by themselves. They seek information from the Internet, colleagues and friends. Using this information, they try to self-diagnose and self-care for their feet [9]. However, the information received and gathered is often incorrect, nonevidence based and outdated [32]. Using this kind of information leads to inadequate self-care activities and, in many cases, to more complications rather than healthy outcomes.

Conclusions

Several ethical issues related to foot health care can be identified. Individuality and body image are central aspects when caring for patients with foot problems. Individuality could be supported by assessing patients' foot health regularly and asking patients about the influence of their feet on their daily life. Many persons with long-term health conditions are active and try to manage with daily activities despite having foot problems. However, patients experience foot problems and bodily changes differently, which is why the discussion about ethical issues in foot health care needs to continue, and ethical sensitivity to reporting and bringing the issues to public awareness must be encouraged.

References

1. Tsung BYS, Zhang M, Fan YB, et al. Quantitative comparison of plantar foot shapes under different weight bearing conditions. J Rehabil Res Dev. 2003;40(6):517–26.
2. Graham AS, Stephenson J, Williams AE. A survey of people with foot problems related to rheumatoid arthritis and their educational needs. J Foot Ankle Res. 2017;10:12. https://doi.org/10.1186/s13047-017-0193-6. eCollection 2017.
3. Stolt M, Suhonen R, Leino-Kilpi H. Foot health in patients with rheumatoid arthritis – a scoping review. Rheumatol Int. 2017;37(9):1413–22.
4. Allan J, Munro W, Figgins E. Foot deformities within the diabetic foot and their influence on biomechanics: a review of the literature. Prosthetics Orthot Int. 2016;40(2):182–92.
5. Bezza A, Niamane R, Amine B. Involvement of the foot in patients with psoriatic arthritis. A review of 26 cases. Joint Bone Spine. 2004;71(6):546–9.
6. Firth J, Nelson E, Briggs M, et al. A qualitative study to explore the impact of foot ulceration on health-related quality of life in patients with rheumatoid arthritis. Int J Nurs Stud. 2011;48(11):1401–8.
7. Loewy EEH. Textbook of healthcare ethics. Dordrecht: Springer; 2005.
8. Blake A, Mandy PJ, Stew G. Factors influencing the patient with rheumatoid arthritis in their decision to seek podiatry. Musculoskeletal Care. 2013;11(4):218–28.
9. Williams AE, Blake A, Cherry L, et al. Patients' experiences of lupus-related foot problems: a qualitative investigation. Lupus. 2017;26(11):1174–81.
10. Stolt M, Suhonen R, Puukka P, et al. Development process and psychometric testing of foot health assessment instrument. J Clin Nurs. 2013;22(9-10):1310–21.
11. Bennett PJ, Patterson C, Wearing S, et al. Development and validation of a questionnaire designed to measure foot-health status. J Am Podiatr Med Assoc. 1998;88(9):419–28.
12. Grogan S. Body image: understanding body dissatisfaction in men, women, and children. 2nd ed. New York: Routledge/Taylor & Francis Group; 2008.
13. Watson B, Fuller-Tyszkiewicz M, Broadbent J, et al. The meaning of body image experiences during the perinatal period: a systematic review of the qualitative literature. Body Image. 2015;14:102–13.
14. Holzer LA, Sevelda F, Fraberger G, et al. Body image and self-esteem in lower-limb amputees. PLoS One. 2014;9:e92943. https://doi.org/10.1371/journal.pone.0092943.
15. Salome GM, de Almeida SA, de Jesus Pereira MT, et al. The impact of venous leg ulcers on body image and self-esteem. Adv Skin Wound Care. 2016;29(7):316–21.
16. Goodacre LJ, Candy FJ. 'If I didn't have RA I wouldn't give them house room': the relationship between RA, footwear and clothing choices. Rheumatology. 2011;50(3):513–7.
17. Branthwaite H, Chockalingam N, Grogan S, et al. Footwear choices made by young women and their potential impact on foot health. J Health Psychol. 2012;18(11):1422–31.

18. Silvester RN, Williams AE, Dalbeth N, et al. Choosing shoes: a preliminary study into the challenges facing clinicians in assessing footwear for rheumatoid arthritis patients. J Foot Ankle Res. 2010;4(43):S1.
19. Hendry GJ, Brenton-Rule A, Barr G, et al. Footwear experiences of people with chronic musculoskeletal diseases. Arthritis Care Res. 2015;67(8):1164–72.
20. Tiggemann M, Andrew R. Clothing choices, weight, and trait self-objectification. Body Image. 2012;9(3):409–12.
21. Naidoo S, Anderson S, Mills J, et al. "I could cry, the amount of shoes I can't get into": a qualitative exploration of the factors that influence retail footwear selection in women with rheumatoid arthritis. J Foot Ankle Res. 2011;4:21. https://doi.org/10.1186/1757-1146-4-21.
22. Johnson M, Newton P, Goyder E. Patient and professional perspectives on prescribed therapeutic footwear for people with diabetes: a vignette study. Pat Educ Counsel. 2006;64(1):167–72.
23. Williams AE, Nester CJ, Ravey MI. Rheumatoid arthritis patients' experiences of wearing therapeutic footwear – a qualitative investigation. BMC Musculoskelet Disord. 2007;8:104. https://doi.org/10.1186/1471-2474-8-104.
24. Williams AE, Nester CJ, Ravey MI, et al. Women's experiences of wearing therapeutic footwear in three European countries. J Foot Ankle Res. 2010;3:23. https://doi.org/10.1186/1757-1146-3-23.
25. Hendry GJ, Gibson KA, Pile K, et al. "They just scraped off the calluses": a mixed methods exploration of foot care access and provision for people with rheumatoid arthritis in South-Western Sydney, Australia. J Foot Ankle Res. 2013;6(1):34. https://doi.org/10.1186/1757-1146-6-34.
26. Neder S, Nadash P. Individualized education can improve foot care for patients with diabetes. Home Healthc Nurse. 2003;21(12):837–40.
27. Juarez M, Price E, Collins D, et al. Deficiencies in provision of integrated multidisciplinary podiatry care for patients with inflammatory arthritis: a UK district general hospital experience. Foot. 2010;20(1):71–4.
28. Graham AS, Williams AE. Foot health education for people with rheumatoid arthritis: '…. A game of chance…' – A survey of patients' experiences. Musculoskeletal Care. 2016;14(1):37–46.
29. Williams AE, Graham AS. 'My feet: visible, but ignored…' A qualitative study of foot care for people with rheumatoid arthritis. Clin Rehabil. 2012;26(10):952–9.
30. Prezio EA, Pagán JA, Shuval K, et al. The Community Diabetes Education (CoDE) program: cost-effectiveness and health outcomes. Am J Prev Med. 2014;47(6):771–9.
31. Nabuurs-Franssen MH, Huijberts MSP, Nieuwenhuijzen Kruseman AC, et al. Health-related quality of life of diabetic foot ulcer patients and their caregivers. Diabetologia. 2005;48(9):1906–10.
32. Abedin T, Ahmed S, Al Mamun M, et al. YouTube as a source of useful information on diabetes foot care. Diabetes Res Clin Pract. 2015;110:e1–4.

Individualised Care and Related Concepts

16

Evridiki Papastavrou

Abstract

The aim of this chapter is to describe and analyse significant evidence of individualised care as related to other concepts, such as care and caring behaviours, patient participation in care, patient satisfaction, nurse satisfaction, patient autonomy, patient empowerment and quality of life. This chapter is based mainly on the results of two international research projects (Care and Individualised Care Projects) that have explored individualised care in relation with caring behaviours and patient satisfaction. Patients were asked to give their own opinion of what they mean by individualised care as well as their experience about the care they received, whether they felt that it was actually individualised according to their own needs and preferences. The results provided evidence that patients and nurses have different perceptions of individualised care, suggesting that both patients' and nurses' evaluations are needed to deliver care according to each individual patient's needs, experiences, behaviours, feelings and perceptions. Other relations are also discussed through smaller-scale studies performed in different countries which underline the internationality and the challenges of exploring the individualised care concept. This chapter could provide useful information to nursing managers and policymakers on introducing nursing approaches and practices based on individualised care so as to improve quality of care, enhance patient dignity, keep people safe and consequently increase patients' satisfaction.

Keywords

Individualised care · Caring behaviour · Satisfaction · Participation

E. Papastavrou
School of Health Sciences, Department of Nursing, Cyprus University
of Technology, Limassol, Cyprus
e-mail: e.papastavrou@cut.ac.cy

16.1   Introduction

Individualised care and caring are both terms found in almost all nursing documents, scientific or not, and despite their widespread use, they are poorly understood, and the relationship between them is unclear but at the same time is synonymous. Caring is a complex phenomenon that although is believed to be in the heart of nursing and is the core construct of many nursing theories, the concept is still not well understood, and there is no consensus of the meaning among the members of the scientific community. The caring literature proposes an operational definition of "caring behaviours" to facilitate the description and measurement of what nurses perceive and what they do, as well as what patients perceive, as caring. Whatever the accepted definition or conceptual framework, a common element of almost every explanation or analysis is that care is:

> the response to the needs of the individual and that care is to recognise patients as unique individuals with unique qualities, experiences and perspectives that are valued and respected.

Aiming to facilitate understanding of related concepts, Finfgeld-Connett [1], although she does not mention the term "individualised care", in her analysis focuses on individual differences and that through care each individual is viewed through the lens of unconditional positive regard and respect. It is clear therefore that care and individualised care are handled as synonymous terms. Respect of individuality is also an important issue stated in contemporary international professional codes of nursing (e.g. The ICN Code of Ethics for Nurses) as well as national. For example, the American Nurses Association (ANA) [2] states clearly that:

> The nurse plans and individualizes care to allow the person to live with as much physical, spiritual, social, and emotional well-being as possible.

According to Gallagher et al. [3], there is a strong theoretical and philosophical base that justifies the provision of individualised care, and much of what is described as contributing to dignity in care could be grouped under the heading of *individualised care*. Other benefits of individualised care include the empirical evidence of positive impact on patient outcomes such as increased satisfaction with nursing care, perceived autonomy and health-related quality of life [4]. Decisional control is another concept that although it has multiple definitions, in nursing, is considered as an important aspect of individualised care and the interaction of the nurse with the patient as a unique individual [5]. However, there is evidence of limited agreement between the perceptions of patients and the perceptions of nurses that care is delivered according to individual needs of patients, and there are differences of opinion on which behaviours convey caring [6] and to what degree the patient is involved in the planning and implementation of care.

The aim of this chapter is to describe and analyse relevant evidence of individualised care as related to similar concepts through the results of two international research projects (Care Project and Individualised Care Projects) that have explored individualised care in relation with caring behaviours, decisional control and patient satisfaction. Patients and nurses from several European countries (and one state from the USA) participated in the studies, and the results showed that the associations between caring behaviours and individualised care for both patients and nurses are positive and significant. Similarly, the results confirmed strong positive correlation between individualised care and patient satisfaction, and actually 45% of the variance in patient satisfaction is explained by the delivery of care that is according to the patients' individual needs. This chapter could provide useful information to nursing managers and policymakers on introducing nursing approaches and practices to care that would improve quality of care, enhance dignity, keep people safe and consequently increase patients' satisfaction.

16.2 Individualised Care and Caring Behaviours

Although care and individualised care are both ubiquitous terms [7], for the purpose of the above study, it was decided to explore them as two different concepts. However, although this could be possible in terms of the research tools used, that is, one measuring individualised care and the other measuring caring behaviours, it was difficult to make a distinction between the two concepts. The most interesting observation in searching for the definition or analysis of the concept of care and caring is that although not explicitly, nursing scholars argue about recognising individual differences, and individualised care needs to ensure the maintenance of respect and integrity in the caring process. The empirical evidence on caring also revealed a wide range of caring behaviours in meeting biopsychosocial and spiritual needs of patients and their families and most emphasises the importance of providing care that is specifically tailored to individual needs following comprehensive health assessment.

A significant influence in the conceptualisation of care comes from the work of McCance and McCormack [8] in their analysis of the concept of care and their subsequent work on the concept of person-centred care. Following the Donabedian's model of structure-process-outcome in analysing care [9, 10], described nurses' attributes as their professional competence, interpersonal skills, commitment to the job and personal, as the structural elements of care including also organisational issues and patient attributes. The processes of care covered a wide range of nursing activities that constituted caring as perceived by patients and included providing for patients' physical needs and psychological needs such as providing information, reassurance, communicating and showing concern, as well as being attentive, getting to know the patient, taking time, being firm, showing respect and the extra touch. The outcomes emanated from the process of caring and included a feeling of emotional and physical well-being and patient satisfaction. In their later work, the authors [11, 12] combined original conceptual frameworks against the person-centred nursing, existing caring literature and focus groups with practitioners to develop a framework of person-centred nursing, underlining that with the emergence of a biopsychosocial approach to person-centred care, nurses are expected to meet the *individual needs* of clients and families.

An essential concept in person-centred nursing care rests on the individualisation of the patient and his/her care as well as respect of the individuality of each patient [13]. In the nursing literature, "individualised care" is described as an essential element of nursing, and the term shared similar conceptual and philosophical directions as "person-centred care". Suhonen et al. [13] in a review of the literature found that there is a limited and incoherent perception of the concept and that definitions are not sufficiently comprehensive to allow for a detailed analysis of the content of the concept. The review has demonstrated that individualised care has become an important concept in philosophical, ethical and empirical nursing research, but it also revealed that patients do not seem to feel they have received individualised care or that they have been treated as individuals. In a following review, the same authors [14], aiming to describe the driving and restraining forces that promote and impede the implementation of individualised nursing care, identified the different understanding of the concept. This is complicated by the nurses' and patients' individual characteristics as well as the work environment provided by the organization. These include structural issues, staffing, the organisation of work, teamwork leadership and management, which are the most frequently stated forces that may hinder the implementation of individualised care.

Many of these issues were explored in the Care Project, designed to explore patients' and nurses' perceptions and experiences of care, individualised care and the professional practice environment in which care is delivered [4, 15]. The Care Project started in 2009 aiming to compare patients' and nurses' perceptions of caring behaviours and individualised care within the environment of care. The study employed a descriptive, comparative study design, and the data were collected from patients admitted to surgical wards and their nurses in five countries: Cyprus, the Czech Republic, Finland, Greece and Hungary. Data were collected from 1659 patients and 1195 nurses from 88 general surgical inpatient wards in 34 hospitals. The hospitals included in the study were chosen based on the specific characteristics and policies of each research partner's health system, the access, proximity and convenience of use. The results from comparing nurses' and patients' views are as follows.

16.2.1 A Comparison of Patients' and Nurses' Perceptions of Caring Behaviours

Patients' and nurses' perceptions were compared according to their responses to the categories of questions of the caring behaviours inventory (CBI). A factor analysis of the CBI resulted in four categories of questions, namely, the (a) knowledge and skills, (b) assurance of human presence, (c) respectful deference to others and (d) patient connection. The highest means of the patients and the nurses, as well as agreement, was observed in the category of questions related to "knowledge and skills". However, independent sample t-tests showed that there were important differences in the first (assurance of human presence, $p < 0.001$) and third category of questions (respectful deference to others, $p < 0.001$), where the nurses' responses had higher means (more answers, towards agree/strongly agree) compared to that of the patients'. For the comparisons between nurses and patients for each country separately, independent sample t-tests showed that important differences between the mean values of patients and nurses and for the whole scale were only observed in Cyprus and the Czech Republic. In both cases, the nurses' means were higher compared to those of the patients.

16.2.2 A Comparison of Patients' and Nurses' Perceptions of Individualised Care

As regards the support of individuality (ICS-A), Cypriot patients gave the highest assessment about the support of patient individuality through nursing activities (ICS-A), and Greek patients gave the lowest. Regarding the ICS-A for nurses, Hungarian nurses assessed that they supported patient individuality through nursing activities well, while Greek nurses gave the lowest assessments. Independent sample t-test showed differences between patients' and nurses' perceptions of the support of patient individuality in each participating country ($p < 0.01$). As regards perceptions of individuality in the care received (ICS-B), patients assessed that the care they received was individualised. Again, Cypriot patients gave the highest assessments, and the Greek patients gave the lowest. In relation to the nurses assessments of the individuality in the care provided, the Hungarian nurses gave the highest assessments about the maintenance of individuality in the care they provided for their patients, while the Greek nurses gave the lowest assessments. In the ICS-B scale, the patients' and nurses' assessments differed significantly in the Czech Republic, Greece and Hungary. In Finland and Cyprus, patients' and nurses' assessments were very similar.

16.2.3 Comparison of Caring Behaviours with Individualised Care

As it is supported by the theoretical literature, another hypothesis of our study was that caring behaviours are related to individualised care, so further tests were done to see if there is a significant positive relationship between these two concepts. The results showed that there is a significant positive relationship between individualised care and caring behaviours as perceived by patients of the whole sample of the study. Similar results were obtained for nurses, which imply a significant positive relation between the perception of caring and caring behaviour of nurses.

This study provided some evidence that individualised care is an integral part of care and that each caring behaviour needs to be tailored according to the individual needs of each patient, adding to the theoretical understanding of caring literature. The results demonstrated that patients and nurses perceived knowledge and skill as the most important aspect of caring behaviours, and this is in agreement with the previous studies supporting that patients evaluate nursing work on the technical aspects of care and professional knowledge [16–20]. Significantly different opinions between patients and nurses were observed in the category "assurance of human presence" [4]. Nursing presence is a concept representative of caring behaviours and a holistic approach to caring in which the nurse encounters the patient as a unique human being in a unique situation and chooses to "'spend' herself on his behalf" [21, 22]. Caring and human presence have many overlapping components in the sense that they both appear to involve interpersonal sensitivity, expert nursing practice and an intimate reciprocal relationship between the patient and the nurse [1]. The category "assurance of human presence" is containing items like "visiting the patient, communicating, encouraging calling, responding to patients calls", and they were given lower ratings by patients compared to nurses [4]. This finding adds to the debate about the difficulties in defining abstract concepts in nursing, the unarticulated similarities among the concepts and failure of the profession to offer the clarity that would facilitate moral thinking and a behaviour that conveys caring and most importantly that is received by the patients as caring. Similarly, the results of the Care Project revealed that there is a clear trend that nurses tend to think that the care they provide is individualised more often than their patients, supporting earlier studies in other topics (e.g. [23–25]). Nurses' higher assessments about individualised care may be attributed to their attitudes to their work, which has been associated with a high morality and the recognition of individuality [26]. In contrast, some nurses may think that care is individualised per se because patients are cared for one at a time. The discrepancy between nurses' and patients' evaluations about the same situation (e.g. [24, 27–30]) does indicate that patients and nurses have different perceptions about healthcare practice.

The cross-country comparison, as expected, revealed many between-country differences which correspond to the results of previous international studies [31–33], and these differences were found mainly on a north–south European axis. It is possible to speculate that these differences may be attributed to organisational factors, different healthcare systems and models of nursing care delivery, different aspects of education and training and cultural differences concerned with prevailing values in the society [32]. Therefore, in addition to the comparative findings, it is necessary for the results to be explained in the context of each country considering political and social atmosphere as well as the different constraints in the practice of nursing and the ideologies and philosophical positions of nurse education.

16.3   Individualised Care and Participation in Decision-Making

Involving patients and citizens in decision-making, recognising they are individuals with their own unique values and preferences, is an important element of care that is promoted in many countries at all the levels of care [34]. Decisional control is embedded in individualised care and means the ability or the power to decide what will be ones' involvement in healthcare decisions [5], and it includes encouragement of the patient to take on responsibilities and control by providing options to choose from and decide on. All definitions recognise client's individuality and need for individualised care that is tailored to suit the patient's preferences as an important aspect of patient participation in nursing care [35]. Patients have decisional control over their care when the individual has expectations of having the power to participate in making decisions to obtain desirable consequences [14]. Thus to practise decisional control, patients usually perform participation activities that are dependent on the level of their characteristics, abilities, readiness and willingness to participate. The benefits of decisional control include better coping with treatment emotions like anxiety and distress, better functional ability, greater satisfaction with care and adherence to treatment recommendations and may influence biomedical outcomes [36].

Tobiano and colleagues [37] in a published integrative review of literature regarding patient participation in nursing care on medical wards found that patients and nurses desire, perceive or enact patient participation passively. Challenging factors for patient participation include patients' willingness and nurses' approach and confusion around expectations and roles. More recently, in a qualitative study, it was found that nurses described their experience of patient participation when they listened to and engaged patients and when they relinquished responsibility and shared power with patients [38].

In our study, decisional control over care was explored as a part of the individualised care, and the results revealed that there are statistically significant differences in perceptions between patients and nurses in all the items of decisional control. The results showed that there are significant differences in the perceptions of patients and nurses in almost all countries regarding all items of the decisional control factor of the ICS-B. More specifically, nurses in all countries reported significantly higher agreement values in ICS-B 14, meaning they perceive that they took into account patients' wishes about their care, but patients do not agree to that ($p < 0.001$). This inconsistency between nurses' and patients' perception of agreement on decisional control remains for the item ICS-B 15 regarding patient participation concerning their care ($p < 0.001$), for item ICS-B 16 relating to the opinions expressed by the patients and the extent to which they were taken into consideration ($p < 0.001$) as well as for the item ICS-B 17 concerning patients' opportunity to make their own decisions on when to wash ($p < 0.001$). For the item ICS-B 17 regarding own decisions on when to wash, patients in all countries reported higher agreement than nurses, and for ICS-B 12 concerning following instructions, patients' reported again higher agreement with the exception of patients in two countries.

The results revealed a lack of understanding and agreement between patients' and nurses' perceptions regarding patients' decisional control over their care, showing that patients do not feel that they are active partners in their own care. However, it remains unclear if this disparity is a result of miscommunication, passivity on behalf of patients or time constraints due to shortage of staff or increased workload. The difference found between the countries that participated concerning patients' as well as nurses' perceptions also supports that decisional control may be influenced by each country's cultural, political, historical and ethnic variations supporting previous research [39].

Our findings are also similar to Florin [23] who found that patients held different views of preferred level of participation and that nurses failed to assess individual patient preferences, adopting rhetoric to patient preferences but not actually involving them in decision-making according to their own perceptions. In this sense decisional control refers to the hypothetical power struggle where healthcare providers in their traditional roles may believe that they know what is best for patients and so retain total decisional control [5]. However, nurses' role is challenging, having to balance patient participation with issues related to patient readiness, safety and complexities of care including nurses' role and expectations. The results of our study may also highlight the great variation in the organisation of surgical care procedures and care in different European countries and highlight the differences in patient experiences of hospital care received in the different hospital systems and the outcomes of care [20, 40] which may also reflect differences in care processes and protocols. Using this information across international boundaries may help to standardise surgical care procedures and nursing care, increasing their transparency between countries and developing international concepts of best practice. However, the aim for person-centred and individualised healthcare services urges that the procedures be flexible and to be adopted and tailored according to individual preferences and characteristics where patient empowerment and independence is of vital importance [41].

16.4   The Patient Outcomes of Individualised Care: Patient Satisfaction, Patient Autonomy and Patient's Health-Related Quality of Life

This section describes the associations of individualised care with selected outcomes, such as patient and nurse satisfaction, patient autonomy and patient health-related quality of life. These outcomes were examined in three different studies, two of them were international through the Care Project [42] and the Individualised Care Project and the other in surgical wards in Finland [43]. The individualised care scale (ICS-A and ICS-B) was used in all studies.

16.4.1 Individualised Care and Patient Satisfaction

Patient satisfaction is a key indicator of quality of care, and the nurse-patient relationship heavily influences patients' satisfaction since nurses spend most of their time providing bedside care. An integrative review of the literature on hospitalised patients' satisfaction with nursing care [44] indicated that patients were highly satisfied with the nurses' level of knowledge and technical skills, especially when the nurses were caring and exhibited good interpersonal skills. However, the results also revealed patients' negative experiences related to the provision of inadequate information provided by nurses such as patient education, treatment plan and pain management as well as inadequate response to patients' needs.

Patient satisfaction as an outcome of individualised care was examined within the framework of the International Care project with the participation of patients from five different European countries [42]. Although there is some evidence of this association, the study assumed a relationship between individualised care and patient satisfaction and aimed to examine this in a broader international level. Data were collected from 72 inpatient wards in 26 general acute hospitals in 5 EU countries, and 1315 questionnaires were eligible for analysis giving a final response of 78%. The measures used included the ICS-A and the ICS-B that examine support of the individualised care (ICS-A) and perceptions in individuality on care (ICS-B). Patient satisfaction was measured with the patient satisfaction scale (PSS), consisting of the following components: technical-scientific, information and interaction/support.

The results showed that surgical patients were satisfied with the care with the highest scores achieved in the technical qualities of care component and the lowest, least satisfied, were with the information care needs. Pearson's correlation coefficients were calculated to define the relationship between the patient satisfaction scale (PSS) and each of the subscales of the individualised care scale (ICS-B) to determine the existence, type and strength of the associations. All the subscales of the ICS-B were significantly related to the PSS, when considered individually, meaning that respondents' perceptions of the maintenance of individualised care are highly positively associated with their satisfaction with nursing care. The predictive ability of the factors of ICS-B showed that patients' perceptions of individualised care explained 45% of the variance in patient satisfaction, and within these perceptions surgical patients were mostly satisfied with the technical qualities of care and least satisfied with the level of information delivered. This finding might demonstrate that technical skills taught in the many kinds of nursing schools are at a similar level and are recognised as such by patients being cared for in different European countries. In contrast, abilities in meeting the informational needs of patients may vary according to the clinical and educational conditions in the participating countries. This difference is important as it has been reported that patients with adequate information become more involved in their own care and their subsequent participation in care leads to greater patient satisfaction. In this study, individualised care has been well correlated with patient satisfaction providing some further evidence that individualised care is a predictor of patient satisfaction. An important contribution of the study is the cross-country comparison that although some differences were detected and explained by the different organisation, culture and management of the healthcare systems, it seems that surgical contexts in the participating countries may have more similarities than their healthcare systems as a whole.

16.4.2 Individualised Care, Quality of Life and Satisfaction with Nursing Care

Individualised care was examined in relation with patient satisfaction with nursing care and health-related quality of life [43]. The authors used the following measures: the individualised care scale (ICS-A and ICS-B) and the patient satisfaction scale (PSS), both described previously in this chapter. The results showed that the more often patients felt they received support for individuality through specific nursing interventions, the higher the individuality of care received. It was also found that the more individualised patients regarded their care, the higher the level of reported patient satisfaction with nursing care. However, patients were least satisfied with the provision of information, a finding that is steady in almost every patient satisfaction study. The correlation between individualised care and health-related quality of life was fairly low, albeit statistically significant, underlining the need for further investigation.

16.4.3 Patient Satisfaction, Autonomy and Health-Related Quality of Life

Aiming to examine the relationship between individualised care and several outcomes, Suhonen et al. [43] tested a hypothetical model that reflected the idea that a patient's individualised care can improve their satisfaction, personal autonomy and perceived health-related quality of life, as these three are the most often described as the outcomes of individualised care. The target population was general hospital patients in acute care, the biggest groups of them being internal medicine, surgical, gynaecological and oncological patients. Patients were recruited consecutively from 35 units within 6 acute hospitals in Southern Finland, and the final sample of 687 properly completed questionnaires was used to test the hypothesis. The measuring instruments included the individualised care scale (ICS-A and ICA-B), patient satisfaction with nursing care (PSS), patient autonomy and perceived health-related quality of life (the 15D). The authors applied a structural equation modelling, a general multivariate statistical modelling technique that is used to analyse structural relationships.

The results showed that individualised nursing care has a positive impact on the three outcomes, and the model explained a great amount of the variance in patient satisfaction and autonomy supporting previous theoretical and empirical literature that demonstrated a positive relationship between individualised care with patient satisfaction, health-related quality of life and patient autonomy. Better quality of life and stress reduction were also found in individualised interventions in cancer patients undergoing radiotherapy [45]. Similarly, attempts to individualise patient education interventions in nurse-led heart failure clinics were found to increase patients' sense of management of the disease and increased their satisfaction [46].

The importance of this study lies on the fact that it provided evidence for the validity of the hypothesised model through testing and added further support for the theoretical framework of individualised care. The model can be used as a guideline for clinical practice, as it supports strongly that individualised care contributes to positive patient outcomes. The items of the ICS can be used to operationalise the concept of individualised nursing care as they give clear examples of nursing interventions that can be tailored to individual patients' needs and preferences.

16.5   The Nurse Outcomes of Individualised Care

Nurse work satisfaction was also examined as an outcome of individualised care. The aim of this study was to examine the association between caregivers' work satisfaction and individualised care by comparing their perceptions of individualised care and work satisfaction in different care settings for older people [47]. Data were collected from 263 carers working in old people's care settings in one healthcare area in Finland. Individualised care was examined with two different measures: (a) the ICS-A-Nurse and the ICS-B-Nurse (described previously) and (b) the individualised care instrument (ICI) that was developed for the measurement of individuality in clinical practice and includes four subscales, the knowing the person, patient/resident autonomy, staff-to-patient/resident communication and staff-to-staff communication. Nurse work satisfaction was examined with the Index of Work Satisfaction (IWS, Part B) that consists of 44 items. The scale requests the respondent's opinion about work satisfaction in their current employment and includes six subscales: pay, autonomy, task requirements, organisational policies, professional status and interaction. The interaction subscale is divided into two separate variables: nurse–nurse interaction and nurse–physician interaction. The findings support the initial hypothesis that perceptions of work satisfaction are positively associated with perceptions of individualised care. Positive statistical correlations were found in the majority of subscales assessing individuality and work satisfaction, meaning that promoting individualised care at an organisational level may contribute to improving satisfaction of workers caring for older people.

Conclusion

The results of the abovedescribed studies revealed that individualised care is an integral part of care and caring behaviour. Good nursing care cannot be delivered if it is not tailored according to each patient's individual needs, own history and experiences, own unique personal characteristics, potentials and expectations. There is also evidence of a positive relation between certain patient outcomes when the care delivered is individualised, and these may include patient satisfaction and quality of life. Nurses also may benefit when they feel that the care they deliver is based on the individual needs, expectations, preferences and experiences of their patients, as studies have found an association between individualised care and job satisfaction. However, more work needs to be done to find the links between many other important outcomes such as patient empowerment, health-related stress and others that contribute to recovery and better coping with the healthcare problems.

References

1. Finfgeld-Connett D. Meta-synthesis of caring in nursing. J Clin Nurs. 2008;17(2):196–204.
2. American Nurses Association, ANA. Code of ethcics for nurses. 2015.
3. Gallagher A, Li S, Wainwright P, et al. Dignity in the care of older people – a review of the theoretical and empirical literature. BMC Nurs. 2008;7:11. https://doi.org/10.1186/1472-6955-7-11

4. Papastavrou E, Efstathiou E, Tsangari H, et al. Patients' and nurses' perceptions of respect and human presence through caring behaviours: a comparative study. Nurs Ethics. 2012;19(3):369–79.
5. Ervin NE, Pierangeli LT. The concept of decisional control: building the base for evidence-based nursing practice. Worldviews Evid-Based Nurs. 2005;2(1):16–24.
6. Papastavrou E, Efstathiou G, Charalambous A. Nurses' and patients' perceptions of caring behaviours: quantitative systematic review of comparative studies. J Adv Nurs. 2011;67(6):1191–205.
7. Finfgeld-Connett D. Concept comparison of caring and social support. Int J Nurs Terminol Classif. 2007;18(2):58–68.
8. McCance T, McCormack B. Person-centred nursing. J Adv Nurs. 2006;56(5):472–9.
9. McCance TV, McKenna HP, Boore JR. Caring: theoretical perspectives of relevance to nursing. J Adv Nurs. 1999;30(6):1388–95.
10. McCance TV. Caring in nursing practice: the development of a conceptual framework. Res Theory Nurs Pract. 2003;17(2):101–16.
11. Joan Yalden B, Mccormack B. Constructions of dignity: a pre-requisite for flourishing in the workplace? Int J Older People Nursing. 2010;5(2):137–47.
12. McCormack B, McCance TV. Development of a framework for person-centred nursing. J Adv Nurs. 2006;56(5):472–9.
13. Suhonen R, Välimäki M, Leino-Kilpi H. "Individualised care" from patients', nurses' and relatives' perspective–a review of the literature. Int J Nurs Stud. 2002;39(6):645–54.
14. Suhonen R, Välimäki M, Leino-Kilpi H. The driving and restraining forces that promote and impede the implementation of individualised nursing care: a literature review. Int J Nurs Stud. 2009;46(12):1637–49. https://doi.org/10.1016/j.ijnurstu.2009.05.012.
15. Suhonen R, Efstathiou G, Tsangari H, et al. Patients' and nurses' perceptions of individualised care: an international comparative study. J Clin Nurs. 2012;21(7–8):1155–67.
16. Widmark-Petersson V, von Essen L, Sjödén PO. Cancer patient and staff perceptions of caring and clinical care in free versus forced choice response formats. Scand J Caring Sci. 1998;12(4):238–45.
17. Zamanzadeh V, Azimzadeh R, Rahmani A, et al. Oncology patients' and professional nurses' perceptions of important nurse caring behaviors. BMC Nurs. 2010;9:10. https://doi.org/10.1186/1472-6955-9-10.
18. Gooding BA, Sloan M, Gagnon L. Important nurse caring behaviors: perceptions of oncology patients and nurses. Can J Nurs Res. 1993;25(3):65–76.
19. Holroyd E, Cheung YK, Cheung SW, Luk FS, Wong WW. A Chinese cultural perspective of nursing care behaviours in an acute setting. J Adv Nurs. 1998;28(6):1289–94.
20. Lawrence J, Delaney CP. Integrating hospital administrative data to improve health care efficiency and outcomes: "The Socrates story". Clin Colon Rectal Surg. 2013;26(1):56–62. https://doi.org/10.1055/s-0033-1333662.
21. Doona MEAD, Chase SK, Haggerty LA. Nursing presence. As real as a milky way bar. J Holist Nurs. 1999;17(1):54–70.
22. Godkin J, Godkin L. Caring behaviors among nurses: fostering a conversation of gestures. Health Care Manage Rev. 2004;29(3):258–67.
23. Florin J. Patient participation in clinical decision making in nursing– a collaborative effort between patients and nurses. 2007. Retrieved from http://www.diva-portal.org/smash/get/diva2:137380/fulltext01. Accessed 28 Mar 2018.
24. Weiss M, Yakusheva O, Bobay K. Nurse and patient perceptions of discharge readiness in relation to postdischarge utilization. Med Care. 2010;48(5):482–6.
25. Zhao SH, Akkadechanunt T, Xue XL. Quality nursing care as perceived by nurses and patients in a Chinese hospital. J Clin Nurs. 2009;18(12):1722–8.
26. Walker L, Porter M, Gruman C, et al. Developing individualized care in nursing homes: integrating the views of nurses and certified nurse aides. J Gerontol Nurs. 1999;25(3):30–5.
27. Chang Y, Lin Y, Chang H, et al. Relationship to level of pain intensity. Cancer Nurs. 2005;28(5):331–9.

28. Gardner A, Goodsell J, Duggan T, et al. "Don't call me sweetie!": Patients differ from nurses in their perceptions of caring. Collegian. 2001;8(3):32–8.
29. McCance T, Slater P, McCormack B. Using the caring dimensions inventory as an indicator of personcentred nursing. J Clin Nurs. 2009;18(3):409–17. https://doi.org/10.1111/j.1365-2702.2008.02466.x.
30. Tuckett A, Hughes K, Gilmour J, Hegney D, Huntington A, Turner C. Caring inresidential aged-care. Qualitative findings from an e-cohort sub-study. J Clin Nurs. 2009;18(18):2604–12. https://doi.org/10.1111/j.1365-2702.2008.02735.x.
31. Leino-Kilpi H, Scott PA, Välimäki M, et al. Perceptions of autonomy in the care of elderly people in five European countries. Nurs Ethics. 2003;10(1):28–38.
32. Watson R, Hoogbruin AL, Rumeu C, et al. Differences and similarities in the perception of caring between Spanish and UK nurses. J Clin Nurs. 2003;12(1):85–92.
33. Suhonen R, Valimaki M, Katajisto J, Leino-Kilpi H. Hospitals' organizational variables and patients' perceptions of individualized nursing care in Finland. J Nurs Manag. 2007;15(2):197–206.
34. Bottacini A, Scalia P, Goss C. Shared decision making in Italy: an updated revision of the current situation. Z Evid Fortbild Qual Gesundhwes. 2017;123–124:61–5. https://doi.org/10.1016/j.zefq.2017.05.023
35. Florin J, Ehrenberg A, Ehnfors M. Clinical decision-making: predictors of patient participation in nursing care. J Clin Nurs. 2008;17(21):2935–44.
36. Ghane A, Huynh HP, Andrews SE, et al. The relative importance of patients' decisional control preferences and experiences. Psychol Health. 2014;29(10):1105–18.
37. Tobiano G, Bucknall T, Marshall A, Guinane J, Chaboyer W. Nurses' views of patient participation in nursing care. J Adv Nurs. 2015;71(12):2741–52. https://doi.org/10.1111/jan.12740.
38. Oxelmark L, Ulin K, Chaboyer W, et al. Registered nurses' experiences of patient participation in hospital care: supporting and hindering factors patient participation in care. Scand J Caring Sci. 2017. https://doi.org/10.1111/scs.12486.
39. Mead H, Andres E, Regenstein M. Underserved patients' perspectives on patient-centered primary care: does the patient-centered medical home model meet their needs? Med Care Res Rev. 2014;71(1):61–84. https://doi.org/10.1177/1077558713509890.
40. Handolin L, Leppäniemi A, Vihtonen K, Lakovaara M, Lindahl J. Finnish trauma audit 2004: current state of trauma management in Finnish hospitals. Injury. 2006;37(7):622–5.
41. Weymann N, Harter M, Petrak F, et al. Health information, behavior change, and decision support for patients with type 2 diabetes: development of a tailored, preference-sensitive health communication application. Patient Prefer Adherence. 2013;7:1091–9.
42. Suhonen R, Papastavrou E, Efstathiou G, et al. Patient satisfaction as an outcome of individualised nursing care. Scand J Caring Sci. 2012;26(2):372–80.
43. Suhonen R, Leino-Kilpi H, Välimäki M. Development and psychometric properties of the individualized care scale. J Eval Clin Pract. 2005;11(1):7–20.
44. Goh ML, Vehviläinen-Julkunen K. Hospitalised patients' satisfaction with their nursing care: an integrative review. Singapore Nurs J. 2016;43(2):11–27.
45. Pollard A, Burchell JL, Castle D, Neilson K, Ftanou M, Corry J, Rischin D, Kissane DW, Krishnasamy M, Carlson LE, Couper J. Individualised mindfulness-based stress reduction for head and neck cancer patients undergoing radiotherapy of curative intent: a descriptive pilot study. Eur J Cancer Care (Engl). 2017;26(2):e12474. https://doi.org/10.1111/ecc.12474.
46. Ross A, Ohlsson U, Blomberg K, Gustafsson M. Evaluation of an intervention to individualise patient education at a nurse-led heart failure clinic: a mixed-method study. J Clin Nurs. 2015;24(11–12):1594–602. https://doi.org/10.1111/jocn.12760.
47. Suhonen R, Charalambous A, Stolt M, et al. Caregivers' work satisfaction and individualised care in care settings for older people. J Clin Nurs. 2013;22(3–4):479–90.

The Organisational Framework for the Delivery of Individualised Care

Minna Stolt and Riitta Suhonen

Abstract

Nursing interventions are aimed at improving nursing care and outcomes for individual patients, groups and citizens. However, studies on nursing interventions and their outcomes are scarce and need further development. This chapter aims to describe research on the individualised care interventions from patients' and healthcare professionals' (nursing professionals') perspective and from other points of view. This section is based on two reviews on the effects of individualised interventions on patient outcomes. An update on literature has been conducted since 2013 where the last review ended.

Keywords

Individualised intervention · Tailored interventions · Nursing interventions

17.1   Introduction

Determining the outcomes of nursing interventions is one of the top research priorities [1–3] in the field of nursing science. Findings from many studies have direct implications for translating existing evidence into practice, underscoring the need

M. Stolt (✉)
Department of Nursing Science, University of Turku, Turku, Finland
e-mail: minna.stolt@utu.fi

R. Suhonen
Department of Nursing Science, University of Turku, Turku, Finland

Turku University Hospital and City of Turku, Welfare Division, Turku, Finland
e-mail: riisuh@utu.fi

for intervention research focused on improving patient outcomes [3]. For example, Bolton et al. [2] stated that the association between nursing care interventions or processes and patient outcomes in acute care settings is limited. In addition to limited literature, there is confusion concerning the use of the terms 'individualised interventions' and 'tailored interventions'. In this chapter, both individualised and tailored interventions are described; the research to describe such interventions is also included.

Individualised nursing interventions have been defined by Lauver et al. [4] as 'highly customised, based on assessment of several characteristics of individuals' (p. 31). They continued that 'guided by general guidelines, interventions evolve in interactions with participants in real time'. This means, for example, that nurses incorporate individual differences into the interventions they perform. Lauver et al. [4] stated that individualised interventions are usually more complex than tailored interventions. Tailored interventions are based on assessment of multiple and individual characteristics, each of which may have many values; the interventions are matched and delivered from a predetermined, specific protocol ([4], p. 31). Thus, tailored interventions are more customised and complex than targeted interventions, which are customised to match a limited number of characteristics shared by a group. Similarly, [4–7] noted that individualised care involves allowing the individuality of a patient to determine interpersonal approaches and nursing interventions. However, in the research literature, the intervention descriptions do not necessarily differentiate these two terms.

Because patients are different, a variety of interventions are required, which defines individualised care [8]. Therefore, the precise content of an individualised intervention is not determined prior to a nurse-patient interaction but develops as a consequence of (or rather during) that interaction ([6], p. 251). In these circumstances, nurses need to work based on general guidelines rather than protocols so that the interventions evolve in interactions with patients in real time ([4], p. 31). On inspecting these two types of interventions, whether synonyms or separate concepts having slight differences, the starting point is similar. Interaction with patients is needed to individualise or tailor the nursing interventions.

17.2 Individualised Interventions and Patient Outcomes

In the review by Suhonen, Välimäki and Leino-Kilpi [9], there was some support, albeit limited, for the assertion that individualised or tailored interactions have a greater impact on patient care than non-individualised or non-tailored interventions [9]. Most of the studies in the review included individualised educational interventions. There is previous evidence especially about the effect of individualised educational interventions on patient outcomes. This review focused on intervention studies conducted up to 2005. Later, Rebelo Botelho et al. [10] reviewed similar literature from 2005 to 2013. An update to literature published since 2013 was conducted to highlight the changes in the foci of individualised interventions on patient outcomes.

In the review by Suhonen, Välimäki and Leino-Kilpi [9], the effects of individualised interventions were categorised into four areas: (1) help-seeking behaviours or utilisation of special type of healthcare services, (2) clinical health status indicators, (3) adherence to the recommended care regimen promoting self-care, and (4) patient perceptions of care quality, such as satisfaction.

17.2.1 Help-Seeking Behaviours or Utilisation of Special Type of Healthcare Services

Individualised or tailored nursing interventions were likely to be effective in health promotion (e.g. [11].), supporting health behaviours through health information [12, 13]. Recent research on the utilisation of care and services suggests the potential benefits of individualised, tailored interventions on service use and thereby, on reduced costs. However, the evidence is still scarce. In addition to the effects of individualised interventions on patient outcomes, the interventions also bring benefits to costs of care by reducing unplanned clinical visits to physicians and to the emergency room and promoting self-care [14]. Olsson et al. [15] found that the recovery trajectory for hip fracture surgery may be shortened if nurses pay more attention to the individual patient's resources and motivation for rehabilitation. The application of an integrated care pathway with individualised care appears to enhance both rehabilitation outcomes and cost-effectiveness. Hamar et al. [16] also pointed out that the effect of individualised support programme participation resulted in significant reductions in hospital admissions (-11.4%, $P < 0.0001$), readmissions (-36.7%, $P < 0.0001$) and bed days (-17.2%, $P < 0.0001$) in patients with chronic diseases. Durfee et al. [17] studied tailored intervention designed to improve care and reduce costs for patients with the highest rates of hospital utilisation. The use of tailored services, including a dedicated intensive outpatient clinic, for super-utilisers within a larger primary care practice transformation reduced mortality and provided significant savings even as total hospitalisations increased.

17.2.2 Clinical Health Status Indicators

Some studies have identified the effects of individualised interventions on patients' clinical outcomes, such as activities of daily living, functional ability or capacity (e.g. [18–20]) and memory functioning [21]. Some intervention studies have been conducted in samples of older people. These showed the effectiveness of individualised or tailored interventions on decreased incontinence (e.g. [22–24].), decreased complications or risks [18], and obtaining balance in chronic conditions [25]. Also shortened recovery after hip fractures [15, 26] was found. Recently, individualised interventions provided by physical therapists were found to have the potential to significantly improve symptom severity and health-related quality of life in women over 65 years of age with different types of urinary incontinence [23]. Individualised patient education interventions were found to be effective in promoting significant changes in the quality of life of cancer patients [27] and heart surgery patients [28]. Individualised interventions were also effective in reducing depression and anxiety in patients undergoing heart surgery [28].

Some studies have been conducted on the effects of individualised interventions on outcomes for people with dementia or who are otherwise in vulnerable condition. Individualised activities for nursing home residents with dementia were more effective in resulting in pleasure, alertness, engagement, positive touch and positive verbal behaviour compared with usual standard activities [29]. Fox et al. [30] suggest that specific acute care for older people interventions including medical review, early rehabilitation and individualised care appears to be optimal for overall outcome achievement and for reducing iatrogenic complications and functional decline in older adults admitted to the hospital for an acute event. Individualised nursing education intervention was also effective in preventing diabetic foot ulceration among diabetic patients with high-risk foot [31].

17.2.3 Adherence to the Recommended Care Regimen Promoting Self-Care

Most of the studies on self-care or self-management and adherence or compliance with care included individualised educational interventions. In recent studies, interventions have been targeted especially on health promotion, supporting health behaviour and changes in health behaviour [28, 32] and prevention [32]. O'Brien and colleagues [33] showed that patient education using motivational interviewing techniques and an individualised approach was successful in altering knowledge, attitudes and beliefs about acute coronary syndrome among a high-risk population. Adherence to recommended care is important for recovery and for returning to a normal way of life after hospitalisation. Such interventions are important as the number of days spent in hospital has decreased significantly thanks to advanced care technology, mini-invasive care options and the change in patients' role. Patients' knowledge of specific issues such as medication [34, 35] and smoking cessation [36, 37] is successfully increased by individualised interventions.

Recent intervention studies have focused on rehabilitation, recovery and self-care. For example, Cossette et al. [38] aimed to determine whether a nursing intervention focusing on patients with acute coronary symptoms and their perceptions of their disease and treatment would increase rehabilitation enrolment after discharge. They found that progressive, individualised interventions by nurses resulted in greater rehabilitation enrolment, thereby potentially improving long-term outcome. Other studies have revealed positive outcomes of individualised interventions on exercise compliance in older people for managing fatigue [39]. Individualised interventions may help support independence, self-management or self-efficacy [16], enhancing patients' active role in self-care [40–42]. A recent review on stroke self-management programmes by Warner et al. [43] concluded that the most prominent strategies identified were goal setting and follow-up and an individualised approach using structured information and professional support. Tailored education implemented by visiting nurses can improve diabetic patients' knowledge of diabetes and foot self-care in particular [44].

17.2.4 Patient Perceptions of Care Quality, Such as Satisfaction

Earlier studies have focused on clinical outcomes in different clinical and community settings. However, other types of patient outcomes are rarely studied. Earlier, only few studies focused on the softer patient outcomes, such as care satisfaction as a result of individualised interventions [13]. Recently, in their review, Rebelo Botelho et al. [10] identified the increase in the number of studies focusing on perceived patient outcomes, such as felt accepted (e.g. [45]), felt respected [46] and felt supported [47, 48].

17.3 Individualised Interventions and Staff Outcomes

There are some studies providing some evidence about individualised care and its effectiveness in producing positive outcomes for professionals as well. Care providers who are able to provide individualised care have been found to be more satisfied and offer a higher quality of care to patients [49, 50]. Moreover, it has been found that adopting a person-centred approach to nursing alters the work environment and increases work satisfaction [50, 51]. Low job satisfaction can affect the provision of individualised care, emphasising the need to promote individualised care at an organisational level as a means of improving work satisfaction [52].

Studies on the effectiveness of individualised or person-centred care have mainly focused on residential aged-care facilities. For example, Brownie and Nancarrow [53] found that staff facility-specific person-centred interventions impacted nurses' sense of job satisfaction and their capacity to meet the individual needs of residents in a positive way.

Individualised care has been found to be one of the rare interventions that also improves the working environment for care providers [54]. Although patient-centred care is ultimately determined by the quality of interactions between patients and clinicians at the practice level, it should be facilitated at organisational level, too [55]. A nationwide 1-year study was conducted aiming to improve patient centeredness, which was operationalised into six subdomains: facilitating self-management support, individualised care plan support, patients' access to medical files, patient education policy, safeguarding patients' interests and formal patient involvement. The intervention consisted of feedback and benchmark and, if requested, a telephone call and/or a consultancy visit. After this intervention, the care groups significantly improved their quality management on patient centeredness (from 47.1 to 53.3%, $p = 0.002$).

Conclusion

This chapter provided some evidence, based mainly on patients' point of views, on the outcomes, possible effectiveness and usefulness of such interventions. The interventions used have mainly been educational in their nature. In these intervention studies, the problem lies in the minimal description of the content, duration and implementation of the individualised interventions. Thus, it is not always possible to describe the exact elements or activities that are individualised or tailored. Rather, the interventions included an approach involving patients strongly in care planning according to their specific needs, preferences and wishes. In addition, some intervention studies were not able to verify any positive outcomes for individualised interventions. For example, Wilson et al. [56] did not find any effect of an individualised preoperative educational intervention on symptoms of patients having total knee arthroplasty operation, such as pain-related interference in activities, pain and nausea.

Regarding the analysis of the effects of individualised interventions, some limitations need to be taken into account. Failure to reveal a significant effect may due to the incomplete understanding of the vague concept, lack of precise description of interventions, inadequate samples (especially sample size) and inability of the instruments to reveal differences in the measured variables. On the other hand, it may be that individualised interventions are not effective in producing certain types of outcomes, such as effects on physical symptoms (see [56]). However, there is considerable evidence available on the possible effects of individualised or tailored interventions on patient outcomes. The number of intervention studies and complex intervention studies is increasing. They may also strengthen the evidence on the effects of individualised interventions on patient outcomes but also on professional or staff outcomes. Interventions aimed to impact staff are lacking from the research literature although some such interventions already exist.

References

1. Barksdale DJ, Newhouse R, Miller JA. The Patient-Centered Outcomes Research Institute (PCORI): information for academic nursing. Nurs Outlook. 2014;62(3):192–200.
2. Bolton LB, Donaldson NE, Rutledge DN, et al. The impact of nursing interventions: overview of effective interventions, outcomes, measures, and priorities for future research. Med Care Res Rev. 2007;64(2 Suppl):123S–1243S.
3. LoBiondo-Wood G, Brown CG, Knobf MT, et al. Priorities for oncology nursing research: the 2013 national survey. Oncol Nurs Forum. 2014;41(1):67–76.
4. Lauver DR, Gross J, Ruff C, et al. Patient-centered interventions: implications for incontinence. Nurs Res. 2004;53(6 Suppl):S30–5.
5. Cox CL. An interaction model of client health behavior: theoretical prescription for nursing. Adv Nurs Sci. 1982;5(1):41–56.
6. Lauver DR, Ward SE, Heidrich SM, et al. Patient-centered interventions. Res Nurs Health. 2002;25(4):246–55.
7. Ryan P, Lauver DR. The efficacy of tailored interventions. J Nurs Sch. 2002;34(3):331–7.
8. Radwin L. Oncology patients' perceptions of quality nursing care. Res Nurs Health. 2000;23(2):179–90.
9. Suhonen R, Välimäki M, Leino-Kilpi H. A review of outcomes of individualised nursing interventions on adult patients. J Clin Nurs. 2008;17(7):843–60.
10. Rebelo Botelho A-M, Fonseca C, Suhonen R, et al. Intervenções de Enfermagem Individualizadas: Uma Revisão da Literatura. Individualised nursing interventions: a literature review (In English). Pensar Enfermagem. 2015;19:47–61.
11. Lusk SL, Eakin BL, Kazanis AS, et al. Effects of booster intervention on factory workers' use of hearing protection. Nurs Res. 2004;53(1):53–8.

12. de Nooijer J, Lechner L, Candel M, et al. Short- and long-term effects of tailored information versus general information on determinants and intentions related to early detection of cancer. Prev Med. 2004;38(6):694–703.
13. Derdiarian AK. Effects of information on recently diagnosed cancer patients' and spouses' satisfaction with care. Cancer Nurs. 1989;12(5):285–92.
14. Inman DM, Jacobson TM, Maxson PM, et al. Effects of urinary catheter education for patients undergoing prostatectomy. Urol Nurs. 2013;33(6):289–98.
15. Olsson L-E, Hansson E, Ekman I, et al. A cost-effectiveness study of a patient-centered integrated care pathway. J Adv Nurs. 2009;65(8):1626–35.
16. Hamar GB, Rula EY, Coberley C, et al. Long-term impact of a chronic disease management program on hospital utilization and cost in an Australian population with heart disease or diabetes. BMC Health Serv Res. 2015;15:174. https://doi.org/10.1186/s12913-015-0834-z.
17. Durfee J, Johnson T, Batal H, et al. The impact of tailored intervention services on charges and mortality for adult super-utilizers. Healthc (Amst). 2017. https://doi.org/10.1016/j.hjdsi.2017.08.004.
18. Lundström M, Edlund A, Lundström G, et al. Reorganisation of nursing and medical care to reduce the incidence of postoperative delirium and improve rehabilitation outcome in elderly patients treated for femoral neck fractures. Scand J Caring Sci. 1999;13(3):193–200.
19. Mulrow CD, Gerety MB, Kanten D, et al. A randomized trial of physical rehabilitation for very frail nursing home residents. J Am Med Assoc. 2004;271(7):519–24.
20. Poulsen T, Elkjaer E, Vass M, et al. Promoting physical activity in older adults by education of home visitors. Eur J Ageing. 2007;4(3):115–24.
21. Moniz-Cook E, Agar S, Gibson G, et al. A preliminary study of the effects of early intervention with people with dementia and their families in a memory clinic. Aging Ment Health. 1998;2(2):199–211.
22. Jirovec MM, Templin T. Predicting success using individualized scheduled toileting for memory-impaired elders at home. Res Nurs Health. 2001;24(1):1–8.
23. Neville CE, Beneciuk J, Bishop M, et al. Analysis of physical therapy intervention outcomes for urinary incontinence in women older than 65 years in outpatient clinical settings. Top Geriatr Rehabil. 2016;32(4):251–7.
24. Schnelle JF, Cruise PA, Alessi CA, et al. Individualized night time incontinence care in nursing home residents. Nurs Res. 1998;47(3):197–204.
25. Frich LM. Nursing interventions for patients with chronic conditions. J Adv Nurs. 2003;44(1):137–53.
26. Hagsten B, Svensson O, Gardulf A. Early individualized postoperative occupational therapy training in 100 patients improves ADL after hip fracture. A randomized trial. Act Orthop Scand. 2004;75(2):177–83.
27. Sajjad S, Ali A, Gul RB, et al. The effect of individualized patient education, along with emotional support, on the quality of life of breast cancer patients – A pilot study. Eur J Oncol Nurs. 2016;21:75–82. https://doi.org/10.1016/j.ejon.2016.01.006.
28. Fredericks S, Yau T. Clinical effectiveness of individual patient education in heart surgery patients: a systematic review and meta-analysis. Int J Nurs Stud. 2017;65(1):44–53.
29. Van Haitsma KS, Curyto K, Abbott KM, et al. A randomized controlled trial for an individualized positive psychosocial intervention for the affective and behavioral symptoms of dementia in nursing home residents. J Gerontol B Psychol Sci Soc Sci. 2015;70(1):35–45.
30. Fox MT, Sidani S, Persaud M, et al. Acute care for elders components of acute geriatric unit care: systematic descriptive review. J Am Geriatr Soc. 2013;61(6):939–46.
31. Ren M, Yang C, Lin DZ, et al. Effect of intensive nursing education on the prevention of diabetic foot ulceration among patients with high-risk diabetic foot: a follow-up analysis. Diabetes Technol Ther. 2014;16(9):576–81.
32. van den Wijngaart LS, Sieben A, van der Vlugt M, et al. A nurse-led multidisciplinary intervention to improve cardiovascular disease profile of patients. West J Nurs Res. 2015;37(8):705–23.
33. O'Brien F, McKee G, Mooney M, et al. Improving knowledge, attitudes and beliefs about acute coronary syndrome through an individualized educational intervention: a randomized controlled trial. Patient Educ Couns. 2014;96(2):179–87.

34. Hayes KS. Randomized trial of geragogy-based medication instruction in the emergency department. Nurs Res. 1998;47(4):211–8.
35. Huang TT, Acton GJ. Effectiveness of home visit falls prevention strategy for Taiwanese community-dwelling elders: randomized trial. Public Health Nurs. 2004;21(3):247–56.
36. Gebauer C, Kwo CY, Haynes EF, et al. A nurse-managed smoking cessation intervention during pregnancy. J Obstet Gynecol Neonatal Nurs. 1998;27(1):47–53.
37. Rowe K, Clark JM. Evaluating the effectiveness of a smoking cessation intervention designed for nurses. Int J Nurs Stud. 1999;36:301–11.
38. Cossette S, Frasure-Smith N, Dupuis J, et al. Randomized controlled trial of tailored nursing interventions to improve cardiac rehabilitation enrollment. Nurs Res. 2012;61(2):111–20.
39. Liu JY, Lai CK, Siu PM, et al. An individualized exercise programme with and without behavioural change enhancement strategies for managing fatigue among frail older people: a quasi-experimental pilot study. Clin Rehabil. 2017;31(4):521–31.
40. Driscoll A, Davidson P, Clark R, et al. Tailoring consumer resources to enhance self-care in chronic heart failure. Aust Crit Care. 2009;22(3):133–40.
41. Huang TT, Li YT, Wang CH. Individualized programme to promote self-care among older adults with asthma: randomized controlled trial. J Adv Nurs. 2009;65(2):348–58.
42. Johansson A, Adamson A, Ejdebäck J, et al. Evaluation of an individualised programme to promote self-care in sleep-activity in patients with coronary artery disease -- a randomised intervention study. J Clin Nurs. 2014;23(19–20):2822–34.
43. Warner G, Packer T, Villeneuve M, et al. A systematic review of the effectiveness of stroke self-management programs for improving function and participation outcomes: self-management programs for stroke survivors. Disabil Rehabil. 2015;37(23):2141–63.
44. Ko IS, Lee TH, Kim GS, et al. Effects of visiting nurses' individually tailored education for low-income adult diabetic patients in Korea. Public Health Nurs. 2011;28(5):429–37.
45. Hayashi A, Kayama M, Ando K, et al. Analysis of subjective evaluations of the functions of tele-coaching intervention in patients with spinocerebellar degeneration. NeuroRehabilitation. 2008;23(2):159–69.
46. Poochikian-Sarkissian S, Wennberg RA, Sidani S. Examining the relationship between patient-centred care and outcomes on a neuroscience unit: a pilot project. Can J Neurosci Nurs. 2008;30(1):14–9.
47. Johnson M, Goodacre S, Tod A, et al. Patients' opinions of acute chest pain care: a qualitative evaluation of Chest Pain Units. J Adv Nurs. 2009;65(2):120–9.
48. Kolcaba K, Schirm V, Steiner R. Effects of hand massage on comfort of nursing home residents. Geriatr Nurs. 2006;27(1):85–9.
49. Rathert C, May DR. Health care work environments, employee satisfaction, and patient safety: care provider perspectives. Health Care Manag Rev. 2007;32(1):2–11.
50. Tellis-Nayak V. A person-centered workplace: the foundation for person-centered caregiving in long-term care. J Am Med Dir Assoc. 2007;8(1):46–54.
51. Slater P, McCormack B, Bunting B. The development and pilot testing of an instrument to measure nurses' working environment: the Nursing Context Index. Worldviews Evid-Based Nurs. 2009;6(3):173–82.
52. Suhonen R, Charalambous A, Stolt M, et al. Caregivers' work satisfaction and individualised care in care settings for older people. J Clin Nurs. 2013;22(3–4):479–90.
53. Brownie S, Nancarrow S. Effects of person-centered care on residents and staff in aged-care facilities: a systematic review. Clin Interv Aging. 2013;8:1–10.
54. Schalk DMJ, Bijl LMP, Halfens RJG, et al. Interventions aimed at improving the nursing work environment: a systematic review. Implement Sci. 2010;5:34. https://doi.org/10.1186/1748-5908-5-34.
55. Campmans-Kuijpers MJ, Lemmens LC, Baan CA, et al. Patient-centeredness and quality management in Dutch diabetes care organizations after a 1-year intervention. Patient Prefer Adherence. 2016;10:1957–66. eCollection 2016.
56. Wilson RA, Watt-Watson J, Hodnett E, et al. A randomized controlled trial of an individualized preoperative education intervention for symptom management after total knee arthroplasty. Orthop Nurs. 2016;35(1):20–9.

Riitta Suhonen, Minna Stolt, and Andreas Charalambous

Abstract

In recent years, individualised care has emerged as the golden standard for healthcare, one that has been promised by policymakers, is desired by patients and families, and has been championed by nurses and allied professionals in an increasing number of countries around the globe. Such demands pose challenges for healthcare management and leadership, especially nursing leadership. Individualised nursing care delivery has been found to be associated with some organisational variables including organisation of work, but especially leadership and management. Previous studies have shown that management and leadership are important factors in supporting the delivery of individualised care. The association of individualised nursing care and leadership goes beyond its supportive role and includes the cultivation of an appropriate patient-centred culture and environment where individualised care can be introduced. This chapter sheds light on the associations between individualised nursing care and leadership as well as presenting the pathway by which leadership can cultivate an individualised caring environment.

R. Suhonen (✉)
Department of Nursing Science, University of Turku, Turku University Hospital, City of Turku, Welfare Division, Turku, Finland
e-mail: riisuh@utu.fi

M. Stolt
Department of Nursing Science, University of Turku, Turku, Finland
e-mail: minna.stolt@utu.fi

A. Charalambous
Department of Nursing, Cyprus University of Technology, Limassol, Cyprus

University of Turku, Turku, Finland
e-mail: andreas.charalambous@cut.ac.cy

© Springer International Publishing AG, part of Springer Nature 2019
R. Suhonen et al. (eds.), *Individualized Care*,
https://doi.org/10.1007/978-3-319-89899-5_18

195

Keywords
Leadership · Management · Nursing leaders

18.1 Leadership and Management

Nurse managers and leaders hold an assigned position within the hierarchy of an organisation. They have decision-making powers and control over certain processes and are expected to carry out specific duties. When we refer to a leader, this person may or may not have recognised authority within the organisation [1]. Both of these situations are included in this chapter. However, it is often the case that a leader possesses a different kind of power, one that comes from the ability to influence others through effective communication and interpersonal skills. Irrelevant to the source of managers' and leaders' power, these two roles have both been associated with the manifestation of a clinical environment that fosters patient outcomes [2] and individualised care [3] and ensures patient safety and quality care [4, 5].

Effective leadership and management of nursing work help to advance the delivery of individualised patient care in various ways [6–8]. Vice versa, inadequate administrative support and the lack of a leading role of nurse managers to support the individualised care delivery have been found to increase nurse turnover and decrease the quality of care in various clinical contexts [9, 10]. A successful example of leadership and management collaboration with healthcare professionals towards achieving an individualised care model has been demonstrated especially in the context of nursing homes [11]. The partnership between staff and management works to change the organisation and focus of nursing home frontline work, supporting a transition towards person-centred care. Person-centred care in nursing homes was found to foster changes in the organisation of frontline work aimed at improving nursing home residents' quality of life and care [11]. The research in the area shows that management practices are essential and influential in developing and initiating a move to a person-centred care culture and environment [7, 12, 13], enabling also individualisation of nursing care.

Nurses who perceive their work place as facilitating a more individualised approach to patient care provide a better quality of care to patients and are overall more satisfied with their work compared to those whose workplaces are perceived as less concerned with individualised care [14–16]. This can be attributed to various reasons; for example, care that lacks an individualised approach tends to be more task-oriented and repetitive as well as deviating from the principles taught and promoted by nursing science, such as the concepts of "total person" and "holistic caring" [17]. This can lead to poor job satisfaction among nurses and an increase in nurse turnover rate, as well as to the provision of poor quality care resulting in poor patient experiences [18].

The importance of individualised nursing care and its effectiveness in producing positive outcomes for patients [19, 20], caregivers [15, 16, 21] and overall clinical pathways has been clearly demonstrated in the literature. However, individualised care frameworks often remain at developmental stages, and nurses do not seem to be universally convinced of their utility in day-to-day practice [22]. Assessments of individualised care by providers or care recipients are neither acknowledged nor integrated (or integrated only to a limited degree) into healthcare development plans [21, 23].

Forbes-Thompson et al. [24] have revealed differences in the performance of nursing care organisations according to how nurse leaders behave. Leaders in high-performing homes behaved congruently with the nursing home's stated and lived mission by fostering connectivity among staff, ample information flow, and the use of cognitive diversity. In contrast, leaders in low-performing nursing homes behaved disharmoniously with the stated mission, which confused and eroded trust and relationships among staff members, contributed to poor communication, and fostered role isolation and discontinuity in resident care. Therefore, it is also of utmost importance to evaluate the role of leadership and management of nursing profession in terms of how they may or may not foster nursing work just by working effectively and representing value-based health and nursing care [24–26].

18.2   The Ways in Which the Organisation of Work Fosters Individualised Care

If individualised care is to develop, the structures and processes of ward organisation need to be adequately resourced [27–29]. Firstly, structural issues of an organisation, such as a well-equipped care environment, have been found to facilitate individualised patient care [8, 30]. It has also been found that there is a need to support new nurses with discussion, led by the nursing managers, to promote the delivery of individualised care [31].

Secondly, care process issues [32, 33], led by nurse managers, are important in the delivery of individualised care. Individualised care is enhanced when staff learns to adapt their routines to accommodate individual patients [34] and make their schedules more flexible. For example, in many older peoples' care settings, the delivery of individualised care is impeded by a traditional nursing culture which focuses on task orientation, rigid hierarchical structures, and the consequent disempowerment of staff [9, 12, 27, 35].

Thirdly, individualised care has been systematically linked to the organisation of nursing work, especially in the primary nursing model [36, 37]. However, when individualised care is defined in the context of interaction between the patient and the nurse, it should be noted that any model of nursing care work organisation may facilitate the delivery of individualised patient care [3, 8]. Using strict routines in nursing care may impede the provision of individualised care [38, 39] as individualised care calls for adjusting or removing many routines that suppress the ability of the nurse to place the patient at the centre of the care. This occurs because such restricting routines affect the nurses' ability to know the patients and provide individualised care [40].

Finally, leadership and management have an impact on how nurses perceive their work, work climate and working environment. The leadership behaviour of managers significantly impacts person-centred care practice and contributes to the psychosocial climate for both staff and residents in aged care [6]. Higher levels of staff satisfaction, lower levels of job strain, lower levels of stress of conscience, higher levels of a supportive psychosocial unit climate, and a higher proportion of staff with continuing education in dementia care were associated with higher levels of person-centred care [41]. Job strain and a supportive psychosocial climate explained most of the variation in person-centred care [41]. This also suggests the importance of nurse competence. However, the number of studies on competence, leading competence, and individualized care is very limited [42].

The next subchapter will provide some explanations for how staffing levels, creating the climate and environment, organisation-specific factors, and leading competence have been found to associate with the delivery of individualised care.

18.2.1 Staffing Levels and Individualised Care

Individualised care is strongly linked to the quality of care [10, 43, 44], and the lack of individualised care has been reported to be one obstacle to low quality of nursing care [45]. The lack of individualised care has been frequently linked with the adequate amount, skill mix and experience of nursing staff [27, 46, 47]. As nurses evidently spend a lot of time with patients, they appear mostly to affect patients' experiences of care [48], and nurses' time need to be meaningfully used with the patients [28]. The more day-to-day contact caregivers have with residents, the more effect nursing staff appear to have on the perceived empowerment and the reported provision of individualised care [12]. However, the amount of time that a nurse can actually spend with each patient may be significantly restricted due to poor staffing levels in the organisation. These circumstances force nurses to prioritise the care delivered to patients; however, this does not necessarily reflect patients' needs and expectations. Ball et al. [49] provided evidence that nurses are more likely to report care being left undone (or 'missed') when they are working on shifts with high numbers of patients per registered nurse, resulting in poor quality of care and poor safety.

18.2.2 Creating a Climate and Culture

Nursing in an individualised and patient-centred context is not a goal that can be achieved with isolated attempts by selective members of an organisation. Any attempt of this kind is not sustainable, and its possibilities of success are likely to be very limited. There is a need for a far more fundamental change in any organisation seeking to adopt an individualised model of care; it involves the creation and maintenance of an appropriate patient-centred culture and care individualisation.

There is an increasing amount of literature reporting a culture change in care facilities, especially in long-term care and care settings for older people [28, 50, 51]. In this cultural change, the aim for more individualised nursing care has clearly been pointed out. Brownie and Nancarrow [52] reviewed the effects of person-centred care on residents and staff as a culture change led by nursing leaders. Especially one person-centred intervention, i.e. the Eden Alternative, was associated with significant improvements in residents' levels of boredom and helplessness. In contrast, facility-specific person-centred interventions were found to impact nurses' sense of job satisfaction and their capacity to meet the individual needs of residents in a positive way. This review highlighted that staff, led by nursing leaders, are key to quality nursing care. Bringing about such fundamental changes takes time and requires a long-term perspective as well as a clear, sustained strategy. These changes require leadership capable of transforming not just the physical environment but also the beliefs and practices of nurses and other healthcare workers providing care in that environment and of those within the healthcare organisations who establish the policies and practices that shape the environment.

Understanding and developing the organisational environment is of global importance [14] as the work environment has an effect on the behaviour of employees in organisations [53, 54], and this has played a substantial role in the successful implementation of patient care provision [26]. More than ever, care providers say they are practising in situations with a lack of congruency between individual patients' needs and the demands of the organisation [55], which produces ethically difficult situations. Conflicts on whether nurses are able to provide individualised care based on an inclusive approach or not have implications for nurses' role and responsibilities in clinical practice [53, 56].

Individualised care has been found to be one of the rare interventions that improve the working environment for care providers as well [19]. Increasing possibilities for nurses' empowerment in the culture change models enable possibilities for individualised nursing care [12]. However, because of their focus on organisations' economy and resources, health system reforms have not taken into account the processes from the client's point of view, and studies on the care environment and interventions are lacking.

The provision of individualised care has been found to be associated with a good working environment [3, 50, 57]. Rathert and May [14] conceptualised person-centred work environments that incorporate benevolent ethical climates and facilitate patient-centred care and quality improvement. Moving into work at the healthcare team level, McCormack et al. [58] highlighted the importance of the development of teamwork, workload, time management, and staff relations to create a culture where there is space for forming person-centred relationships. In developing patient-centred initiatives in nursing homes, Crandall et al. [7] found that units differ in their culture; depending on their work culture, some units were better than others in enhancing patient-centred orientation.

18.2.3 Organisation-Related Specifics

Some specific organisation-related issues have been linked to the delivery of individualised nursing care. The size of the hospital and ward has been found to be associated with patients' perceptions of individualised care [37]. The bigger the hospital and ward, the less individuality was perceived in the care provided. This may be explained by the fact that in units with many nurses, there is a lack of consistency in the nurses that the patients meet during their stay in the hospital. Therefore, the necessary time for building a therapeutic relationship and trust between nurse and patient is not provided, resulting in poor quality of care linked to nurses not becoming familiar with the needs of their patients [59]. As an integral part of a therapeutic relationship, the communication between nurses and patients also suffers from barriers resulting from the care being delivered with poor nurse-patient ratios [60]. All aspects of care and nursing are of high importance in communication with patients as patients consider interaction with nurses key to their treatment [61]. Patient-centred care encompasses the individual experiences of a patient, the clinical service, the organisational and the regulatory levels of healthcare [62]. Healthcare organisations that are patient-centred engage patients as partners and hold human interactions as a pillar of their service.

As organisations, healthcare systems within a European as well as an international context present similarities but, most importantly, many country-specific differences. Prospectively, these differences might explain, either positively or negatively, the delivery of individualised care. Between-country differences in both patients' [20] and nurses' [63] perceptions of individualised patient care have been found in international comparative studies, suggesting that the systems or organisations may also have a role in these differences. Furthermore, the speciality of the ward has been found to be associated with perceptions of individualised care from both patients' [20] and nurses' [63, 64] point of view. It has been found that nurses in the mental health area perceive that they deliver individualised patient care while nurses in long-term care settings perceive lower levels of ability to provide individualised care for the patients [64].

18.2.4 Leading Competence

Patient-centredness and the care provided according to it have been stated to be one of the core competencies in nursing [65] and the education of nurses [42], but they have also gained an important role when implementing safe and quality care for patients. Nurse leaders have an utmost important role in leading competence, especially in supporting staff to update their knowledge, train skills and adopt evidence-based or evidence-informed practice development activities [42, 62]. Understanding nurses' competency for patient-centred care is necessary in order to facilitate the transition towards patient-centred care in clinical practice [42].

Today, educational programmes in faculties of medicine, schools of nursing and schools of allied health incorporate cultural competence training in their curricula. Despite the increasing focus in education and clinical practice on providing patient-centred care, individualisation and culturally sensitive care, challenging situations can arise when patients wish to perform practices that do not fit within institutional or clinical norms. In many such situations, healthcare providers and hospital administrators adapt institutional or clinical norms and structures [66].

18.3   Nurses and Leadership

The administrative role of nurse leadership and management was described earlier in this chapter. Another important notion is the leadership role of every individual nurse working with patients. Studies have shown that the choices nurses make about their practice tend to comply more often with prevailing norms than with those championed by person-centred care [25].

Within the context of work, Charalambous et al. [67] found several factors relevant to team dynamics that were associated with the provision of individualised care. Such factors included the problem-solving approach to handling disagreements and conflict, control over practice and relationships with physicians. These findings coincided with those of preceding studies stressing the pivotal role of control over practice [26, 32] and autonomous practice [68] for providing individualised care. Autonomous practice gives nurses the necessary freedom for decision-making based on the individual needs expressed by the patient. On the contrary, centralised decision-making limits the ability of the nurse to adjust the care according to the needs expressed by the patient [69].

Dwyer [70] reviewed registered nurses' role in clinical leadership. Dwyer considered this leadership role of individual nurses as crucial to the clinical governance and management of care given in the patient-nurse relationship. The results by Dwyer [70] pointed out that nurses reported the negative experiences of nurses in residential aged care and geriatrics more frequently compared to many other settings, especially acute care settings. Nurses will continue to be devalued if there is no professional identity and support for their roles, and they need to have a career pathway when making the decision to enter into aged and geriatric practice. Clinical leadership training is required for nurses to transition through practice into specialised roles such as registered nurse team leader and geriatric nurse practitioner. Dwyer suggested highlighting the specific independent and autonomous role of nurses: providing a career structure and choice for the nurse to become a clinical leader or manager of health services will improve recruitment and retention.

One example of advancing the leadership role of nurses is leadership supporting interventions to develop the working environment. Caspar et al. [51] developed and tested the responsive leadership intervention for practices by team leaders and found it to be a feasible method for improving responsive leadership practices and individualised care in the care settings for older people. In another study, Caspar et al. [13] pointed out that contextual- and individual-level factors exert considerably less influence on individualised care than factors associated with staff's perceptions of empowerment. They concluded that interventions aimed at increasing individualised care in long-term care settings should carefully consider staff's access to structural empowerment.

Conclusion

In today's multicultural, complex, and diverse healthcare context, the provision of individualised care needs to be nurtured and promoted with the necessary resources, appropriate mind-shifting, and, most importantly, adequate ongoing patient-centred education. In its complexity, patient-centred care culture, including individualisation of patient care, involves commitment on behalf of the person delivering the care but also on behalf of the persons who manage and lead those who care. Therefore, any introduction of patient-centred care culture and every effort in individualisation of care in the clinical context can only be sustainable if both bottom-to-top and top-to-bottom strategies are adopted. Literature points out a clear need of a culture change in nursing care, and this change is currently ongoing in many countries and healthcare organisations. Value-based healthcare calls for prioritising the environment, culture, culture change and the quality and safety of patient care to produce individualised care, services and environments for different patients. The role of nurse managers is to have stronger visibility in the development of nursing care, services and environment within healthcare and service systems.

References

1. Page A (2004) Transformational leadership and evidence-based management. Institute of Medicine (US) committee on the work environment for nurses and patient safety. Washington (DC): National Academies Press. https://www.ncbi.nlm.nih.gov/books/NBK216194/. Accessed 28 Mar 2018.
2. Cummings C. Perspectives on nursing research. The call for leadership to influence patient outcomes. Nurs Leadersh. 2011;24(1):22–5.
3. Suhonen R, Välimäki M, Leino-Kilpi H. The driving and restraining forces that promote and impede the implementation of individualised nursing care: a literature review. Int J Nurs Stud. 2009;46(12):1637–49.
4. Ausserhofer D, Schubert M, Desmedt M, et al. The impact of the work environment of nurses on patient safety outcomes: a multi-level modelling approach. Int J Nurs Stud. 2013;50(2):240–552.
5. Kirwan M, Matthews A, Scott PA. The impact of the work environment of nurses on patient safety outcomes: a multi-level modelling approach. Int J Nurs Stud. 2013;50(2):253–63.
6. Backman A, Sjögren K, Lindkvist M, et al. Towards person-centredness in aged care–exploring the impact of leadership. J Nurs Manag. 2016;24(6):766–74.
7. Crandall LG, White DL, Schuldheis S, et al. Initiating person-centered care practices in long-term care facilities. J Gerontol Nurs. 2007;33(11):47–56.
8. Redfern S. Individualised patient care: its meaning and practice in a general setting. NT Res. 1996;1(1):22–33.
9. Walker L, Porter M, Gruman C, et al. Developing individualised care in nursing homes: integrating the views of nurses and certified nurse aides. J Gerontol Nurs. 1999;25(3):30–5.
10. Waters KR, Easton N. Individualized care: is it possible to plan and carry out? J Adv Nurs. 1999;29(1):79–87.
11. Leutz W, Bishop CE, Dodson L. Role for a labor-management partnership in nursing home person-centered care. Gerontologist. 2010;50(3):340–51.
12. Caspar S, O'Rourke N, Gutman GM. The differential influence of culture change models on long-term care staff empowerment and provision of individualized care. Can J Aging. 2009;28(2):165–7.
13. Caspar S, Cooke HA, O'Rourke N, et al. Influence of individual and contextual characteristics on the provision of individualized care in long-term care facilities. Gerontologist. 2013;53(5):790–800.
14. Rathert C, May DR. Health care work environments, employee satisfaction, and patient safety: care provider perspectives. Health Care Manag Rev. 2007;32(1):2–11.

15. Suhonen R, Charalambous A, Stolt M, et al. Caregivers' work satisfaction and individualised care in care settings for older people. J Clin Nurs. 2013;22(3–4):479–90.
16. Tellis-Nayak V. A person-centered workplace: the foundation for person-centered caregiving in long-term care. JAMDA. 2007;8(1):46–54.
17. McEvoy L, Duffy A. Holistic practice–a concept analysis. Nurse Educ Pract. 2008;8(6):412–9.
18. You LM, Aiken LH, Sloane DM, et al. Hospital nursing, care quality, and patient satisfaction: cross-sectional surveys of nurses and patients in hospitals in China and Europe. Int J Nurs Stud. 2013;50(1):154–61.
19. Schalk DMJ, Bijl LMP, Halfens RJG, et al. Interventions aimed at improving the nursing work environment: a systematic review. Implement Sci. 2010;5:34. https://doi.org/10.1186/1748-5908-5-34.
20. Suhonen R, Berg A, Idvall E, et al. Individualised care from the orthopaedic and trauma patients' perspective: an international comparative survey. Int J Nurs Stud. 2008;45(11):1586–97.
21. Wilson D, Neville S. Nursing their way not our way: working with vulnerable and marginalised populations. Contemp Nurse. 2008;27(2):165–76.
22. Dewing J. Concerns relating to the application of frameworks to promote person-centeredness in nursing with older people. J Clin Nurs. 2004;13(3a):39–44.
23. Costello J. Nursing older dying patients: findings from an ethnographic study of death and dying in elderly care wards. J Adv Nurs. 2001;35(1):59–68.
24. Forbes-Thompson S, Leiker T, Bleich MR. High-performing and low-performing nursing homes: a view from complexity science. Health Care Manag Rev. 2007;32(4):341–51.
25. Rushton C, Edvardsson D. Reconciling conceptualizations of ethical conduct and person-centred care of older people with cognitive impairment in acute care settings. Nurs Philos. 2017;19(2). https://doi.org/10.1111/nup.12190.
26. Suhonen R, Stolt M, Gustafsson ML, et al. The associations between the ethical climate, the professional practice environment and individualised care in care settings for older people: a cross-sectional survey. J Adv Nurs. 2014;70(6):1356–68.
27. Curry L, Porter M, Michalski M, et al. Individualized care: perceptions of certified nurse's aides. J Geront Nurs. 2000;26(7):45–51.
28. Hartmann CW, Snow AL, Allen RS, et al. A conceptual model for culture change evaluation in nursing homes. Geriatr Nurs. 2013;34(4):388–94.
29. Suhonen R, Stolt M, Puro M, et al. Individuality in older people's care–challenges for the development of nursing and nursing management. J Nurs Manag. 2011;19(7):883–96.
30. Zimmerman S, Anderson WL, Brode S, et al. Systematic review: effective characteristics of nursing homes and other residential long-term care settings for people with dementia. J Am Geriatr Soc. 2013;61(8):1399–409.
31. Jones A, Kamath PD. Issues for the development of care pathways in mental health. J Nurs Manag. 1998;6(1):87–95.
32. Carey N, Courtenay M. A review of the activity and effects of nurse-led care in diabetes. J Clin Nurs. 2007;16(11c):296–304.
33. Larsson IE, Sahlsten MJ. The staff nurse clinical leader at the bedside: Swedish registered nurses' perceptions. Nurs Res Pract. 2016;2016:1797014. https://doi.org/10.1155/2016/1797014.
34. Teeri S, Leino-Kilpi H, Välimäki M. Long-term nursing care of elderly people: identifying ethically problematic experiences among patients, relatives and nurses in Finland. Nurs Ethics. 2006;13(2):116–29.
35. Tonuma M, Winbolt M. From rituals to reason: creating an environment that allows nurses to nurse. Int J Nurs Pract. 2000;6(4):214–8.
36. Athlin E, Furåker C, Jansson L, et al. Application of primary nursing within a team setting in the hospice care of cancer patients. Cancer Nurs. 1993;16(3):388–97.
37. Suhonen R, Välimäki M, Katajisto J, et al. Hospitals' organizational factors and patients' perceptions of individualized nursing care. J Nurs Manag. 2007;15(2):197–206.
38. Lundh L, Rosenhall L, Törnkvist L. Care of patients with chronic obstructive pulmonary disease in primary health care. J Adv Nurs. 2006;56(3):237–46.
39. Suhonen R, Alikleemola P, Katajisto J, et al. Nurses' perceptions of individualised care in long-term care institutions. J Clin Nurs. 2012;21(7–8):1178–88.

40. Gutierrez KM. Critical care nurses' perceptions of and responses to moral distress. Dimens Crit Care Nurs. 2005;24(4):229–41.
41. Sjögren K, Lindkvist M, Sandman PO, et al. To what extent is the work environment of staff related to person-centred care? A cross-sectional study of residential aged care. J Clin Nurs. 2015;24(9–10):1310–9.
42. Hwang JI. Development and testing of a patient-centred care competency scale for hospital nurses. Int J Nurs Pract. 2015;21(1):43–51.
43. Rantz MJ, Mehr DR, Hicks L, et al. Entrepreneurial program of research and service to improve nursing home care. West J Nurs Res. 2006;28(8):918–34.
44. Suhonen R, Stolt M, Berg A, et al. Cancer patients' perceptions of quality-of-care attributes-associations with age, perceived health status, gender and education. J Clin Nurs. 2018;27(1–2):306–16.
45. Deutchman M. Redefining quality and excellence in the nursing home culture. J Gerontol Nurs. 2001;27(8):28–36.
46. Lang TA, Hodge M, Olson V, et al. Nurse-patient ratios: a systematic review on the effects of nurse staffing on patient, nurse employee, and hospital outcomes. J Nurs Admin. 2004;34(7–8):326–37.
47. Schmidt LA. Patients' perceptions of nurse staffing, nursing care, adverse events, and overall satisfaction with the hospital experience. Nurs Econom. 2004;22(3):295–306.
48. Kieft RA, de Brouwer BB, Francke AL, et al. How nurses and their work environment affect patient experiences of the quality of care: a qualitative study. BMC Health Serv Res. 2014;14:249. https://doi.org/10.1186/1472-6963-14-249.
49. Ball JE, Murrells T, Rafferty AM, et al. Care left undone during nursing shifts: associations with workload and perceived quality of care. BMJ Qual Saf. 2013;23(2):116–25.
50. Caspar S, Cooke HA, Phinney A, et al. Practice change interventions in long-term care facilities: what works, and why? Can J Aging. 2016;35(3):372–84.
51. Caspar S, Le A, McGilton KS. The responsive leadership intervention: improving leadership and individualized care in long-term care. Geriatr Nurs. 2017;38(6):559–66.
52. Brownie S, Nancarrow S. Effects of person-centered care on residents and staff in aged-care facilities: a systematic review. Clin Interv Aging. 2013;8:1–10. https://doi.org/10.2147/CIA.S38589.
53. McGilton KS, Boscart VM, Brown M, et al. Making trade-offs between the reasons to leave and reasons to stay employed in long-term care homes: perspectives of licensed nursing staff. Int J Nurs Stud. 2014;51(6):917–26.
54. Olson LL. Hospital nurses' perceptions of the ethical climate of their work setting. Image: J Nurs Scholars. 1998;30(3):345–9.
55. Hart SE. Hospital ethical climates and registered nurses' turnover intentions. J Nurs Scholars. 2005;37(2):173–7.
56. Tønnessen S, Nortvedt P, Førde R. Rationing home-based nursing care: professional ethical implications. Nurs Ethics. 2011;18(4):386–96.
57. Cohen-Mansfield J, Parpura-Gill A. Practice style in the nursing home: dimensions for assessment and quality improvement. Int J Geriatr Psychiatry. 2008;23(4):376–86.
58. McCormack B, Dewing J, Breslin L, et al. Developing person-centred practice: nursing outcomes arising from changes to the care environment in residential settings for older people. Int J Older People Nursing. 2010;5(1):93–107.
59. Sheldon LK, Barrett R, Ellington L. Difficult communication in nursing. J Nurs Scholars. 2006;38(2):141–7.
60. Tay LH, Ang E, Hegney D. Nurses' perceptions of the barriers in effective communication with inpatient cancer adults in Singapore. J Clin Nurs. 2012;21(17–18):2647–58.
61. Norouzinia R, Aghabarari M, Shiri M, et al. Communication barriers perceived by nurses and patients. Global J Health Sci. 2016;8(6):65–74.
62. Newell S, Jordan Z. The patient experience of patient-centered communication with nurses in the hospital setting: a qualitative systematic review protocol. JBI Database System Rev Implement Rep. 2015;13:76–87.

63. Suhonen R, Papastavrou E, Efstathiou G, et al. Nurses' perceptions of individualised care: an international comparison. J Adv Nurs. 2011;67(9):1895–907.
64. Suhonen R, Gustafsson M-L, Katajisto J, et al. Nurses' perceptions of individualised care. J Adv Nurs. 2010;66(5):1035–46.
65. Cronenwett L, Sherwood G, Barnsteiner J, et al. Quality and safety education for nurses. Nurs Outlook. 2007;55(3):122–31.
66. Hunt MR. Patient-centered care and cultural practices: process and criteria for evaluating adaptations of norms and standards in health care institutions. HEC Forum. 2009;21(4):327–39.
67. Charalambous A, Katajisto J, Välimäki M, et al. Individualised care and the professional practice environment: nurses' perceptions. Int Nurs Rev. 2010;57(4):500–7.
68. Thompson IE, Melia KM, Boyd KM, et al. Nursing ethics. 5th ed. Edinburgh: Elsevier-Churchill Livingstone; 2006.
69. Lake ET, Friese CR. Variations in nursing practice environments: relation to staffing and hospital characteristics. Nurs Res. 2006;55(1):1–9.
70. Dwyer D. Experiences of registered nurses as managers and leaders in residential aged care facilities: a systematic review. Int J Evid Based Healthc. 2011;9(4):388–402.

The Importance of the Physical Environment to Support Individualised Care

19

Susanna Nordin and Marie Elf

Abstract

The physical environment is an important part of individualised care. Creating care environments tailored towards the individual person's needs is essential for high-quality care and is increasingly recognised as being associated with improved health and well-being among older people. Today, care should be holistic and view the person behind the disease, taking that person's perspective and treating the patient as a unique individual. Despite the emerging focus on individualised care approaches, the physical environment is still not considered as an integral part of care, and relatively little attention has been paid to environmental aspects. However, the physical environment has a great potential to facilitate or restrict care processes in a broad range of care settings, not least in residential care facilities for older people. The present chapter focuses on ways to support the individual in terms of the physical environment.

Keywords

Care environment · Design · Health outcomes · Individual needs · Older people · Residential care facilities

S. Nordin (✉)
School of Education, Health and Social Studies, Dalarna University, Falun, Sweden
e-mail: snr@du.se

M. Elf
School of Education, Health and Social Studies, Dalarna University, Falun, Sweden

School of Architecture, Chalmers University of Technology, Gothenburg, Sweden
e-mail: mel@du.se

© Springer International Publishing AG, part of Springer Nature 2019   207
R. Suhonen et al. (eds.), *Individualized Care*,
https://doi.org/10.1007/978-3-319-89899-5_19

19.1   The Care Environment as Part of Individualised Care

For individuals with a high degree of frailty, an inadequate care environment that is not adapted to individual needs can have severe impacts and result in health decline and reduced well-being. Therefore, it is time to view the environment as far more than simply decorative and aesthetically appealing and to consider the environment as an integral part of individualised care by being aware of its potential to facilitate or hinder care processes [1, 2].

Previous studies have indicated that individualised care is associated with improved health and well-being among patients as well as with higher satisfaction with care [3–5]. Individualised care for older individuals requires an interdisciplinary approach in which the person's needs, resources and preferences are central and in which the care should be based on her or his perspectives. The following four critical attributes have been previously applied to individualised care: knowing the person, relationships, choice in terms of decision-making and risk-taking, and participation [6]. In addition, enhancing independency in daily life has often been prioritised [7].

The living environment is considered vitally important to a person's identity, health and well-being. It constitutes a safe base where the most fundamental needs can be met and is also a platform from which social relationships are created [8–10]. While this is universal and relevant for most people, it is particularly true for older persons who spend a majority of their time within facilities due to chronic conditions and physical and cognitive frailties [8].

A highly essential part of individualised care is the environment in which the care is provided, and by adapting the environment, individual needs can be met [1]. Importantly, the care environment has an essential role in facilitating social interactions, activities and a sense of home for older persons in residential care facilities [11–13]. For example, clear walking paths, access to outdoor spaces, and information on the purpose of the room can enhance individualised care and support older persons' sense of self [14], whereas institutional characteristics such as endless double-banked corridors have the opposite effect [15]. Despite the recognition of the importance of environmental aspects for supporting older individuals with frail health, the care environment is an underused resource in elderly care and could explain variations as to the extent to which care is adapted to the individual [2, 16, 17].

19.2   Definition of Care Environments

The care environment consists of physical aspects (i.e. the built environment) and psychosocial aspects, both playing an important role in achieving individualised care. In addition, the care environment is multidimensional, including people, processes, resources and equipment [1] together with information and technology. Aspects of the physical environment can be classified as architectural, ambient or related to interior design. Examples of architectural aspects are the spatial layout, room size or distance between spaces. Ambient aspects involve lighting, noise levels and temperature. Meanwhile, interior design aspects include furnishings and colours [18]. The psychosocial environment can be defined as an individual's perceptions of being in the care environment [19]. These perceptions vary from person to person, and previous experiences, values and health status will affect the psychosocial environment [20].

The physical environment cannot be separated from the psychosocial environment as aspects of the physical environment convey messages to those in the facility, and the care atmosphere can contribute to a sense of identity and can support previous interests and habits [11, 12, 21]. For example, familiar and pleasant elements such as art and flowers can have a positive influence on people and promote a sense of control and feelings of homeliness [11, 12].

19.3   Theories on the Person: Environment Relationship

The theoretical basis for understanding the relation between people and their environment can be found in psychologist Kurt Lewin's "field theory", in which human interactions are assumed to be driven by the persons and the environment surrounding them [22]. Lewin developed an ecological equation, which states that behaviour is a function of the person and his or her environment, $B = f(P, E)$, where B is behaviour, P denotes personal characteristics, and E denotes environmental characteristics. This person-environment fit (P-E fit) was further developed and applied to the ageing process by Powell Lawton and Lucille Nahemow in 1973 [23]. Their ecological theory on ageing has been used worldwide for the past few decades and has had a major influence in gerontological research. According to this theory, the interaction between an older individual and the environment is central. The individual is regarded to have a set of competencies such as physical and cognitive health [24], whereas the environment can be viewed in terms of demands. When there is a balance between the person's competencies and environmental demands, positive outcomes can occur. On the other hand, an imbalance can result in negative outcomes [23, 25]. The ecological theory on ageing was an elaboration of the environmental docility hypothesis from 1968 by Lawton and Simon:

> The more competent the organism—in terms of health, intelligence, ego strength, social role performance, or cultural evolution—the less will be the proportion of variance in behaviour attributable to physical objects or conditions around him… With high degrees of competence he will, in common parlance, rise above his environment. However, reduction of competence, or deprived status, heightens his behavioural dependence on external conditions. ([25], p. 108)

In other words, people with lower competencies (e.g. frail health) are more sensitive to demands from the environment compared to those with higher competencies. This means that a supportive healthcare environment can compensate for decreasing functional abilities [23, 25].

19.4   The Physical Care Environment: A Historical Backdrop

The built environment has always been formed based on the prevailing norms in society. Already in the mid-1800s, the importance of the environment was emphasised for people with frail health in order to achieve good healthcare outcomes. Florence Nightingale, a British nurse, was a pioneer in many ways, and her systematic work during the Crimean War was of great importance for our understanding of the physical environment and its impact on people with frail health. She realised that the lack of sanitation was the primary cause of high mortality among soldiers who were patients, and by improving factors in the physical environment, such as the sewage system, the water supply, and ventilation, the mortality rate declined significantly. In addition, Nightingale brought forwards ideas that environmental aspects such as fresh air and daylight could affect patient health, safety, and recovery. Her work had an enormous impact and contributed to several changes regarding environmental design and care practises in hospitals [26]. Approximately 100 years later, a new era emerged in which technical and rational aspects were emphasised [27], as the healthcare system was inspired by industry and its focus on results and productivity [28]. As a consequence, many hospitals were designed to be clinically efficient, with specialised units for different medical conditions and diagnoses, leading to the risk of patient objectification [29]. This is still the prevailing model in many healthcare facilities, designed to serve the organisation before supporting the persons in need of care [30].

In recent years, the pendulum seems to have swung again in the other direction, and Nightingale's environmental theory has gained new interest [31]. Although the physical environment is still regarded as something separated from care, awareness of the importance of healthcare environments has evolved, reflected both in social debates and in the growing number of international research articles on the topic.

19.5   The Link Between the Physical Environment and Health Outcomes

Research has shown that the physical environment impacts health and well-being [32–34]. Previous research within residential care facilities has demonstrated that aspects of the physical environment such as lighting, noise levels and access to nature can improve older people's sleep and orientation. Moreover, these environmental aspects have been found to increase engagement in activities and positively affect overall well-being [15, 35]. A Swedish study has shown that several factors in the physical environment, such as the layout of the building and space size, can affect older residents' activities and social interactions. For example, an open-plan solution with automatic door opening and with access to elevators in common spaces seems to facilitate the ability to move around in the facility, whereas closed doors have the opposite effect and limit use of the facility. Moreover, when older individuals have access to daylight and large windows, they can follow the daily life activities occurring outside the facility [36].

Safe handrails, proper flooring materials, adequate lighting and cues in the environment can support mobility and orientation [37], whereas monotonous physical environments negatively influence older persons and can cause difficulties for them in finding their way around [38, 39]. Moreover, well-designed physical environments can reduce psychiatric disturbance and increase well-being among people with cognitive disabilities such as dementia [40, 41]. Several studies have shown that spatial design and cues in the environment such as colours and signage can support the ability to navigate in those with dementia [38, 39, 42], and personalised cues such as photographs and personal items have been found to be of great help for these individuals [39]. Furthermore, specific environmental aspects such as cognitive supportive features have been found to be associated with older persons' social well-being. Consequently, an environment that is easy to interpret and that has a logical layout, reference points and cues can enhance well-being in terms of social activities and interactions [43].

The physical environment is also important for emotional connectedness and can influence an individual's feelings of being at home in the facility [44]. For example, by having personal belongings and furniture, a sense of normalness is supported, as unknown facilities become more familiar for the resident. This can be of great value for retaining personal identity [9, 10]. In other words, aspects in the physical environment can facilitate a person's sense of identity and enhance privacy and integrity [45]. Therefore, when moving into residential care, it can be tremendously important to have a private room or apartment [46, 47].

19.6   Evidence-Based Design

To increase the likelihood that new environments for older people will generate expected outcomes and support individualised care, decisions about the design must be evidence-based. Evidence-based design (EBD) principles make use of information from research when making design decisions that are ultimately expected to lead to improvements in the organisation's clinical performance, economic performance, productivity, and terms of use [48]. EBD is part of a continuous improvement in quality model which requires that care goals be defined by the best possible research, knowledge and experience and that clear goals should be presented at the beginning of a project to enable evaluation when the project is completed and in use. EBD is defined as a critical and reflective process where decision-making is based on current evidence, analysis, and experience from already built environments and not least on structured user experience analysis [49]. In regard to residential care facilities and supporting individualised care for older individuals, knowledge about their situations, including how the physical environment can facilitate or restrict individualised care, has to be identified early in the process of planning new facilities. This also means that the work with planning and designing care environments for older persons requires an interdisciplinary collaboration in which various knowledge and perspectives are acknowledged [50].

19.7   Environmental Quality Assessments

Given the importance of the physical environment for individualised care, methods that can be used to evaluate environmental quality are required. According to a systematic review of instruments assessing the quality of the physical environment in healthcare facilities, many instruments have been developed for residential care facilities for older people. However, valid and reliable instruments are lacking, and many of the instruments are old and lack theoretical basis. Moreover, the perspective of the individual is relatively invisible in these instruments [51]. The review has resulted in the identification of a British instrument that has been regarded as applicable to Swedish care facilities for the elderly, the Sheffield Care Environment Assessment Matrix (SCEAM) [33]. This instrument has a strong theoretical foundation and was developed for use in care facilities for older people with a wide range of frailties, including physical and cognitive disabilities. It is derived from the idea that high-quality environments should support the needs of the residents as frailty increases. Recently, this instrument was translated and culturally adapted for use in Swedish residential care facilities, resulting in a version called the Swedish version of the Sheffield Care Environment Assessment Matrix, S-SCEAM [52].

The S-SCEAM contains over 200 items, and each of these items relates to a location within the facility (e.g. overall layout, entrance and external area, garden, lounge, dining area, private apartments) [52]. The instrument is built on several domains theorised to be highly important for older people living in care facilities: cognitive support, physical support, safety, normalness, openness and integration, privacy, comfort, and choice. The following is a short description of each of these domains. The cognitive support domain involves elements considered to contribute to visual clarity and logical layout in order to promote independence for residents with cognitive disabilities. The features in the physical support domain can facilitate the everyday life for persons with physical disabilities and aid accessibility regardless of their level of functioning. The safety domain features contribute to risk reduction in the care home and promote a sense of safety and security for the residents, while the normalness domain is concerned with residents' feelings of homeliness and sense of familiarity. The features in the openness and integration domain enable residents' participation in and awareness of community life. The privacy domain involves elements to support residents in their everyday life without intrusion or observation by others, while the comfort domain contains features that can contribute to a pleasant, stimulating, and sustainable facility. Finally, the features within the choice domain concern residents' use of the facility based on their own wishes and preferences [2].

The first study using S-SCEAM for assessing environmental quality in care facilities for older people showed that there was substantial variation between and within care facilities. In general, safety features were of high quality, whereas cognitive support and privacy were of lower quality. When using S-SCEAM to assess different areas of the facilities, private apartments and dining areas had high environmental scores, while gardens and outdoor areas had lower scores. Despite high-standard requirements, there were large variations with regard to the quality of the physical environment, indicating that there is potential to improve environmental aspects in order to meet the needs of older people living in these facilities [2].

Conclusion

Although much work remains with regard to integrating the physical environment into care, there is an increasing interest in and awareness of environmental aspects and the way in which these aspects affect health outcomes for older people. Today, this is especially important as we are facing a growing elderly population with chronic conditions and high levels of physical and cognitive frailties. To meet their needs, high-quality care facilities are required. However, previous research shows variation in terms of the quality of the physical environment of residential care facilities for older people. Thus, it is reasonable to assume that the potential to apply individualised care will differ among care facilities, given the important role of environmental aspects in supporting residents' individual needs. In summary, both the physical environment and psychosocial environment need to be taken into account in the design of care facilities, and environmental aspects must go hand in hand with the organisation of healthcare. Thus, a prerequisite for achieving truly individualised care is to adopt a holistic approach based on cooperation across professional boundaries.

References

1. McCormack B, McCance T. Person-centred nursing: theory, models and methods. Oxford: Wiley-Blackwell Publishing; 2010.
2. Nordin S, McKee K, Wijk H, et al. Exploring environmental variation in residential care facilities for older people. HERD. 2016;10(2):49–65.
3. Epstein RM, Fiscella K, Lesser CS, et al. Why the nation needs a policy push on patient-centered health care. Health Aff (Millwood). 2010;29(8):1489–95.
4. Mead N, Bower P. Patient-centred consultations and outcomes in primary care: a review of the literature. Patient Educ Couns. 2002;48(1):51–61.
5. Sjogren K, Lindkvist M, Sandman PO, et al. Person-centredness and its association with resident well-being in dementia care units. J Adv Nurs. 2013;69(10):2196–205.
6. Happ MB, Williams CC, Strumpf NE, et al. Individualized care for frail elders: theory and practice. J Gerontol Nurs. 1996;22(3):6–14.
7. Innes A, Macpherson S, McCabe L. Promoting person-centred care at the front line. York: Joseph Rowntree Foundation; 2006.
8. National Board of Health and Welfare. Bostad i särskilt boende är den enskildes hem (in Swedish) [Housing in a residential care facility is the home of the individual]. Stockholm: Socialstyrelsen; 2011.
9. Rowles GD, Bernard M. Environmental gerontology: making meaningful places in old age. New York: Springer; 2013.
10. Rubinstein RL. The home environments of older people: a description of the psychosocial processes linking person to place. J Gerontol. 1989;44(2):S45–53.
11. Edvardsson D, Sandman P-O, Rasmussen B. Swedish language person centred climate questionnaire–patient version: construction and psychometric evaluation. J Adv Nurs. 2008;63(3):302–9.
12. Edvardsson D, Winblad B, Sandman P-O. Person-centred care of people with severe Alzheimer's disease: current status and ways forward. Lancet Neurol. 2008;7(4):362–7.
13. Fazio S. Person-centered care in residential settings: taking a look back while continuing to move forward. Alzheimer's Care Today. 2008;9(2):155–61.
14. Zeisel J. Improving person-centered care through effective design. Generations. 2013;37(3):45–52.
15. Joseph A (2006) Health promotion by design in long-term care settings. The Center for Health Design. http://www.healthdesign.org/research/reports/longtermcare.php Accessed 28 Mar 2018.

16. Papastavrou E, Acaroglu R, Sendir M, et al. The relationship between individualized care and the practice environment: an international study. Int J Nurs Stud. 2015;52(1):121–33.
17. Suhonen R, Stolt M, Gustafsson M-L, et al. The associations among the ethical climate, the professional practice environment and individualized care in care settings for older people. J Adv Nurs. 2014;70(6):1356–68.
18. Harris PB, McBride G, Ross C, et al. A place to heal: environmental sources of satisfaction among hospital patients. J Appl Soc Psychol. 2002;32(6):1276–99.
19. Browall M, Koinberg I, Falk H, et al. Patients' experience of important factors in the healthcare environment in oncology care. Int J Qual Stud Health Well-Being. 2013;8:20870. https://doi.org/10.3402/qhw.v8i0.20870.
20. Williams AM, Dawson S, Kristjanson LJ. Exploring the relationship between personal control and the hospital environment. J Clin Nurs. 2008;17(12):1601–9.
21. Edvardsson JD, Sandman PO, Rasmussen BH. Sensing an atmosphere of ease: a tentative theory of supportive care settings. Scand J Caring Sci. 2005;19(4):344–53.
22. Lewin K. Field theory and experiment in social psychology. Am J Sociol. 1939;44(6):868–96.
23. Lawton MP, Nahemow L. Ecology and the aging process. In: Lawton CEMP, editor. The psychology of adult development and aging. Washington, DC: American Psychological Association; 1973. p. 619–74.
24. Scheidt R, Norris-Baker C, Wahl H. The general ecological model revisited: evolution, current status, and continuing challenges. In: Aging in context: socio-physical environments, Annual review of gerontology and geriatrics, vol. 23. New York: Springer; 2003. p. 34–58.
25. Lawton MP, Simon B. The ecology of social relationships in housing for the elderly. Gerontologist. 1968;8(2):108–15.
26. Nightingale F. Notes on nursing what it is, and what it is not. London: Churchill Livingstone; 1860/1980.
27. Dirckinck-Holmfeld K. Sansernes hospital. Copenhagen: Arkitektens Forlag; 2007.
28. Taylor FW. The principles of scientific management. New York: Dover; 1998.
29. Fridell S. Rum för vårdens möten: om utformning av fysisk vårdmiljö för god vård [Architectural space for caring relationships: on the design of the physical environment for care and nursing]. Doctoral dissertation, Kungliga Tekniska Högskolan. Institutionen för arkitektur och stadsbyggnad. 1998.
30. McCormack B. Person-centredness in gerontological nursing: an overview of the literature. J Clin Nurs. 2004;13(1):31–8.
31. Medeiros ABA, Enders BC, Lira ALBDC. The Florence Nightingale's environmental theory: a critical analysis. Escola Anna Nery. 2015;19(3):518–24.
32. Huisman ERCM, Morales E, van Hoof J, et al. Healing environment: a review of the impact of physical environmental factors on users. Build Environ. 2012;58(1):70–80.
33. Parker C, Barnes S, McKee K, et al. Quality of life and building design in residential and nursing homes for older people. Ageing Soc. 2004;24(6):941–62.
34. The World Health Organization Quality of Life Assessment (WHOQOL) Group. The World Health Organization Quality of Life Assessment (WHOQOL): development and general psychometric properties. Soc Sci Med. 1998;46(12):1569–85.
35. Brawley EC. Environmental design for Alzheimer's disease: a quality of life issue. Aging Mental Health. 2001;5(2):79–83.
36. Nordin S, McKee K, Wallinder M, et al. The physical environment, activity and interaction in residential care facilities for older people: a comparative case study. Scand J Caring Sci. 2017;31(4):727–38.
37. Joseph A, Choi YS, Quan X. Impact of the physical environment of residential health, care, and support facilities (RHCSF) on staff and residents. A systematic review of the literature. Environ Behav. 2015;48(10):1203–41.
38. Marquardt G. Wayfinding for people with dementia: a review of the role of architectural design. HERD. 2011;4(2):75–90.
39. Marquardt G, Bueter K, Motzek T. Impact of the design of the built environment on people with dementia: an evidence-based review. HERD. 2014;8(1):127–57.

40. Cohen-Mansfield J. Non-pharmacological interventions for agitation in dementia: various strategies demonstrate effectiveness for care home residents; further research in home settings is needed. Evid Based Nurs. 2016;19(1):31. https://doi.org/10.1136/eb-2015-102059.

41. Day K, Carreon D, Stump C. The therapeutic design of environments for people with dementia: a review of the empirical research. Gerontologist. 2000;40(4):397–416.

42. Cohen-Mansfield J. Nonpharmacologic interventions for inappropriate behaviors in dementia: a review, summary, and critique. Am J Geriatr Psychiatr. 2001;9(4):361–81.

43. Nordin S, McKee K, Wijk H, et al. The association between the physical environment and the well-being of older people in residential care facilities: a multilevel analysis. J Adv Nurs. 2017;73(12):2942–52.

44. Wiles J. Conceptualizing place in the care of older people: the contributions of geographical gerontology. J Clin Nurs. 2005;14(S2):100–8.

45. Rubinstein RI, Parmelee PA. Attachment to place and the representation of the life course by the elderly. In: Altman I, Low SM, editors. Place attachment. New York: Springer; 1992. p. 139–63.

46. Rijnaard M, van Hoof J, Janssen B, et al. The factors influencing the sense of home in nursing homes: a systematic review from the perspective of residents. J Aging Res. 2016;2016:6143645. https://doi.org/10.1155/2016/6143645.

47. van Hoof J, Janssen M, Heesakkers C, et al. The importance of personal possessions for the development of a sense of home of nursing home residents. J Housing Elderly. 2016;30(1):35–51.

48. Hamilton DK, Watkins DH. Evidence-based design for multiple building types. Hoboken: John Wiley & Sons; 2009.

49. Stankos M, Schwarz B. Evidence-based design in healthcare: a theoretical dilemma. Interdisciplinary Design and Research e-Journal. 2007;1(1):1–14.

50. Elf M, Frost P, Lindahl G, et al. Shared decision making in designing new healthcare environments-time to begin improving quality. BMC Health Serv Res. 2015;15:114. https://doi.org/10.1186/s12913-015-0782-7.

51. Elf M, Nordin S, Het al W. A systematic review of the psychometric properties of instruments for assessing the quality of the physical environment in healthcare. J Adv Nurs. 2017;73(12):2796–816. https://doi.org/10.1111/jan.13281.

52. Nordin S, Elf M, McKee K, et al. Assessing the physical environment of older people's residential care facilities: development of the Swedish version of the Sheffield Care Environment Assessment Matrix (S-SCEAM). BMC Geriatr. 2015;15:3. https://doi.org/10.1186/1471-2318-15-3.

Stavros Vryonides and Evridiki Papastavrou

Abstract

The achievement of the main goals of the nursing profession, including the provision of quality and individualised nursing care to patients, often requires improvements in the working environment of nurses, while there are various research evidences to support such a need. However, it is additionally recognised in the scientific community that the ethical climate of an organisation is actually an important component of the overall working environment that is related to employees' shared perceptions of what is ethically correct behaviour and how ethical issues should be handled in organisations. Moreover, both the nurses' practice environment and the ethical climate that exist in healthcare settings specifically, as it is perceived by nurses themselves, had been linked in some studies to various important professional variables and patient outcomes including individualised nursing care. Having this in mind, the aim of this chapter is to discuss the literature regarding the ethical climate as it is perceived by nurses themselves with a focus on the association between ethical climate and individualised nursing care. In this light the chapter attempts to demonstrate the existing body of relevant knowledge and the possible knowledge deficits that need exploration with further research studies.

Keywords

Ethical climate · Professional environment · Nurses · Individualised nursing care · Quality · Missed care

S. Vryonides (✉) · E. Papastavrou
School of Health Sciences, Department of Nursing, Cyprus University
of Technology, Limassol, Cyprus
e-mail: svrionii@cytanet.com.cy; e.papastavrou@cut.ac.cy

20.1   The Nursing Profession and Individualised Care

This chapter begins with the widely adopted argument that nursing is a scientific discipline, as well as a learned profession [1, 2]. Thus, the nursing entity is built on a unique body of knowledge [2] that is gained from a nursing assessment of the subjective experiences of healthcare consumers, families, communities and populations [1] and the assessment of the working experiences of healthcare employees, as well as on the assessment of the objective outcomes of nursing interventions and the provided nursing care. In addition, it is built on specific skills that are based on principles of the biological, physical, behavioural and social sciences [1], as well as in certain broadly accepted attitudes towards people and the members of the society in general.

Moreover, the ethical foundations of nursing create clear obligations to nurses towards the directions of respecting human rights, of preserving human life, of promoting safety and of preventing harm to all people and especially to patients [3]. Additionally, these ethical foundations call the nurses for providing high-quality, [4] dignified [5–7], compassionate [7, 8], comprehensive [7] and individualised care [9–14] with justice and without any discrimination [7]. This alliance of knowledge, skills, attitudes and moral obligations jointly reflects the components of nursing as a science and as an art.

Thus, nurses as scientists and as professionals should use critical judgment and reflecting thinking [2] in order to apply the best available objective data, research evidence, knowledge, skills and attitudes to their practice, as well as in order to sustain their moral identity. At the same time, they should also continually evaluate the quality and the effectiveness of the provided nursing care [1, 2] and seek to optimise its outcomes, on a continual basis, as to ensure the integrity and sustainability of nursing practice in all current and future healthcare systems. However, stakeholders and organisations in healthcare [15], as well as lay people, emphasise that the desired health outcomes are associated with healthcare that is responsive to people's personal and individual needs.

In this light, "individualised nursing care" had been considered essential and as an indicator for quality care [14, 15], while the need for the provision of this type of care to the patients had been revealed in several and cross-cultural nursing studies [14]. Nevertheless, there is also some evidence in the literature [9, 16–18] supporting that nursing practice does not always achieve the provision of individualised nursing care for each person, for several reasons, most of which are related to nurses' professional practice environment where the care takes place [18, 19].

Indeed, nursing practice and the resulting nursing care that is provided to patients, including individualised nursing care, do not occur in a vacuum and are not solely influenced by individual nurse's decisions (micro level) but are additionally influenced by organisational factors (meso level) and the broader socio-political framework (macro level) [20] in which this practice is taking place. The following parts of this chapter discuss the role of some organisational factors and specifically the ethical climate that may exist in an organisation which in turn influence the professional nursing practice and the provision of nursing care. The emphasis however of this discussion is given to the association of individualised nursing care with the working environment of nurses and more specifically on the association of individualised nursing care with the ethical climate of nurses' working environment which is considered as an important part of this environment.

20.2   Professional Goals, Nurses' Working Environment and Ethical Climate

The nurses' working environment is very important for the achievement of the goals of nursing profession [21] as this environment has an influence on the behaviour of nurses working in healthcare organisations [22] and plays a substantial role in the successful provision of quality care to the patients [16, 23]. However, this environment may include structural factors, social factors, behavioural factors and the existing climate or atmosphere [18, 24].

Thus, the existing communication systems, the available human and material resources, the level of teamwork, the social relations, the leadership and the management of a particular working environment may all influence the practice of nurses either positively or else negatively. For example, a good working environment may allow nurses to work effectively in interdisciplinary groups, to mobilise resources quickly and appropriately [25] and to have a control over their practice, and all these could improve their practice. Additionally, there is some research evidence that factors in the working environment of nurses (e.g. the practice style of care and the organisation of work) influence their ability to know the individual needs of their patients and thus to provide individualised care [18].

In this light, one can argue that certain organisational-related factors, in the working environment of nurses, can influence nursing practice and that the achievement of the main goals of the nursing profession, including the provision of individualised nursing care to patients, may require improvements in this environment. Moreover, there is also sufficient research evidence supporting these arguments since the nurses' perceptions of their working environment have been found to be associated with important outcomes for the patients as well as the nurses themselves [9, 11, 16, 19, 21, 23, 25–28].

For example, the nurses' working environment has been associated, among others, with nurse-related outcomes, such as the nurses' professional empowerment and the establishment of effective work teams [29], the nurses' work performance [30], the nurses' satisfaction or dissatisfaction with their work [25, 26, 31], their rates of burnout from their job [31, 32], their intention to stay at or quit their jobs and their subsequent retention in this job or their turnover [30], as well as their professional behaviour [22].

As regards the patient-related outcomes, the perceptions of nurses of their working environment have been associated with patients' satisfaction with the care they have received [31], the levels of missed nursing care [33, 34], the patients' safety and quality of care [16, 23, 26, 35–40] and the mortality rates [26, 39] as well as with the provision of individualised nursing care to patients [9, 11, 18, 19].

In this light and as Tellis-Nayak [28] emphasises, when the environment in the workplace adds quality to the life of nurses, nurses can then add quality to the life of their patients [28]. Having in mind all the above discussion, as well as the information discussed in the previous chapters of this book, one can argue that the provision of individualised nursing care can add quality to the life of patients, and as it is revealed in some studies [9, 11, 18, 19], the organisational climate that exists in the workplace of nurses can seriously assist towards the achievement of this important effort. The organisational climate had been described as a group of measurable characteristics (e.g. the processes of decision-making, the leadership styles and the norms) existing in the working environment of a specific organisation and that become perceived as such, either directly or indirectly, by the members of this organisation [41].

However, it is additionally widely recognised in the scientific literature [42, 43] including the nursing literature [11, 44–46] that the ethical climate of an organisation is actually an important component of the overall organisational climate and in this light can play an important role in the provision of nursing care including the individualised nursing care. In fact, as an identifiable [43] dynamic part of the overall working environment of nurses [11, 47], the ethical climate can be modified [48] according to evaluations, to improve the workplace of nurses [22, 49–51] and to guide nurses' working behaviours towards the achievement of professional goals and the satisfaction of the patients' individual needs.

In this realm of nursing literature, the ethical climate had been mainly described as the nurses' perceptions of how care issues with ethical implications (e.g. patient care dilemmas, difficult interrelationships, etc.) are handled [45] in order to achieve better patient outcomes as well as how these issues are reflected in the organisational values, beliefs, norms, habits, policies and practices of the nurses' workplace [51]. Therefore, the investigation of ethical climate is nowadays considered as an important part of quality assessment in healthcare [11, 45, 46], and as a result the relevant research studies are gradually increasing in the nursing literature.

Moreover, both the nurses' practice environment and the ethical climate that exist in healthcare settings specifically, as it is perceived by nurses themselves, had been linked to various nurse-related and patient-related outcomes, including individualised nursing care. This chapter further discusses the existing body of relevant knowledge regarding the ethical climate in the working environment of nurses as it is perceived by nurses themselves and its associations with other organisational variables with a focus on the association between ethical climate and individualised nursing care. Knowledge deficits in the literature regarding the association of ethical climate with individualised nursing care that need exploration with further research studies are also discussed.

20.3 The Investigation of Ethical Climate in Nursing

Ethical climate was initially conceptualised in the business literature by Victor and Cullen [42] as "the shared perceptions of what is ethically correct behavior and how ethical issues should be handled in organizations" ([42], pp. 77–78). On the basis of this conceptualisation, several nurse scholars in the later years [22, 49] have argued that the ethical climate that exists in the nurses' workplace is related to their ethical beliefs and attitudes and thereby may serve as a reference of their decisions, as well as a reference of their actual behaviour [11, 47, 52, 53]. In this light, it had been sufficiently investigated in the nursing literature [11, 45, 47, 49, 51, 52, 54, 55], especially during the last 15 years.

A positive ethical climate is characterised by benevolent and utilitarian ideals and is guided by the compliance and respect in ethical principles, rules, laws, standards and codes of conduct [46] as well as the humanistic values of caring, the connectedness and the mutual support in the workplace [56]. Obviously, such a positive ethical climate that recognises the patients' rights and enables the patients' holistic needs to be met [56] may result in less care omissions [46] and thus in the provision of care of better quality. On the other hand, a negative ethical climate or one climate that focuses on egoistic tendencies and personal morality [46] may be linked to unsafe care such as medical errors [55] or more care omissions [46]. Therefore, the ethical climate that may exist in nurses' workplace may, in a way, shape nurses' practice and have an impact on the provided care and its quality [11, 45, 47].

Guided by these recognitions, the nurses' overall perception about the ethical climate in their working setting had been examined in the nursing literature. In most of these studies, the nurses perceived the ethical climate in their workplace as mainly positive [22, 55, 57–59], in some studies as neutral [60] and in other studies as negative [53, 54]. Positive associations were additionally found between a positively perceived ethical climate and several working variables, such as the nurses' ethical practices [45], their perceived organisational support [52], their intention to retain their current job [50, 52, 55], their job satisfaction [52, 61, 62], their commitment to the organisation [52, 61, 62], their professional competence [63], the reporting of less medical errors [55] as well as the provision of individualised nursing care [11]. On the other hand, inverse relationships had been found between a positively perceived ethical climate and the nurses' moral distress [58, 64, 65], but in other studies no significant correlation had been found between the two variables [60].

These associations led some researchers to focus their attention to the factors that may improve the ethical climate of nurses' working environment such as the supportive administration [48, 57, 62, 66, 67], the leadership styles [61], the nurses' shared responsibility and teamwork [67], the shared mission of the hospital among staff members [57], the interdisciplinary cooperation and communication in care settings [54], the organisational practices enriched with the principles of caring relationships [61] and the patient-focused initiatives from managers [57]. Other researchers have called for improvements in ethical climates in order to minimise the negative consequences of moral distress (e.g. high turnover) [55] although a previous literature review [51] revealed that there was not enough evidence supporting a clear impact of ethical climate on nurses' moral distress or on nurses' turnover.

The antecedents that affect nurses' perception of ethical climate such as the nurses' demographic characteristics [57], the type of working setting that nurses are employed (e.g. hospital type, ownership status, geographical region, teaching status, department level, type of care units) [49, 61, 62, 68, 69], the nurses' type of work (e.g. work group, job position, tenure) [49], the type of management and leadership styles in their working setting [61] and the differences in professional roles [53] had been also examined in the nursing literature.

Some of the studies that can be found in nursing literature have examined ethical climate within a single continuum using the ethics environment questionnaire (EEQ) [70]. Other studies have examined the nurses' perception of ethical climate by using the hospital ethical climate survey (HECS) developed by Olson [45] that encompasses five factors and examines the ethical climate in terms of nurses' perceived relation with the physicians, the managers, the peers, the patients and the hospital [11, 47, 71].

Additionally other researchers had examined ethical climate using the two-dimensional typology of ethical climate proposed by Victor and Cullen [42] that takes into consideration that different types of ethical climate existing in organisations may be related in a different manner to selected organisational outcomes. At the intersections of the two dimensions of their typology, Victor and Cullen [42] suggested nine hypothesised types of ethical climate. However, empirical testing indicated the existence for only six of them [42], while only five (i.e. instrumental, caring, rules, law and code, independence) appear frequently in the literature [43, 72, 73] including the nursing care [46, 49, 52, 74]. Caring ethical climates are based on benevolent ideals and the welfare for others [73, 74] and encourage behaviours that yield the most positive result for the greatest number of people [46, 49, 73]. Instrumental ethical climates are promoting self-interest and encouraging decision-making from a selfish standpoint [46, 49, 73, 74]. Ethical climates are guided by a clear expectation to follow the local standards, rules, procedures, codes of good practice and policies of the organisation strictly [46, 72–74]. However, in the type of ethical climate that is called as "laws and codes", the compliance to external influences such as laws, external rules, professional standards and codes of conduct is required from everyone, over and above other factors [46, 61, 73–75]. Finally, in independence ethical climates, employees are following their personal moral beliefs to make decisions with minimal impact from external influences [46, 73–75].

However, it is out of the scope of this chapter to discuss further these research approaches and the details from these studies except when their findings are related by any means to individualised nursing care. For an overall picture of most studies focusing on ethical climate in the nursing environment, one can refer to a useful scoping review [44] that had been published very recently in the nursing literature.

20.4 Ethical Climate and Individualised Care

From the discussion in this chapter, so far, it is revealed that individualised nursing care is closely connected with the general philosophy of the nursing profession, as well as the ethical obligations, which are expected from nurses in their practice. In addition, one can conclude that the nurses' working environment can play a substantial role in the successful achievement of the goals of nursing, including the provision of individualised nursing care to patients. Moreover, it is obvious that there is an agreement in the scientific community that the ethical climate of an organisation is actually an important component of the overall organisational environment.

In this light, the ethical climate that reflects the policies, procedures and practices, regarding the ethical issues in the nurses' working environment [63], can play an important role in the satisfaction of the patients' individual needs. In fact, values, norms, beliefs and habits shared by nurses in their working environment are associated with their decisions when they provide nursing care to their patients, which should be based on the assessment of the patients' individual needs. These ethical elements in the workplace that can lead to a common understanding of what is the ethically correct behaviour and how ethical issues should be managed in fact constitute the ethical climate [11, 42, 43, 45, 46] of the environment, where nurses provide care to patients. Previous studies have showed some association between organisational factors in hospitals and the patient perceptions of individualised care [76]. Other studies have associated the individualised care with the nurses' working environment [9, 11, 18, 19]. Having in mind that the ethical climate is an important part of the employees' working environment, several scholars had appeared in the nursing literature, either to argue or to support empirically that the ethical climate of healthcare organisations can play its part in the provision of individualised nursing care to patients.

For example, it has been argued that the feeling that a good ethical climate exists in the nurses' working environment can produce the energy for the provision of individualising nursing care to patients [9, 28], while the perception that an ethical climate is not present in this environment, may decrease the individuality in care that is provided to patients [77]. Thus, certain ethical elements that may exist in the nurses' working environment, such as the attitudes of staff and their values, have been found to be the most important facilitating forces of this type of care [24]. Since the individual values of nurses reflect collectively the broader value-based system of the organisation where these nurses work [22], one can argue that some organisation-related factors and especially those factors that deal with the ethical elements of the organisation can facilitate the development of such an environment or climate in the workplace that can sustain person-centred care to patients [78].

Similarly, McCormack et al. [79] had given a great emphasis on the development of teamwork and the improvement of relationships among the working staff in healthcare organisations and suggested that these are necessary conditions in order to create a working climate where there would be space for the formation of person-centred relationships [79] in the environment of care provision. The person-centred nursing philosophy as it is conceptualised in the model of McCormack and McCance [80] comprises four constructs. These constructs are the prerequisites (which focus on the attributes of the nurse), the care environment (which focuses on the context in which care is delivered), the person-centred processes (which focus on delivering care through a range of activities) and the expected outcomes (which are the results of the effective person-centred nursing) [80]. The person-centred working environment had been also conceptualised by Rathert and May [81] as the one that incorporates benevolent ethical climates, facilitates the patient-centred care and promotes in a continual basis the improvement of quality in the care that is provided [81]. According to these conceptualisations and in order for person-centred care to be delivered effectively to patients, it seems that the development of nurses' personal attributes, as well as the development of the environment where care is provided, is a necessary prerequisite for providing this type of care through a range of person-centred processes and activities.

The perceptions of nurses regarding the aspects or characteristics of the practice environment that can contribute to their ability to provide individualised nursing care had been examined also in other studies. Charalambous et al. [9], for example, found that motivation from work, the relationships with other professionals and the cultural sensitivity in the workplace are related among others to the level of individuality in provided care [9]. Similarly the degree of staff motivation had been associated with the provision of individualised care [11, 24, 28]. Takase et al. [30] on the other hand found that nurses' job performance was facilitated in a working environment that highlights their personal values as well as the ethics of the working group [30]. More recently Papastavrou et al. [19] found significant associations between aspects of the nurses' professional practice environment and the nurses' views of the level of care of individualisation in seven countries [19]. Based on the findings of their study, these scholars suggested that developing professional care environment, especially internal work motivation, cultural sensitivity, teamwork and control over practice, would enhance care individualisation [19].

On the other hand, several shortcomings in the nurses' work environments had been found to be related to reduce quality of provided care, although the healthcare systems were different between countries [23, 27]. These studies suggested that there is an increasing need to develop the environment of care and especially an increasing need to focus on the staffing and the appropriate skill mix of the workplace. However, based on the findings of their own study that have examined some of the organisational variables of hospitals in relation to the patients' perceptions of individualised nursing care, Suhonen et al. [76] suggested that there is also a need to improve the quality of the nurse-patient interactions in order to facilitate individualised nursing care [76].

Other studies have identified some of the factors or characteristics in the environment of care that make individualised care more difficult, while there is sufficient evidence to support that the provided nursing care does not always correspond to the individual needs of each patient [9, 16–18]. Similarly some characteristics of the nurses' practice environment had been found to be related to omissions in nursing care or to a lack of individuality of care that is provided [34]. In this light, nurses reported that the individual needs of the patients and the requirements of the organisation are not always congruent [50].

Such factors that can be considered obstacles or barriers for the provision of individualised nursing care as they were revealed in relevant studies are the negative attitudes of staff regarding this type of care, the poor skill mix or inappropriate staffing [24], the absence of interdisciplinary teams, the problems and poor communication between the members of the healthcare team [9, 24], the inability of nurses to have control over their practice [9] and the traditional nursing culture, which have its focus on task orientation and rigid hierarchical structures that are dominated by ward routines that pay little attention to the individual needs of the patients [17]. Some of these barriers had been also found in a review of qualitative studies [82], where an ethical dimension of nursing care omissions had been revealed.

Some of the characteristics of the workplace described above as to be related to the provision of individualised nursing care are also included in the "caring" type of ethical climate, while some of the characteristics that had been found to act as obstacles for the provision of individualised nursing care are included in the "instrumental" and "independence" types of ethical climate, as these types of ethical climate had been conceptualised by Victor and Cullen [42] and briefly discussed earlier in this chapter. In a recent study [46], these types of ethical climate had been found to be related to the level and frequency of missed nursing care. Thus, when nurses had perceived that the ethical climate in their working place was guided by benevolent and utilitarian ideals (i.e. a caring ethical climate), then they had reported less omissions in nursing care, whereas when they had perceived the ethical climate in their organisation as one that focuses in egoistic tendencies (i.e. an instrumental ethical climate) or as ane that is guided by personal morality (i.e. an independence ethical climate), they had reported more omissions in nursing care [46]. In this sense, the type of ethical climate which is labelled as "caring" could also be related to the ability to provide individualised nursing care, whereas "independence" and "instrumental" ethical climates could be associated with the inability to provide individualised nursing care to patients.

However, to the best of our knowledge, no studies examined the individualised nursing care in terms of the typology of ethical climate developed by Victor and Cullen [42]. Moreover, only few studies have examined the associations among individualised nursing care and the ethical climate in the nurses' working environment [11, 28], while the only study that clearly aimed to investigate the associations among the ethical climate, professional practice environment and individualised nursing care [11] was carried out using the hospital ethical climate survey (HECS) in care settings for older people. Nevertheless, statistically significant correlations were found in this study [11] among ethical climate (HECS) and individualised nursing care and between individualised nursing care and the three subscales of the professional practice environment (i.e. the internal work motivation, the control over practice and the leadership and autonomy) [11]. While 16% of the variance in the individuality in care provided was explained by all these four factors, the ethical climate alone accounted for the largest percentage of this variance (13%) [11]. Based on the findings of their study, these scholars argued that individualised nursing care cannot be imposed, but it can only be facilitated through appropriate cultivation of norms, beliefs and behaviours among nurses [11].

Having in mind the results of this study [11] as well as the discussion of the ethical elements and characteristics of the workplace that can either facilitate or prevent the provision of individualised nursing care, as discussed earlier, it seems that the developing of the ethical climate of the nurses' working environment could enhance individualised nursing care. However, the efforts to increase the level of individualised care by improving the ethical climate in the nurses' working environment require the support of nursing leaders, nurse managers and nurse educators. For example, nurse managers may be able to assist in the improvement of ethical climate of their organisation by actively listening to the nurses; by behaving to all of them with respect, equality and justice; and by showing caring attitudes towards all of them as well as towards the patients. Additionally, they may facilitate the collaboration and the interpersonal relations among nurses, in order to strengthen the team functioning within their organisation. These improvements in turn may have an impact on the provision of individualised nursing care. In addition, the preparation of nurses in terms of theoretical and clinical knowledge, skills and professional attitudes, on what constitutes a positive ethical climate, may assist in their effort to recognise the individuality of each patient and to enhance individualised approaches to patient care.

Conclusions

The preceding literature demonstrated some preliminary associations between the ethical climates and individualised nursing care but also the scarcity of research exploring these associations in some extent. Thus, and despite the fact that there are some arguments in the literature as well as some research indications that the ethical climate in the nurses' working environment is related to the provision of individualised nursing care, the research studies that clearly demonstrate such a relationship are very scarce. In this chapter, the elements in the literature that suggest that there is a correlation between ethical climate and individualised nursing care had been discussed. However, these elements also clearly show that there is a significant need for further research focused on international level and in various clinical areas, in order to find more robust evidence to clarify this relationship.

References

1. American Nurses Association. Nursing: scope and standards of practice second edition, Silver Spring, Maryland; 2010. http://www.worldcat.org/title/nursing-scope-and-standards-of-practice/oclc/646388479. Accessed 28 Mar 2018.
2. Finkelman A, Kenner C. The essence of nursing: knowledge and caring. In: Finkelman A, Kenner C, editors. Professional nursing concepts. 2nd ed. Burlington: Jones & Bartlett Learning; 2013. p. 53–84.
3. International Council of Nurses. The ICN code of ethics for nurses (revised 2012). ICN; 2012. http://www.icn.ch/images/stories/documents/about/icncode_english.pdf. Accessed 28 Mar 2018.
4. Commission of the European Communities. Together for health: a strategic approach for the EU 2008–2013. Commission staff working document, Document accompanying the White Paper. 2007. http://ec.europa.eu/health/ph_overview/Documents/strategy_wp_en.pdf. Accessed 28 Mar 2018.
5. Baillie L, Gallagher A, Wainwright P. Defending dignity: challenges and opportunities for nursing. 2008. https://www.scie-socialcareonline.org.uk/defending-dignity-challenges-and-opportunities-for-nursing/r/a11G0000001806zIAA. Accessed 28 Mar 2018.

6. Gallagher A, Li S, Wainwright P, et al. Dignity in the care of older people – a review of the theoretical and empirical literature. BMC Nurs. 2008;7:11. https://doi.org/10.1186/1472-6955-7-11.

7. Lanara V. Heroism as a nursing value: a philosophical perspective. 2nd ed. Athens: G Papanikolaou Graphic Arts; 1996.

8. Blomberg K, Griffiths P, Wengström Y, et al. Interventions for compassionate nursing care: a systematic review. Int J Nurs Stud. 2016;62(1):137–55.

9. Charalambous A, Katajisto J, Välimäki M, et al. Individualised care and the professional practice environment: nurses' perceptions. Int Nurs Rev. 2010;57(4):500–7.

10. Suhonen R, Välimäki M, Leino-Kilpi H, et al. Individualised care from the orthopaedic nurses' point of view: a cross-cultural comparative survey. J Orthop Nurs. 2009;13(4):214.

11. Suhonen R, Stolt M, Gustafsson M-L, et al. The associations among the ethical climate, the professional practice environment and individualized care in care settings for older people. J Adv Nurs. 2014;70(6):1356–68.

12. Suhonen R, Papastavrou E, Efstathiou G, et al. Nurses' perceptions of individualized care: an international comparison. J Adv Nurs. 2011;67(9):1895–907.

13. Suhonen R, Papastavrou E, Efstathiou G, et al. Patient satisfaction as an outcome of individualised nursing care. Scand J Caring Sci. 2012;26(2):372–80.

14. Suhonen R, Efstathiou G, Tsangari H, et al. Patients' and nurses' perceptions of individualised care: an international comparative study. J Clin Nurs. 2012;21(7–8):1155–67.

15. Organisation for Economic Co-operation and Development OECD. Towards high-performing health systems. OECD health project, Paris: OECD Publications; 2004. 2. http://www.oecd.org/els/health-systems/towardshigh-performinghealthsystems.htm. Accessed 28 Mar 2018.

16. Hall LM, Doran D. Nurse staffing, care delivery model, and patient care quality. J Nurs Care Qual. 2004;19(1):27–33.

17. Kirkley C, Bamford C, Poole M, et al. The impact of organisational culture on the delivery of person-centred care in services providing respite care and short breaks for people with dementia. Health Soc Care Community. 2011;19(4):438–48.

18. Suhonen R, Välimäki M, Leino-Kilpi H. The driving and restraining forces that promote and impede the implementation of individualised nursing care: a literature review. Int J Nurs Stud. 2009;46(12):1637–49.

19. Papastavrou E, Acaroglu R, Sendir M, et al. The relationship between individualized care and the practice environment: an international study. Int J Nurs Stud. 2015;52(1):121–33.

20. Gallagher A. Moral distress and moral courage in everyday nursing practice. Online J Issues Nurs. 2010;16(2):8.

21. Rathert C, May DR. Health care work environments, employee satisfaction, and patient safety: care provider perspectives. Health Care Manag Rev. 2007;32(1):2–11.

22. Olson LL. Hospital nurses' perceptions of the ethical climate of their work setting. Image J Nurs Sch. 1998;30(4):345–9.

23. Rafferty AM, Clarke SP, Coles J, et al. Outcomes of variation in hospital nurse staffing in English hospitals: cross-sectional analysis of survey data and discharge records. Int J Nurs Stud. 2007;44(2):175–82.

24. Walker L, Porter M, Gruman C, et al. Developing individualized care in nursing homes: integrating the views of nurses and certified nurse aides. J Gerontol Nurs. 1999;25(3):30–5.

25. Lake ET. The nursing practice environment: measurement and evidence. Med Care Res Rev. 2007;64(2 Suppl):104S–22S.

26. Aiken LH, Clarke SP, Sloane DM, et al. Effects of hospital care environment on patient mortality and nurse outcomes. JONA. 2008;38(5):223–9.

27. Aiken LH, Clarke SP, Sloane DM, et al. Nurses' reports on hospital care in five countries. Health Aff. 2001;20(3):43–53.

28. Tellis-Nayak V. A person-centered workplace: the foundation for person-centered caregiving in long-term care. JAMDA. 2007;8(1):46–54.

29. Laschinger HK, Havens DS. Staff nurse work empowerment and perceived control over nursing practice, Conditions for work effectiveness. J Nurs Adm. 1996;26(9):27–35.

30. Takase M, Maude P, Manias E. Explaining nurses' work behaviour from their perception of the environment and work values. Int J Nurs Stud. 2005;42(8):889–98.
31. Copanitsanou P, Fotos N, Brokalaki H. Effects of work environment on patient and nurse outcomes. Br J Nurs. 2017;26(3):172–6.
32. Van Bogaert P, Clarke S, Roelant E, et al. Impacts of unit-level nurse practice environment and burnout on nurse-reported outcomes: a multilevel modelling approach. J Clin Nurs. 2010;19(11–12):1664–74.
33. Ausserhofer D, Zander B, Busse R, et al. Prevalence, patterns and predictors of nursing care left undone in European hospitals: results from the multicountry cross-sectional RN4CAST study. BMJ Qual Saf. 2014;23(2):126–35.
34. Papastavrou E, Andreou P, Tsangari H, et al. Rationing of nursing care within professional environmental constraints: a correlational study. Clin Nurs Res. 2014;23(3):314–35.
35. Schubert M, Clarke SP, Glass TR, et al. Identifying thresholds for relationships between impacts of rationing of nursing care and nurse- and patient-reported outcomes in Swiss hospitals: a correlational study. Int J Nurs Stud. 2009;46(7):884–93.
36. Aiken LH, Sermeus W, Van den Heede K, et al. Patient safety, satisfaction, and quality of hospital care: cross sectional surveys of nurses and patients in 12 countries in Europe and the United States. BMJ. 2012;344(2):e1717. https://doi.org/10.1136/bmj.e1717.
37. Van Bogaert P, Clarke S, Vermeyen K, et al. Practice environments and their associations with nurse-reported outcomes in Belgian hospitals: development and preliminary validation of a Dutch adaptation of the Revised Nursing Work Index. Int J Nurs Stud. 2009;46(1):54–64.
38. Duffield C, Diers D, O'Brien-Pallas L, et al. Nursing staffing, nursing workload, the work environment and patient outcomes. Appl Nurs Res. 2011;24(4):244–55.
39. Schubert M, Clarke SP, Aiken LH, et al. Associations between rationing of nursing care and inpatient mortality in Swiss hospitals. Int J Qual Health Care. 2012;24(3):230–8.
40. Wong CA, Cummings GG, Ducharme L. The relationship between nursing leadership and patient outcomes: a systematic review update. J Nurs Manag. 2013;21(5):709–24.
41. Zhang J, Liu Y. Organizational climate and its effects on organizational variables: an empirical study. Int J Psychol Stud. 2010;2(2):189. https://doi.org/10.5539/ijps.v2n2p189.
42. Victor B, Cullen JB. A theory and measure of ethical climate in organizations. In: Fredrick WC, Preston L, editors. Business ethics: research issues and empirical studies. Bingley: Emerald Group Publishing Limited; 1987. p. 77–98.
43. Victor B, Cullen JB. The organizational bases of ethical work climates. Adm Sci Q. 1988;33(1):101–25.
44. Koskenvuori J, Numminen O, Suhonen R. Ethical climate in nursing environment. Nurs Ethics. 2017. https://doi.org/10.1177/0969733017712081.
45. Olson L. Ethical climate in health care organizations. Int Nurs Rev. 1995;42(3):85–90.
46. Vryonides S, Papastavrou E, Charalambous A, et al. Ethical climate and missed nursing care in cancer care units. Nurs Ethics. 2016. https://doi.org/10.1177/0969733016664979.
47. Suhonen R, Stolt M, Katajisto J, et al. Validation of the Hospital Ethical Climate Survey for older people care. Nurs Ethics. 2015;22(5):517–32.
48. Rathert C, Fleming DA. Hospital ethical climate and teamwork in acute care: the moderating role of leaders. Health Care Manag Rev. 2008;33(4):323–31.
49. Filipova AA. Licensed nurses' perceptions of ethical climates in skilled nursing facilities. Nurs Ethics. 2009;16(5):574–88.
50. Hart SE. Hospital ethical climates and registered nurses' turnover intentions. J Nurs Scholarsh. 2005;37(2):173–7.
51. Schluter J, Winch S, Holzhauser K, et al. Nurses' moral sensitivity and hospital ethical climate: a literature review. Nurs Ethics. 2008;15(3):304–21.
52. Abou Hashish EA. Relationship between ethical work climate and nurses' perception of organizational support, commitment, job satisfaction and turnover intent. Nurs Ethics. 2015;24(2):151–66.
53. Bartholdson C, Sandeberg MA, Lutzen K, et al. Healthcare professionals' perceptions of the ethical climate in pediatric cancer care. Nurs Ethics. 2015;23(8):877–88.

54. Hui EC. A survey of the ethics climate of Hong Kong public hospitals. Clin Ethics. 2008;3(3):132–40.
55. Hwang J-I, Park H-A. Nurses' perception of ethical climate, medical error experience and intent-to-leave. Nurs Ethics. 2014;21(1):28–42.
56. Silén M, Kjellström S, Christensson L, et al. What actions promote a positive ethical climate? A critical incident study of nurses' perceptions. Nurs Ethics. 2012;19(4):501–12.
57. Bahcecik N, Oztürk H. The Hospital Ethical Climate Survey in Turkey. JONAS Healthc Law Ethics Regul. 2003;5(4):94–9.
58. Pauly B, Varcoe C, Storch J, et al. Registered nurses' perceptions of moral distress and ethical climate. Nurs Ethics. 2009;16(5):561–73.
59. Silén M, Svantesson M, Kjellström S, et al. Moral distress and ethical climate in a Swedish nursing context: perceptions and instrument usability. J Clin Nurs. 2011;20(23–24):3483–93.
60. Allari R, Abu-Moghli F. Moral distress among Jordanian critical care nurse and their perception of hospital ethical climate. J Nat Sci Res. 2013;3(5):144–53.
61. Goldman A, Tabak N. Perception of ethical climate and its relationship to nurses' demographic characteristics and job satisfaction. Nurs Ethics. 2010;17(2):233–46.
62. Huang C-C, You C-S, Tsai M-T. A multidimensional analysis of ethical climate, job satisfaction, organizational commitment, and organizational citizenship behaviors. Nurs Ethics. 2012;19(4):513–29.
63. Numminen O, Leino-Kilpi H, Isoaho H, et al. Ethical climate and nurse competence – newly graduated nurses' perceptions. Nurs Ethics. 2015;22(8):845–59.
64. Hamric AB, Blackhall LJ. Nurse-physician perspectives on the care of dying patients in intensive care units: collaboration, moral distress, and ethical climate. Crit Care Med. 2007;35(2):422–9.
65. Lützén K, Blom T, Ewalds-Kvist B, et al. Moral stress, moral climate and moral sensitivity among psychiatric professionals. Nurs Ethics. 2010;17(2):213–24.
66. Storch J, Rodney P, Pauly B, et al. Enhancing ethical climates in nursing work environments. Can Nurse. 2009;105(3):20–5.
67. Storch J, Rodney P, Varcoe C, et al. Leadership for ethical policy and practice (LEPP): participatory action project. Nurs Leadersh. 2009;22(3):68–80.
68. Filipova AA. Ethical climates in for-profit, nonprofit, and government skilled nursing facilities: managerial implications for partnerships. JONAS Healthc Law Ethics Regul. 2011;13(4):125–33.
69. Filipova AA. Relationships among ethical climates, perceived organizational support, and intent-to-leave for licensed nurses in skilled nursing facilities. J Appl Gerontol. 2011;30(1):44–66.
70. McDaniel C. Development and psychometric properties of the ethics environment questionnaire. Med Care. 1997;35(9):901–14.
71. Suhonen R, Stolt M, Katajisto J, et al. Review of sampling, sample and data collection procedures in nursing research – an example of research on ethical climate as perceived by nurses. Scand J Caring Sci. 2015;29(4):843–58.
72. Martin KD, Cullen JB. Continuities and extensions of ethical climate theory: a meta-analytic review. J Bus Ethics. 2006;69(2):175–94.
73. Simha A, Cullen J. Ethical climates and their effects on organizational outcomes – implications from the past, and prophecies for the future. Acad Manag Perspect. 2012;26(4):20–34.
74. Borhani F, Jalali T, Abbaszadeh A, et al. Nurses' perception of ethical climate and organizational commitment. Nurs Ethics. 2014;21(3):278–88.
75. Tsai M-T, Huang C-C. The relationship among ethical climate types, facets of job satisfaction, and the three components of organizational commitment: a study of nurses in Taiwan. J Bus Ethics. 2008;80(3):565–81.
76. Suhonen R, Välimäki M, Katajisto J, et al. Hospitals' organizational variables and patients' perceptions of individualized nursing care in Finland. J Nurs Manag. 2007;15(2):197–206.
77. Gutierrez KM. Critical care nurses' perceptions of and responses to moral distress. Dimens Crit Care Nurs. 2005;24(5):229–41.

78. McCormack B, Dewing J, McCance T. Developing person-centred care: addressing contextual challenges through practice development. Online J Issues Nurs. 2011;16(2):3.
79. McCormack B, Dewing J, Breslin L, et al. Developing person-centred practice: nursing outcomes arising from changes to the care environment in residential settings for older people. Int J Older People Nursing. 2010;5(2):93–107.
80. McCormack B, McCance TV. Development of a framework for person-centred nursing. J Adv Nurs. 2006;56(5):472–9.
81. Rathert C, May DR. Person-centered work environments, psychological safety, and positive affect in healthcare: a theoretical framework. Org Ethics. 2008;4(2):109–25.
82. Vryonides S, Papastavrou E, Charalambous A, et al. The ethical dimension of nursing care rationing: a thematic synthesis of qualitative studies. Nurs Ethics. 2015;22(8):881–900.

Challenges and Future Directions

A wealth of literature has been written and a number of studies have been conducted on the topic of indiviualised nursing care from different perspectives. In the future, it is possible to synthesise the knowledge and direct research and theoretical work on several aspects of the topic. For example, based on the existing knowledge, it is possible to collect the steps in theory generation regarding the construct towards the middle range theory of individualised care and factors related. Conceptual and empirical work needs to be directed on the examination of the concepts associated with the individualised care, to reveal the common underlying contents and to determine the differing contents.

The Individualised Care Scale has proven validity and reliability and plenty of evidence exists about its usability and sensitivity in different cultural contexts. Future research should focus on intervention studies using individualised care as an outcome of differing nursing interventions. The role of the patient or client has changed dramatically the in 2010s healthcare. Therefore, it is useful to study the concept of individualised care in association with health promotion, patient education and councelling and empowerment. Selfcare, self-management and activities of individuals have received much stronger recognition in the healthcare systems. How we look at individual patients has dramatically changed since 1990s.

The Individualised Care Scale was developed for the measurement of first, patients' and second, nurses' perceptions about the support and maintenance of individualised nursing care in the in-patient care settings. Future research activities may be focused on the development of an instrument for out-patient care settings, and a more sensitive instrument to be used in the care setting of older people. Such instruments need to focus on revealing the slight nuances in deeper perceptions of individuality, especially focusing on patient's personal life situation. Future research would also show whether it is necessary to weight the personal life situation subscale, as it has turned to provide the most explanatory power for explaining individuality in care provided. The Individualised Care Scale was developed starting in the 1990s and it would be beneficial to analyse the content in the future, whether the content of the concept has changed over time. Also, it would be of value to include other health and social care professionals as samples while measuring the individualised patient care.

The importance and demand for individualised care has risen in the care delivery and nursing leadership and management. This highlights the new coming and importance of value-based healthcare systems, services and patient care. In addition to ethical elements of care, evidence-based healthcare and practices calls for the research on perceptions of patients, but especially the outcomes of nursing care and, thus, intervention studies. Some evidence exists in the research literature about the important role of the physical environment, but also social and symbolic environment, the organizational context, leadership and management. Therefore, more research on these issues in relation to perceptions of individualised care needs to be initiated. Only a few examples exist pointing out that economical issues may have a role in the delivery of individualised patient care, but also pointing out possible savings for the society.